AFFECT, CREATIVE EXPERIENCE, AND PSYCHOLOGICAL ADJUSTMENT

THE SERIES IN CLINICAL AND COMMUNITY PSYCHOLOGY

CONSULTING EDITORS
Charles D. Spielberger and Irwin G. Sarason

Bedell Psychological Assessment and Treatment of Persons with Severe Mental Disorders
Burchfield Stress: Psychological and Physiological Interactions
Burstein and Loucks Rorschach's Test: Scoring and Interpretation
Diamant Homosexual Issues in the Workplace
Diamant Male and Female Homosexuality: Psychological Approaches
Erchul Consultation in Community, School, and Organizational Practice: Gerald Caplan's Contributions to Professional Psychology
Fisher The Science of Psychotherapy
Hobfull Stress, Social Support, and Women
Kassinove Anger Disorders: Definition, Diagnosis, and Treatment
Krohne and Laux Achievement, Stress, and Anxiety
London The Modes and Morals of Psychotherapy, Second Edition
Muñoz Depression Prevention: Research Directions
Reisman A History of Clinical Psychology, Second Edition
Reitan and Davison Clinical Neuropsychology: Current Status and Applications
Rickel, Gerrard, and Iscoe Social and Psychological Problems of Women: Prevention and Crisis Intervention
Rofé Repression and Fear: A New Approach to the Crisis in Psychology
Russ Affect, Creative Experience, and Psychological Adjustment
Savin-Williams Gay and Lesbian Youth: Expressions in Identity
Spielberger and Diaz-Guerrero Cross Cultural Anxiety, Volume 3
Spielberger and Vagg Test Anxiety: Theory, Assessment, and Treatment
Spielberger, Diaz-Guerrero, and Strelau Cross Cultural Anxiety, Volume 4
Suedfeld Psychology and Torture
Veiel and Baumann The Meaning and Measurement of Social Support
Williams and Westermeyer Refugee Mental Health in Resettlement Countries

THE SERIES IN CLINICAL AND
COMMUNITY PSYCHOLOGY

AFFECT, CREATIVE EXPERIENCE, AND PSYCHOLOGICAL ADJUSTMENT

by
Sandra W. Russ
Case Western Reserve University

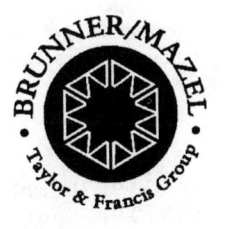

BRUNNER/MAZEL
Taylor & Francis Group

USA	Publishing Office:	BRUNNER/MAZEL *A member of the Taylor & Francis Group* 325 Chestnut Street, Suite 800 Philadelphia, PA 19106 Tel: (215) 625-8900 Fax: (215) 625-2940
	Distribution Center:	BRUNNER/MAZEL *A member of the Taylor & Francis Group* 47 Runway Road, Suite G Levittown, PA 19057-4700 Tel: (215) 269-0400 Fax: (215) 269-0363
UK		BRUNNER/MAZEL *A member of the Taylor & Francis Group* 1 Gunpowder Square London EC4A 3DE Tel: 171 583 0490 Fax: 171 583 0581

AFFECT, CREATIVE EXPERIENCE, AND PSYCHOLOGICAL ADJUSTMENT

Copyright © 1999 Taylor & Francis. All rights reserved. Printed in the United States of America. Except as permitted under the United States Copyright Act of 1976, no part of this publication may be reproduced or distributed in any form or by any means, or stored in a database or retrieval system, without the prior written permission of the publisher.

1 2 3 4 5 6 7 8 9 0

Printed by Braun-Brumfield, Ann Arbor, MI, 1998.

A CIP catalog record for this book is available from the British Library.
♾ The paper in this publication meets the requirements of the ANSI Standard Z39.48-1984 (Permanence of Paper)

Library of Congress Cataloging-in-Publication Data

Affect, creative experience, and psychological adjustment/edited by
   Sandra R. Russ.
       p.   cm.—(The series in clinical and community psychology.
   ISSN 0146-0846)
   Includes bibliographical references and index.
   ISBN 0-87630-917-1 (hardcover: alk. paper).—ISBN 0-87630-918-X
(pbk.: alk. paper)
   1. Creative ability. 2. Affect (Psychology) 3. Adjustment
(Psychology) I. Russ. Sandra Walker. II. Series.
BF408.A34   1999
153.3'5—dc21   98-22837
                                                                                                CIP

ISBN: 0-87630-917-1 (hardcover)
ISBN: 0-87630-918-X (paperback)

Dedication

To all investigators of new realms in the creative process.

Contents

Contributors		ix
Foreword		xv
Introduction		xix
Acknowledgments		xxv

PART ONE
AFFECT AND THE CREATIVE EXPERIENCE

Chapter 1	On the Relationship Between Affect and Creative Problem Solving	3
	Alice M. Isen	
	Why Does Positive Affect Facilitate Creative Problem Solving? Some Myths Debunked	9
	The Dopamine Hypothesis	12
	Conclusion	13
Chapter 2	Mood and Creativity Research: The View From a Conceptual Organizing Perspective	19
	Suzanne Vosburg and Geir Kaufmann	
	What Is Meant by "Creativity"?	19
	Sorting Mood Concepts	20
	A Framework for Mood and Creativity Research	22
	Review of the Research on Mood and Creativity	25
	A Theory of Mood Effects on Creative Problem Solving	32
	Conclusion	34

vii

Chapter 3	The Emotional Resonance Model of Creativity: Theoretical and Practical Extensions *Isaac Getz and Todd I. Lubart*	41
	The Emotional Resonance Model for Generating Associations	43
	Creative Metaphor: A Way to Express Emotion-Based Associations	47
	Accounting for Mood Influences on Creativity	48
	Improving Creativity in Ordinary People	49
	Conclusion	53
Chapter 4	Play, Affect, and Creativity: Theory and Research *Sandra W. Russ*	57
	Affect and Creativity	57
	Play, Affect, and Creativity	58
	Positive and Negative Affect in Creativity	66
	Play, Creativity, and Coping in Children	71
	Conclusion	72
Chapter 5	Intrinsic Motivation, Affect, and Creativity *Beth A. Hennessey*	77
	Proposed Mechanisms of Decreased Motivation with Reward Expectation	80
	The Work–Play Study	82
	An Alternative Affective Explanation	83
	The Immunization Studies: Indirect Evidence to Support the Affective Work–Play Hypothesis	84
	The Affect/Creativity Link	86
	Conclusion	88

PART TWO
AFFECT AND CREATIVE EXPRESSION

Chapter 6	Affect In Artistic and Scientific Creativity *Gregory J. Feist*	93
	Theory on Affect and Creativity	94
	Research on Affect and Creativity	97
	Conclusion	104

CONTENTS

Chapter 7	Affect in Artists and Architects: Images of Self and World Stephanie Z. Dudek	109
	The 20th-Century Social Scene	112
	Personality and Creation	114
	The Present Study	115
	Conclusion	126
Chapter 8	Feeling Creativity Through *Deep Listening* Kimberly A. McCarthy	129
	The Power of Sound: Deep Listening and CARE	131
	Awareness of Experience Through Affect and Attention	136
	Affect and Attention in Creativity Through Deep Listening	142
	Conclusion	143
Chapter 9	On the Role of Affect in Scientific Discovery Melvin P. Shaw	147
	The Model	149
	The Handling of the Data	151
	Results	153
	Implications, Applications, and Conclusions	157

PART THREE
CREATIVITY, PSYCHOPATHOLOGY, AND ADJUSTMENT

Chapter 10	Tension, Adaptability, and Creativity Mark A. Runco	165
	Experience, Tension, and Creativity	167
	Adulthood	171
	Marginality	174
	Top-Down Processing	175
	Creativity as Interpretation	178
	Defining "Problem"	181
	Discussion	183
	Creativity as Adaptability: Necessity is Not the Mother of Creativity	185

Chapter 11	The Subtle Attraction: Beauty as a Force in Awareness, Creativity, and Survival *Ruth Richards*	195
	Characteristics of Aesthetic Appreciation	197
	An Evolution of Information	204
	An Example—Aesthetic, Appreciation, Adversity, and Creative Possibility	207
	The Sublime	210
	Conclusion	215
Chapter 12	Creativity, Bipolarity, and the Dynamics of Style *David Schuldberg*	221
	Empirical Work on Creativity and Psychopathology Traits	222
	Specific Affects and Creativity	224
	A Model of the Dynamics of Affect and Cognitive Meaning in Creativity	228
	Conclusion	234
Index		239

Contributors

Stephanie Dudek is currently a Professor Emerita at the University of Montreal. She has published extensively in the areas of primary process, art, and creativity, and is an active member of the American Psychological Association. She has also served as the President of Division 10 of APA, Psychology and the Arts.

Gregory J. Feist is an assistant professor of psychology at the College of William and Mary, Williamsburg. Virginia.

Isaac Getz is an associate professor of information science and psychology at Groupe ESCP—Paris School of Management. He has published on expertise, learning, and information systems and, more recently, on creativity, emotion, and metaphors. Getz has recently held visiting appointments at the University of Massachusetts, Amherst; Cornell University; Stanford University, Paris; and Helsinki School of Economics and Business Administration.

Beth Hennessey is an associate professor of psychology at Wellesley College, Wellesley, Massachusetts. She was a recipient of a Spencer Post Doctoral Fellowship/National Academy of Education Grant and has published research and theoretical articles on the social psychology of motivation and creativity. She is the coauthor (with Teresa Amabile) of *Creativity and Learning: What Research says to the Teacher.*

Alice M. Isen is a professor of psychology at Cornell University, Ithaca, New York. Her current research concerns the influence of affect on social interaction; thought processes; problem solving; and decision making, including medical decision making. She is the coauthor (with A. H. Hastorf) of *Cognitive Social Psychology* and *Affect and (with B. Moore) Social Behavior* and is the editor of the journal *Motivation and Emotion.*

Geir Kaufmann is a professor of psychology and the chairperson of the Psychology Department at the Norwegian School of Management, Oslo/Norway. He is the author of several research articles and books in the area of problem solving, symbolic representations, affect, and creativity. Kaufmann serves on the editorial board of a number of international journals, has been a keynote speaker at major international conferences, and has been a Fulbright scholar and visiting professor at the University of California, San Diego, and State University of New York, Buffalo.

Todd I. Lubart is currently an assistant professor of psychology at the University of Paris V, France. His research focuses on creativity, with emphases on individual differences, the development of creativity, and the role of emotion in creativity. He is coauthor of *Defying the Crowd: Cultivating Creativity in a Culture of Conformity.*

Kimberly A. McCarthy, music composer and psychologist, has studied with Pauline Oliveros for several years through the *Deep Listening* certification program. A professor of creativity, psychology, and interdisciplinary humanities at Columbia College, she has focused her research on the role of creativity and affect in *Deep Listening,* theater, and community development in diverse or risky environments (e.g., Skid Row, Los Angeles, and Uptown, Chicago).

Ruth Richards is a professor of psychology and faculty cochair at Saybrook Graduate School and Research Institute and an associate clinical professor in the Department of Psychiatry at the University of California, San Francisco. She is also a research affiliate at McLean Hospital and lecturer at Harvard Medical School. Dr. Richards is on the editorial board of the *Creativity Research Journal,* on the Executive Advisory Board for *The Encyclopedia of Creativity,* and coeditor (with Marc Runco) of *Eminent Creativity, Everyday Creativity, and Health.*

Mark Runco is currently a professor of psychology at California State University at Fullerton, editor of the *Creaative Research Journal,* and president of Division 10 (Psychology and the Arts) of the American Psychological Association.

Sandra W. Russ is a professor of psychology and the chair of the Psychology Department at Case Western Reserve University, Cleveland, Ohio. Her research area is children's play and creativity; she recently summarized her work for her book *Affect and Creativity: The Role of Affect and Play in the Creative Process.* Russ has served as president of the Section on Clinical Child Psychology in Division 12 of the American Psychological Association and is currently president-elect of the Society for Personality Assessment.

David Schuldberg is a professor of psychology in the Clinical Psychology program at the University of Montana, Missoula, Montana. His research interests include schizophrenic symptomatology, automated assessment, psychological well-being, and the measurement of creativity. He has done research funded by the National Institute of Mental Health on positive aspects of adjustment in putatively at-risk young adults. He is currently at work on a book on nonlinear dynamical-systems approaches to the theory of physical and psychological health.

Melvin P. Shaw is a psychologist and psychotherapist in private practice in Birmingham, Michigan. He maintained a second career as a physicist through 1996 and is presently a professor emeritus of electrical and computer engineering at Wayne State University, Detroit, Michigan. He has published more than 80 papers in scientific and professional journals, coauthored three physics books, and coedited one psychology book.

Suzanne Vosburg includes her coauthored chapter (with Kaufmann) as part of her doctoral thesis, which has been submitted to the University of Bergen, Bergan, Norway. Her research interests are problem solving and affect and creativity. She is currently affiliated with the New York Hospital—Cornell Medical Center.

Foreword

In 1764 when Samuel Johnson's great friend Sir Joshua Reynolds established the Literary Club, it was for the express purpose to "give him (Johnson) unlimited opportunities for talking." When Sandra Russ invited speakers to her American Psychological Association symposium in 1994, it must have been in the same spirit: participants, all recognized scholars, were given an opportunity to present their own research and, perhaps not quite Johnsonian, pay attention to the other speakers. Out of these presentations and exchanges, Russ has fashioned a book of importance: This is a book about serious things. Nor is it one simply for other scholars. It is a book important to teachers, psychotherapists, day-care givers, and, of course, parents whose interests go beyond the playground and Toys R Us. The focus of this book, and I am sure the editor's original instruction to participants conveyed this, was to avoid isolating their particular topics and to explore the common boundaries of their interests. There is no reason for us to act as if these interfaces will or should fit snugly together or do not generate tensions of their own. Parts of the book show them and reflect a research maturity. Another recurrent characteristic throughout the book is authors' intentions and efforts to put their work and that of others in a credible framework, that is, one long on data and short(er) on speculations. "Theory", "model", "hypothesize", "interrelation" are not just buzz words but stand for cogent constructions we see these authors struggling with. Almost all chapters present the author's working "model" to readers' benefit. It is difficult to imagine the reader who comes away from this book with the same mind-set he or she began the book.

Author after author show an awareness that things regarding creativity are never as simple as they appear no matter the age of the subject or how emotionally vibrant (e.g., manic), or flattened (e.g., depressed), or "neutral" the individual. As one who was raised to believe that a little mania (hypomania) was "not a bad thing to have for creativity," as one famous speaker put it, and that depression is the sinkhole of creativeness, it is encouraging to find that this group of authors know how overstated this is and that some research paradigms, clear as they may be, could not help but give overly simple answers to questions that are never simple or clear. Chapter after chapter, regardless of their particular topic, show us that things, when it comes to affect and creativity, are complex and at times counter-intuitive no matter where creativeness takes shape and comes to lodge in us. Take for example Richards' chapter "The Subtle Attraction: Beauty as a Force in Awareness, Creativity, and Survival" and Schuldberg's "Creativity, Bipolarity, and the Dynamics of Style." They complement one another at times and in doing so indicate how much our health depends on our daily aesthetic appreciation and how influenced the "assignment of meaning" to our lives *and* the stylistic composition of "any" artistic product ("any" may be offering too much from my perspective) is by where one's everyday experiences lie along dynamic, interacting affective and cognitive dimensions. These dimensions represent processes that are deeply set within each of us and what we experience in ourselves are not simply "symptoms" or "styles" but real-life instances of biological and environmental interactions (spoken of as phenotypes in evolutionary psychology). It is no stretch (to use Darwin's term) to accept a conclusion suggested by Richards and Schuldberg that the pursuit of beauty and creative effort are complementary survival mechanisms available to the non-eminent just as much as they are to the (over-studied?) eminent. It is clear that considering evolution theory can only enrich our understanding of creativity from a broader perspective than of individuals, eminent or not (Albert, in press).

Reading these two chapters help clarify a question for me. When, if ever, do personal moods and talents operating together override cultural and historical "interests" and parameters? There is more than the issue of priority of influence involved here; involved in the question is whether or not the set of specific traits and emotional factors we often see involved in creativeness are cultural constructions, according to cultural determinism. The fact that many can be traced far back in time and across cultural boundaries leaves the matter unclear (see Albert, 1994, for discussion). A more specific question might help the reader. Surely there were as many "depressed" as there were "manic" artists during the Romantic period (circa late 1700–1800s), so how did those depressed and emotionally flattened individuals interface with the rich, existing intellectual culture around them? (Certainly not all went into business?)

What happens to talented children, to say nothing of the men and women whose emotional thermostats are not set to go "up" or past "OK" according to their culture? And on more recent terms, what is happening now with the non-computer oriented, less mathematical-engineering inclined boy and girl? Several of the book's chapters discuss this question.

Along with the intellectual stimulation, another of the book's bonuses is that the research presented throughout this book should lead naturally to the next generation of research in the areas of affect, creative experience and psychological adjustment. Contributors have laid down the linkages, many of them fundamental, among these areas.

Readers who come to this book with some background in any two of the three prime areas of concern—affect, creative experience, and psychological adjustment—will understand when I say that for the most part the centerpiece among the three has been "creativity". A lot of psychology has been transported by it across the years.

I won't list the book's variations on the creativity theme (don't make me count the ways!), but it is interesting to see how little space is set aside by the authors for identifying *the* creative individual or creative people as if they were a sub-species. The psychologist as taxonomist seems to be quickly fading, and judging by this book, everyday moody, uncreative, infrequent, or exceptional behavior, seems to be coming into its own. Where exceptional persons were once the object of our affections (at least mine) when it came to creativity, persons of everyday worth and achievement now receive their proper share of research attention, although I must add I think subjects captive in daycare centers, classrooms, business, and clinics still seem to be over-represented in the literature. Yet here again several authors recognize this, wisely noting the sometimes truncated results of their own research. By doing this, they sharpen even more the reader's attention to their message. We all gain in our research maturity.

This holds true for anyone who carefully reads this book.

REFERENCES

Albert, R. S. (1994). The contribution of early family history to the achievement of eminence. In N. Colangelo, S. G. Assoulin, and D. L. Ambroson (Eds.), *Talent development,* vol. 11 (pp. 311–360). Dayton, OH: Ohio Psychology Press.

Albert, R. S. (in press). The achievement of eminence: an evolutionary strategy. In M. A. Runco (Ed.), *The creativity research handbook,* vol. 2, Cresshill, NJ: Hampton Press.

Robert S. Albert, Ph.D.
Pitzer College
Claremont, CA 91711

Introduction

Sandra W. Russ
Case Western Reserve University, Cleveland, Ohio

The role of affect in creativity is increasingly being recognized as an important and exciting area to investigate. Research in the creativity area has focused primarily on cognitive processes and personality traits important in creativity, to the relative neglect of the area of affect and creativity (Feist & Runco, 1993; Russ, 1993; Shaw & Runco, 1994). Today, a growing body of research is identifying the affective processes important in creativity.

The field of creativity has long been aware of the importance of affect to the creative process. Interviews with creative individuals, classic tales of literature, everyday folklore, and psychoanalytic theory have all attested to the crucial role of affect in creativity. For example, psychoanalytic theorists have long hypothesized that openness to emotions and to thoughts and images that contain emotional content facilitates creativity. Although descriptions of the affective and cognitive processes of creative individuals support this theory, there has been relatively little research on affect and creativity. A major problem has been the measurement of affect. Recent advances in measurement and methodology have enabled such research to be carried out and alternative theories to emerge to explain the underlying mechanisms.

AN EMERGING FIELD

During the last 15 years, there has been a resurgence of research on the role of affect in creativity. As it should be in any science, the research is theoretically driven: theories are being tested, measures and methods are being refined, and new lines of investigation are opening up.

The complexity of the area is becoming apparent. For example, research with adults has demonstrated that inducing positive affect facilitates creativity. These experimental findings are consistent with research that demonstrates relationships between affect in fantasy and creativity in adults and children. An interesting question is whether negative affect facilitates creativity. Although a number of studies indicate it does, other work suggests that it does not. This important question is discussed throughout this book. Another important trend in creativity research is the awareness that different types of affect contribute to different domains of creativity. The arts are probably different from the sciences in terms of how affect influences the creative process, and within the arts, affect appears to play a different role in artistic production than in musical composition.

Another important area of creativity research is the study of creativity in children. One question is how to study affect and creativity in children. For example, research has found that good pretend play is predictive of creativity. Good players are more creative. Studying affect in children's play may be a good method for investigating affect and creativity in children.

Both measurement and manipulation of affect are necessary for good research on affect and creativity, and both are a challenge to the field. Measurement forces investigators to face the question, What is affect? What dimensions of affect are important in creativity? How do we reliably and validly measure these dimensions? The manipulation of affect is complex. The complexity of that manipulation is being recognized and is addressed throughout this book.

Psychological adjustment is a related area of investigation in affect and creativity research. It is natural to ponder the question of how affect, creativity, and psychological adjustment relate. Therefore, clinical populations are studied, and coping and adjustment measures are incorporated into affect and creativity research. The broad question of whether creativity is an advantage or disadvantage and whether it emerges from comfortable or difficult surroundings and experiences are being investigated in a variety of ways. To date, the answer appears to be "it depends." The authors in this book articulate their opinions about research findings.

The study of affect and creativity necessarily involves scholars and researchers from a variety of fields and subfields within psychology—cognitive, developmental, social, clinical, physiological, and educational. This breadth of scholarship results in an interdisciplinary perspective in viewing the area. Having a variety of perspectives is a plus that should strengthen the research base of the field. Many of these disciplines are represented in this book.

THE SPIRIT OF A SYMPOSIUM

To facilitate interaction among different researchers in the affect and creativity area, I organized a symposium on affect and creativity at the annual meeting of the American Psychological Association in 1994. The symposium gave leading scholars in the field an opportunity to present and discuss cutting-edge research and new theoretical developments that have evolved from it. All of the symposium participants were selected to provide comprehensive coverage of the field, and all of them updated their symposium presentations for this book. In addition, leading researchers who did not participate in the symposium have contributed chapters to the book.

In keeping with the spirit of the symposium from which it grew, this book provides an arena where new theories and concepts can be presented, research findings compared and discussed, methodological issues wrestled with, and future research directions outlined. The chapters provide an overview of the current state of the field, research findings, theoretical and methodological issues, and guidelines for the future. The array of ideas and research findings presented reflects the excitement of the field. The current thinking of the major researchers in the field of affect and creativity is offered in this book.

Key questions in the area of affect and creativity focus on (a) identifying specific affective processes that are most important in creativity; (b) discovering the underlying mechanisms that account for the relationships between affect and creativity; (c) exploring differential effects of various types of affect, such as positive and negative affect, on creativity; and (d) understanding how affect and creativity relate to psychological adjustment. Understanding the development of affect and creativity will also facilitate application of research findings to child-rearing practices, educational approaches, and work environments. The authors in this volume address these questions according to their areas of expertise and present their current thinking about the issues. Most of the chapters have an empirical focus. A few present concepts and syntheses of current work that can be empirically investigated in future work.

OVERVIEW OF CHAPTERS

This book consists of three sections. Part I, "Affect and the Creative Experience," presents some of the major research topics in affect and creativity: mood induction, positive and negative affect, play, and intrinsic motivation. Part II, "Affect and Creative Expression," reviews the role of affect in different domains of creativity in the arts and sciences. Part III, "Creativity, Psychopathology, and Adjustment," focuses on the role of affect in creativity, mental illness, and adaptive functioning.

Part I opens with a chapter by Alice Isen that presents her current thinking about affect and creativity. Isen's seminal work on affect and creativity, which is referred to repeatedly throughout this book, was a catalyst for the affect and creativity area. Here, she brings us up to date on her research program and her thoughts about possible mechanisms underlying the influence of positive affect on creativity.

In Chapter 2, Suzanne Vosburg and Geir Kaufmann present an overview of the mood and creativity research area, discussing some of the possible reasons for mixed results. They present a conceptual framework that categorizes types of creativity tasks and processes and focuses on the interaction of different types of mood states with types of creativity tasks. Their framework and discussion highlight the complexity of the affect and creativity area and provide guidelines for future research.

It is essential that researchers develop theoretical models that account for the data, and in Chapter 3, Isaac Getz and Todd Lubart present an important new model of affect and creativity—the emotional resonance model. This model explains why and how emotions contribute to the access and association of cognitively remote concepts, so important in creativity. They also report ingenious research on improving creativity that is in line with their model.

In Chapter 4, Sandra Russ discusses the role of play in the development of affective processes important in creativity. After reviewing theory and research in the area, she discusses her research program with the instrument she developed for measuring emotion in play, the Affect in Play Scale. Her discussion focuses on the question of positive and negative affect and primary process affect and creativity.

Beth Hennessey presents an overview of the research in the intrinsic motivation area in Chapter 5, focusing on the mechanisms underlying the principle of intrinsic motivation and creativity. She offers an explanation that negative affect may be associated with reward expectation or evaluation and thereby interfere with creativity. Her discussion points to a possible fruitful line of inquiry: affect and intrinsic motivation.

Part II, which focuses on affect and different domains of creativity, opens with Gregory Feist's review of the theoretical and empirical work on affect in the artistic and scientific creative process. Feist provides a broad theoretical overview of the affect and creativity area and categorizes affect states, affect traits, and aesthetic emotions and creativity. He discusses his own research in the area of artistic and scientific creativity and gives guidelines for future research.

In Chapter 7, Stephanie Dudek explores the affective and perceptual process of creative artists and architects. She has studied these individuals for a long period, and her qualitative analysis of the Rorschach responses of these individuals sheds light on the differences between them that fit with their chosen professions. Dudek's rich interpretations reflect her deep understanding of creativity in the arts and of the individuals who gravitate to them.

Kimberly McCarthy takes a different approach in Chapter 8 and presents a model for increasing creativity in music improvisation through a process known as "deep listening." She discusses the role of affect in listening to music and some of the underlying physiological processes involved in affect and the musical experience.

In Chapter 9, Melvin Shaw discusses his structural model for integrated affective and cognitive components of creative thinking in science and engineering. In a study of 12 internationally known research scientists and engineers, he listened to what these creative individuals said about the feeling states that accompany creative thinking. Quotes from these scientists about their various types of affective experiences offer a direct sense of what is involved.

Part III grapples with the overall picture of affect, creativity, and mental health. Although some of the previous chapters address this issue, the three chapters in this section focus specifically on the interrelationships among affect, creativity, and adjustment.

Mark Runco, in Chapter 10, discusses the important role of tension and the experience of cognitive disequilibrium in the creative process. He integrates ideas from a wide variety of literatures and develops a sophisticated view of negative affect, the creative experience, and adaptability.

, In Chapter 11, Ruth Richards stresses the importance of aesthetic experiences in growth and adaptation. On the basis of her research on everyday creativity, Richards views the creative process as an adaptive one that contributes to a joyful and meaningful life. Here, she captures the mature gestalt of creativity and describes the complex integration of affect and cognition involved.

Finally, David Schuldberg gives a thorough review of the area of affective disorders and creativity in Chapter 12. He reviews his own research and presents a dynamic model of the interaction of cognition and affect. This is an exciting model that can be tested in a variety of domains of creativity.

At the beginning of any new line of research investigation, there is a fermenting of hunches, speculations, ideas, research findings, methodological issues, and tests of theoretical models that evolves into a clear vision of heuristic theoretical models and the most important research questions. This book is intended to contribute to that process in the area of affect and creativity.

REFERENCES

Feist, G. J., & Runco, M. A. (1993). Trends in the creativity literature. An analysis of the research in the *Journal of Creative Behavior* (1967–1989). *Creative Research Journal, 6,* 271–286.

Russ, S. (1993). *Affect and creativity: The role of affect and play in the creative process.* Hillsdale, NJ: Lawrence Erlbaum.

Shaw, M. P., & Runco, M. A. (1994). *Creativity and affect.* Norwood, NJ: Albex.

Acknowledgments

I wish to express my deep appreciation to Charles Spielberger for encouraging me to develop this book from a symposium on Affect and Creativity at a meeting of the American Psychological Association. His suggestions for the structure and evolution of the book were extremely helpful. The editorial staff at Taylor and Francis have been great to work with. Special thanks goes to Bernadette Capelle for overseeing this process so efficiently.

Finally, I wish to thank my husband, Tom Brugger, for his loving support of my work.

Part One:

Affect and the Creative Experience

On the Relationship Between Affect and Creative Problem Solving

Alice M. Isen
Cornell University, Ithaca, New York

A growing body of research indicates that positive affect is associated with greater cognitive flexibility and improved creative problem solving across a broad range of settings. This relationship has been found with both induced and naturally occurring positive affect (or "positive affectivity") and not only with college student samples, but also in organizational settings, in consumer contexts, in negotiation, in the literature on coping and stress, in a sample of practicing physicians asked to solve a diagnostic problem, and among children and young adolescents (e.g., Aspinwall & Taylor, 1997; Carnevale & Isen, 1986; Estrada, Isen, & Young, 1997; Estrada, Young, & Isen, 1994; Fiske & Taylor, 1991; George & Brief, 1996; Greene & Noice, 1988; Hirt, Melton, McDonald, & Harackiewicz, 1996; Isen, 1987, 1993; Isen & Baron, 1991; Isen, Daubman, & Nowicki, 1987; Isen, Johnson, Mertz, & Robinson, 1985; Isen & Williams, 1988; Kahn & Isen, 1993; Mano, in press; Showers & Cantor, 1985; Staw & Barsade, 1993; Staw, Sutton, & Pelled, 1994; Taylor & Aspinwall, 1996).

Several studies have indicated that positive affect increases a person's ability to organize ideas in multiple ways and access alternative cognitive perspectives. This has been proposed as a process by which positive affect facilitates creative problem solving. For example, three studies showed that positive affect, induced in any of a variety of simple ways, such as watching 5 min of a comedy film or receiving a small, unanticipated gift, led people to have a broader range of first associates to neutral words (but not to negative words) compared with controls (Isen et al., 1985). That is, people in the positive-affect condition, as a group, had more unusual and more diverse first associates than did people in a neutral-affect control condition. Another study, involving young adolescents (eighth graders), similarly showed increased verbal fluency in the positive-affect condition (Greene & Noice, 1988). When the children were asked to name as many members of a given category as they could, those in the positive-affect condition gave more category words, and more unusual examples of the category, than did controls.

A compatible result with adult participants was obtained recently by Hirt et al. (1996), who found that the effects of positive affect on persistence and performance depended on whether the processing goals assigned to participants focused on enjoyment or "sufficiency" of performance on the task. When people were told to work on the task as long as they were enjoying it, people in the positive-affect condition persisted longer and did more than controls; when the participants were instructed to stop working on the task when they felt they had "done enough," people in the positive-affect condition stopped earlier than controls and did less work. These results are compatible with recent findings and formulations that suggest that the impact of positive affect on cognitive processing and task performance depends on processing demands and goals, and in part on the nature of the materials and the importance or interestingness or enjoyability of the task (e.g., Bodenhausen, Kramer, & Susser, 1994; Forgas, 1995; Isen, 1993; Martin, Ward, Achee, & Wyer, 1993). More important for the purposes of this chapter, the results showed that participants in the positive-affect condition gave more creative responses than controls in all conditions, regardless of the processing goal they were using.

Several other studies have shown that people in positive-affect conditions are able to classify material more flexibly, seeing ways in which nontypical members of categories can be viewed as members of the categories (e.g., Isen & Daubman, 1984; Isen, Niedenthal, & Cantor, 1992; Kahn & Isen, 1993). Through the use of a rating task like that employed by Rosch (1975), creative or flexible classification of nontypical category members has been found for items in natural categories (Isen & Daubman, 1984); for products in the class of snack foods (Kahn & Isen, 1993); and for person types in positive, but not negative, person categories (Isen et al., 1992). Flexible classification has even been found for perception and classification of human social groups: Recent work on social-group perception has shown that induced positive affect results in a tendency to integrate and perceive a socially distinct out-group as part of a superordinate group of which the perceiver is also a member (Dovidio, Gaertner, Isen, & Lowrance, 1995). Thus, positive affect has been shown to enable people to classify not only items, but also people more flexibly, and in particular to see potential relatedness and commonalities among them, and classify them as members of the same group.

It has also been found that if experimental participants are specifically asked to focus on differences and to find ways in which items differ from one another, positive affect can result in more perceived difference (Isen, 1987, p. 234; Murray, Sujan, Hirt, & Sujan, 1990). It has been suggested that this is because positive affect gives rise to cognitive elaboration (e.g., Isen et al., 1985). Elaboration, or the presence in mind of more information, has been found to increase either perceived similarity or perceived difference, depending on contextual factors such as the question that participants are asked to address (Tversky & Gati, 1978). Together, these studies also can be interpreted as indicating that positive affect promotes cognitive flexibility: People who are feeling happy, compared with those in a neutral feeling state, become more able to make associations among ideas and see multiple relations among stimuli. The details of the result of this process (e.g., increased perceived similarity or perceived difference) may depend on factors in the task context (e.g., the processing goal or the question posed); the relevant point for the present discussion is that these results show still another way that positive affect enables flexible consideration of different aspects of concepts, or alternative cognitive perspectives.

Several other studies illustrate additional ways in which positive affect facilitates flexible cognitive processing of neutral or positive material. In a study of the impact of positive affect on job perceptions, people in whom positive affect had been induced judged an interesting task that they had been assigned, but not a dull one, as richer and more varied than did control participants (Kraiger, Billings, & Isen, 1989). In the organizational behavior literature, a task is said to be rich if it is relatively complex and interesting and affords a sense of choice or variety. Again, then, the influence of positive affect on perceived task richness can be seen as reflecting an ability on the part of the positive-affect participants to see additional associations and aspects, particularly of interesting things.

At the same time, the interaction between affect and the type of task, like interactions between affect and the nature of the stimulus materials (e.g., the positive or negative valence of the materials) in the aforementioned studies, indicates that a substantive process related to elaboration and thinking is responsible for the observed effects of positive feelings. This is in contrast with alternative hypotheses about how positive affect may exert influence, which sometimes propose an artifact such as nonsystematic processing or a response bias to perceive everything more positively. The reason that the observed statistical interactions between affect and type of task or stimulus material signify a substantive process, rather than just a bias, is that any nonspecific effect, such as bias or tendency to process non-systematically, should affect all stimuli equivalently. However, interactions between affect and the stimulus materials or task requirements, which have been observed repeatedly, indicate specific processes that are fostered by positive affect.

Another study that supports the point that positive affect promotes cognitive flexibility is Carnevale and Isen's (1986) finding that positive affect, induced by means of receipt of a small gift and by reading funny cartoons, facilitated participants' taking a problem-solving approach in an integrative bargaining task, which resulted in improved outcomes for both parties in the negotiation. An integrative bargaining task is one in which, in order to reach the optimal agreement, people must make trade-offs on different issues, of differing value to them, about which they are bargaining. Reaching agreement on such a task requires seeing possibilities, thinking innovatively, and reasoning flexibly about possible trade-offs. In such a task, neither obvious compromises nor simply yielding to the other party's demands results in satisfactory outcomes (for greater detail, see, e.g., Pruitt, 1983).

In this study, people in the positive-effect condition who bargained face-to-face were significantly less likely to break off negotiations, and more likely to reach agreement and to reach the optimal agreement possible in the situation, than were face-to-face bargainers in the control condition, in which positive affect had not been induced (Carnevale & Isen, 1986). They were also less likely to engage in aggressive tactics during the negotiations and reported more enjoyment of the session. Finally, they were better able than control participants to figure out the other person's payoff matrix (schedule of profit for each component of the agreement) in the negotiation, which differed for the two bargainers. Although the findings include the fact that people in the positive-affect condition enjoyed the session more and were less likely than control participants to behave aggressively, the results of the study suggest that such factors were not responsible for the improved outcome of the negotiation. Rather, the results suggest that positive affect enables flexible thinking and improves people's ability to see ways of relating aspects of the situation to one another to come up with a good solution to the problem.

Another series of studies reflecting positive affect's influence on flexibility and cognitive organization indicates that positive affect promotes creative or innovative responding, measured through tasks typically considered indicators of classic creativity or innovative problem solving (Isen et al., 1987). In one of these methods, the "candle problem" (Duncker, 1945), a person is presented with a candle, a box of tacks, and a book of matches and is asked to affix the candle to the wall so that it will burn without dripping wax on the table or floor. To solve the problem, the person has to empty the box of tacks, tack the box to the wall, and place the candle in the box so that the candle can be lit and won't drip wax onto the table or floor. Thus, the person must "break set" and use one of the items (the box) in a nontypical way. In three studies, from two different labs, using two different age range populations (college students and eighth-grade students), people in whom positive affect had been induced performed significantly better than controls on this task (e.g., Greene & Noice, 1988; Isen et al., 1987). Solving this problem in this way involves cognitive flexibility or the ability to put ideas together in new and useful ways, a classic definition of creativity (e.g., Koestler, 1964). In the early problem-solving literature, it was also referred to as "breaking set" or overcoming "functional fixedness" (Duncker, 1945; Wertheimer, 1945).

A task derived from the Remote Associates Test (M. T. Mednick, Mednick, & Mednick, 1964) has also been used to study the influence of positive affect on cognitive flexibility or creativity. This test, which is based on S. A Mednick's (1962) theory of creativity, has been validated, in its full form, as a measure of individual differences in creativity. In it, participants are presented with three words and a blank line and are asked to provide a fourth word that relates to each of the three words given in the problem. For example,

MOWER   ATOMIC   FOREIGN   _____

In this example, POWER is the correct answer. When the task is used to study the influence of affect on creativity, seven items of moderate difficulty are used. Several studies in which this dependent measure of cognitive flexibility or creativity was used confirm that positive affect increases such ability. These studies employed different populations of participants, including college students and practicing physicians (e.g., Estrada, et al., 1994; Isen et al., 1987).

In another line of investigation, three studies (Kahn and Isen, 1993) indicate that positive affect promotes variety seeking among safe, enjoyable products (though it does not foster risk taking or seeking of danger). These studies reported that when given the opportunity to make several choices in a food category (e.g., soup or snacks), people in whom positive affect had been induced, showed more switching among alternatives than did controls and included a broader range of items in their choice sets, as long as the circumstances did not make unpleasant or negative potential features of the items salient. In contrast, when a negative, but not risky, feature (e.g., the possibility that a low-salt product would be less tasty than the regular) was salient, there was no difference between affect groups in variety seeking, or the tendency to switch around among the items in making choices. Thus, there is evidence that positive affect promotes enjoyment of variety and of a wider range or possibilities but that this occurs only when the situation does not prompt the person to think of unpleasant outcomes.

To summarize the work described so far, more than 25 studies, from several different topic areas, that have examined the effects of different affect inductions and various measures of cognitive flexibility in diverse populations indicate that when positive affect is induced in participants randomly assigned to conditions, it improves their ability to see more aspects of concepts or stimuli and to adopt multiple cognitive perspectives. Further, it should be noted that several studies on the effects of naturally occurring positive affect (or positive affectivity) have shown, compatibly, that positive affect is associated with creative problem solving in work settings (e.g., George & Brief, 1996; Staw & Barsade, 1993; Staw et al., 1994), and with flexible and effective coping skills (e.g., Aspinwall & Taylor, 1997; Taylor & Aspinwall, 1996) and similar measures in other applied contexts. Thus, in both laboratory and field studies, using varied measures, positive feelings have been shown to lead to cognitive elaboration and flexibility, resulting in people's having more thoughts and more nontypical (though relevant) thoughts. It should be noted that positive affect promotes flexible thinking, so that both usual *and* unusual aspects and sense of concepts can be expected to occur to people.

It is important to note that the effects described here are not easily attributable to a global process, such as response bias, increased (or decreased) motivation, decreased motivation to process systematically, or carelessness. This is because the effects appear specific to creative problem solving, and whereas they occur with interesting or important tasks, they tend not to extend to routine tasks and are not observed when the task is both unimportant and unpleasant or uninteresting. For example, among the aforementioned investigations of the impact of induced affect, several showed significant interactions between positive affect and the task materials or conditions, such that affect increased flexibility only when the situation was engaging, involving, or neutral or positive in emotional content. Recall that the study of job perceptions showed an influence of affect only on an enriched task and not on a dull one (Kraiger et al., 1989); for two more illustrations, recall that positive affect led to more unusual associates to neutral words but not to negative words (Isen et al., 1985) and to more flexible categorization into positive but not negative person categories (Isen et al., 1992). These interactions indicate that the impact of positive affect should not be attributed to simple response bias on the part of people in the positive-affect conditions, because simple response bias would tend to have an equivalent impact on all stimuli or situations. Rather, the findings suggest that positive affect fosters flexible thinking about topics that people find interesting, expect to be able to enjoy, or want (or need) to think about.

However, it should also be noted that the studies provide evidence that people in the positive-affect conditions want to think about a wide range of serious tasks, not just games or fun. For physicians and medical students, for example, this includes diagnostic problems (e.g., Estrada et al., 1997; Isen, Rosenzweig, & Young, 1991). In studies with college student samples, the effects were observed on problem-solving tasks, product choice tasks, categorization tasks, and face-to-face negotiations that were complex and difficult and that, in the control situation but not in the positive-affect condition, became full of anger and hostility (e.g., Carnevale & Isen, 1986; Isen et al., 1987; 1985; Kahn & Isen, 1993). Thus, the influence of positive affect on cognitive flexibility, while not extending to all tasks, does apply to a broad range of tasks and is not limited to those that could be considered fun.

Other evidence does indicate that people who are feeling happy do evaluate neutral or positive things (but not negative stimuli) more positively (e.g., Forgas & Bower, 1987; Isen & Shalker, 1982; Isen, Shalker, Clark, & Karp, 1978), and thus many relatively neutral tasks may in fact become more pleasant or more painlessly accomplished under conditions of positive affect. Or, as was observed in the negotiation study, situations of potential interpersonal hostility may be handled more pleasantly so that hostility is averted (Carnevale & Isen, 1986). However, this is a separate matter, and it does not mean that under conditions of positive affect all tasks would be seen as interesting, fun, or pleasant.

Despite the tendency for people who are feeling happy to improve their evaluations and handle situations smoothly and kindly, my colleagues and I have identified many tasks and stimuli that are not facilitated by positive affect. Performance on these tasks is not impaired by positive affect, but it is not improved, either. Besides those already mentioned (in which the materials are not interesting or enjoyable and the task is not presented as important), these tasks include simple routine tasks such as letter cross-out and arithmetic operations such as multiplication and long division (Isen, Berg, & Chen, 1991; see Isen, 1993, for discussion). In these studies, people in the positive-affect conditions did not differ from control participants on the routine tasks, but they did differ from controls on creative-problem-solving tasks such as the Remote Associates Test.

Positive Affect and Systematic Processing

It has been suggested by some authors that positive affect improves creative problem solving because it facilitates heuristic processing (and, some say, interferes with systematic processing) (e.g., Mackie & Worth, 1991; Schwarz & Bless; see Isen, 1993 for a contrasting view). There are at least two problems with this position. One is that it assumes that creative problem solving relies on or is accomplished by use of heuristics or nonsystematic thought processes, but that has not been demonstrated. The other centers on the assumption that positive affect fosters use of heuristics or interferes with systematic thinking.

In fact, creativity is one of our most prized, sought-after, rare abilities, and all efforts are made to foster or discover it. Moreover, tasks requiring creative problem solving, ingenuity, or innovation can be among the most complex. It seems unlikely, then, that creativity and creative problem solving would be easily achieved merely by the application of quick and simple heuristics. If that were so, innovation and creativity would be common, not rare.

On reflection, it seems even less likely that these sought-after solutions would result from application of simplistic, flawed, nonsystematic processes, which some have proposed characterize thinking under conditions of positive effect (e.g., Mackie & Worth, 1991; Schwarz & Bless, 1991). For this reason, it seems inappropriate to say that positive affect by its nature typically interferes with systematic or careful cognitive processing (especially since an important component of the "evidence" for this is that positive affect fosters creative problem solving!). Furthermore, the data simply do not support such a conclusion. Fuller consideration of this topic is beyond the scope of this chapter, but suffice it to say that a body of evidence is now accumulating that questions that proposition and shows that positive affect facilitates careful, thorough (as well as creative) thinking and problem solving, provided that the task is interesting or important, just as might be expected from the creative-problem-solving findings (e.g., Bodenhausen, et al., 1994; Hirt, et al., 1996; Isen et al., 1991; Smith and Shafter, 1991; see Isen, 1993, for discussion).

Positive Affect, Risk Taking, and Creativity

It is often assumed that positive affect promotes risk taking, and in the context of creativity there is a further assumption that willingness to take risks facilitates or even is essential for, creativity. As plausible as both of those assumptions seem, they are not true—or at least not in a simple way.

In fact, the evidence regarding the influence of positive affect on risk taking suggests something quite different: Although people who are feeling happy may seem more risk prone in a hypothetical risk situation, where the risk is slight and would not result in a meaningful loss, people in positive-affect conditions in the context of a genuine risk, have actually been found to be risk averse, not risk prone, in comparison with controls (e.g., Isen & Geva, 1987; Isen & Patrick, 1983). Further, the evidence suggests that this may occur because positive affect increases the subjective potential negative impact of the loss that is under consideration (Isen, Nygren, & Ashby, 1988). That is, the loss seems worse to someone in whom positive affect has been induced. So, although positive affect improves people's estimates of the likelihood of good outcomes (e.g., Johnson & Tversky, 1982), it also makes any potential genuine loss that is under consideration seem worse. The end result is that people in the positive-affect conditions may worry more if a genuine risk is brought to mind and in that situation are less likely to take the risk than controls (Isen & Geva, 1987). Thus, people who are feeling happy appear to be protective of their happy feeling states and not inclined to take large or meaningful risks.

Similarly, since positive affect does lead to flexible thinking and creative problem solving, a tendency toward risky behavior per se (at least as represented in the studies reported) must not be a necessary part of the creative process. Rather, what we think of as risky behavior in creative situations—willingness to try something new, explore, or put forth one's opinion—may not actually involve risk taking. Instead, it may entail stimulation seeking (among safe stimuli), variety seeking, or exploration in situations in which the person may not anticipate any real danger. This was illustrated, for example, in the variety-seeking studies (Kahn & Isen, 1993) described earlier. Recall that in those studies, as long as potential negatives in the products were not made salient, people in the positive-affect conditions showed greater preference for variety than did controls, as measured by an increased amount of switching, an increased number of varieties included in the consideration set, a broader range of varieties considered, and a lower "market share" of the most preferred brand. However, this difference between affect and control conditions disappeared when potential negatives in the nontypical varieties were made salient. Thus, willingness to take a risk or encounter danger may not be the same factor that is involved in the process of creative discovery.

Positive Affect and Arousal

Historically, affect and arousal have sometimes been considered synonymous (e.g., Duffy, 1934, 1941); and especially in the context of creative problem solving, it may seem that it is arousal, rather than positive affect, that leads to innovation or creativity. However, accumulating evidence suggests that it is more appropriate to think of affect and arousal as distinct. Several kinds of data show a disparity between aroused and positive states, including a difference in their ability to foster creativity.

First, there is the theoretical reason not to expect arousal to promote innovation, and that is that arousal is thought to facilitate the *dominant* response in a person's response repertoire, not a novel one (e.g., Berlyne, 1967; Easterbrook, 1959; Hilgard & Bower, 1967; Matlin & Zajonc, 1968; Zajonc, 1965). Second, there are the data from self-reports of experienced emotions or feelings states: People report different levels of affect (valence) and arousal as components of affective states (e.g., Lewinsohn & Mano, 1993; Mano, 1992). Thus, affect and arousal are not likely to be identical. Moreover, Mandler (1984) has suggested that arousal, although central in emotion, is not a factor in common mood states (p. 277). Third, it has long been known that the relationship between arousal and the type of affect experienced is curvilinear (e.g., Berlyne, 1967; Yerkes & Dodson, 1908). That is, very low levels and very high levels of arousal are usually experienced as unpleasant, whereas moderate levels of arousal are associated with pleasant affect. In view of these points, there have been reconceptualizations of arousal that suggest that it may not be a unitary construct and may need to be investigated differently from the way it has been addressed in the past (e.g., Lacey, 1967, 1975; Lacey, Kagan, Lacey, & Moss, 1963; Neiss, 1990; Venables, 1984).

Fourth, and most important, studies showing an impact of positive affect on cognitive flexibility also indicate that positive affect is distinct from negative affect and affectless arousal and is distinct in facilitating flexible responding, in particular (e.g., Isen et al., 1987). That is, in experiments designed to determine whether negative affect, or arousal, facilitates creative problem solving as positive affect does, differences were observed in the effects of these various conditions. In the studies reported here that examined the influence of negative affect and affectless arousal on creative problem solving, one way in which negative affect was induced was by having participants view a few minutes of the film *Night and Fog,* a French documentary about the World War II German death camps. Affectless arousal was induced by having people step up and down on a cinderblock for 2 min, so that heart rate was increased by 60%. Unlike people in the positive-affect conditions, people in either of these two conditions did not perform better than controls on the Duncker candle task or the Remote Associates Test items (Isen et al., 1987).

Negative Affect and Creativity

Both of these conditions, exercise and negative-affect film, were included to represent arousal. However, another question that was addressed in this work was whether negative affect fosters creative problem solving. This is a suggestion for which there is more anecdotal argument than actual data but that nonetheless, is raised every so often, especially in the popular press. Therefore it is worth noting that in the studies described here, negative affect did not facilitate creative problem solving as positive affect did; nor did people's self-reported affect indicate a reliable relationship between negative affect (or arousal) and increased cognitive flexibility (Isen & Daubman, 1984; Isen et al., 1987). Similarly, in some studies that investigated arousal but manipulated it through some type of anxiety (e.g., Matlin & Zajonc, 1968), there is also potential evidence against the notion that negative affect promotes novel responding. In the study by Matlin and Zajonc (1968), for example, people who had to respond in the presence of others gave fewer novel responses than did people who responded alone. There still many be some circumstances under which negative affect may be found to promote unusual responses, but it is likely that this represents a process different from that involved in positive affect's influence on creative problem solving.

The foregoing discussion raises several definitional issues, not only as regards affect and arousal, but also regarding creativity itself. When we say that positive affect facilitates creative problem solving or performance on tasks requiring innovation, but not performance on routine tasks, what do we mean? What defines a task as one involving creativity, and is creativity unitary? Like most complex concepts, creativity is probably not unitary. Just as Sternberg's (1988) triarchic theory of intelligence suggests that there are different types of intelligence, there may be different types of creativity. Thus, different types of tasks may benefit differentially from positive affect. The data reviewed thus far have shown this; my colleagues' and my work on identifying the nature of the tasks facilitated by positive affect is continuing.

The Dopamine Hypothesis

One common thread among the tasks that are facilitated by happy feelings may be the role that cognitive flexibility, that is, the ability to take different perspectives, plays in them. In this context, a recent theory proposing that the impact of positive affect on creative problem solving may be mediated by release of the neurotransmitter dopamine (Ashby, Isen, & Turken, 1998) may help to solve the definitional problem, as well as to increase our understanding of the influence of positive affect more generally. This theory proposes that dopamine, which is known to be released when an organism experiences reward or pleasantness, facilitates flexible deployment of attention and selection of cognitive perspectives, enabling multiple perspectives, and in this way enhances cognitive flexibility and promotes creative problem solving. There is substantial evidence that dopamine is associated with set switching, flexible selection of cognitive perspective, and direction of attention (see Ashby et al., 1998, for discussion). Although much remains to be investigated with regard to this hypothesis, it suggests several intriguing possibilities.

This is not to say that the feeling states, the operations that induced them, their cognitive and behavioral effects, and the circumstances under which they have different effects, are less important than the neurotransmitters in either eliciting the effects that have been observed or leading to an understanding of these relationships. Rather, I suggest that these approaches be used together to further understanding. For example, identification of the neurotransmitters called into play, and the interactions among them, in different circumstances may illuminate crucial distinctions in otherwise vague constructs or may allow more precise predictions for outcomes in different contexts.

Consider, for instance, the different impact positive affect has in a safe, positive context versus a dangerous or threatening context: It leads to increased exploration, variety seeking, and optimism in the former but increased self-protection, risk aversion, and concern with possible loss in the latter (Isen & Geva, 1987; Isen & Kahn, 1992; Kahn & Isen, 1993). These different consequences and behaviors may occur because of different actions of neurotransmitters in the two types of circumstances. In accord with hypotheses such as Damasio's (1994) and LeDoux's (1996), negative and positive events or contexts may be tagged by reactions in the amygdala. This general tag may influence the subsequent action of neurotransmitters released in response to later events in these contexts.

Nonetheless, an understanding of the everyday events that somehow influence the release and uptake of these various neurotransmitters, and the possible processes that link these events, behaviors, cognitions, or feelings to the neurotransmitters, remains equally crucial. I do not suggest that the neuropsychological level of analysis be substituted for the psychological, cognitive, and behavioral levels, but rather that researchers use both of these sources of understanding to advance knowledge and guide investigations of the role that affect may play in thought processes and behavior.

CONCLUSION

Consideration of the evidence suggests the following points:

1. Positive affect tends to facilitate creative problem solving if the task is of interest or needs to be done.
2. The facilitative effect of happy feelings is specific to creativity and does not extend to routine tasks.

3   However, performance on such algorithmic tasks is not disrupted by positive affect, either; people in positive-affect conditions do not regularly perform worse than controls on tasks such as addition, multiplication, or long division.
4   An increased tendency to use heuristics has not been demonstrated as the likely mediator of affect's influence on creativity.
5   An increased willingness to take genuine, meaningful risks has not been found to result from positive affect and therefore is not the likely mediator of its influence on creative problem solving.
6   Positive affect has been distinguished from arousal (and negative affect) in the studies showing a facilitating impact of positive affect on creative problem solving.
7   A possible mediator of the influence of positive affect on creative problem solving may involve release of the neurotransmitter dopamine, because dopamine is associated with reward and also with cognitive set switching, flexible selection of cognitive perspective, and flexible deployment of attention.

All of this work suggests some exciting avenues for continued investigation. There is much still to be uncovered about the impact of feelings on creative problem solving and the ways these effects may be mediated and maintained.

REFERENCES

Ashby, F. G., Isen, A. M., & Turken, A. U. (1998). *A neuropsychological theory of positive affect and its influence on cognition*. Unpublished manuscript, University of California at Santa Barbara.

Aspinwall, L. G., & Taylor, S. E. (1997). A stitch in time: Self-regulation and proactive coping. *Psychological Bulletin, 121*, 417–436.

Berlyne, D. E. (1967). Arousal and reinforcement. In *Nebraska Symposium on Motivation: Vol. 15.* (pp. 1–110). Lincoln: University of Nebraska Press.

Bodenhausen, G. V., Kramer, G. P., & Susser, K. (1994). Happiness and stereotypic thinking on social judgment. *Journal of Personality and Social Psychology, 66*, 621–632.

Carnevale, P. J. D., & Isen, A. M. (1986). The influence of positive affect and visual access on the discovery of integrative solutions in bilateral negotiation. *Organizational Behavior and Human Decision Processes, 37*, 1–13.

Damasio, A. R. (1994). *Descartes' error*. New York: Avon Books.

Dovidio, J. F., Gaertner, S. L., Isen, A. M., & Lowrance, R. (1995). Group representations and intergroup bias: Positive affect, similarity, and group size. *Personality and Social Psychology Bulletin, 21*, 856–865.

Duffy, E. (1934). Emotion: An example of the need for reorientation in psychology. *Psychological Review, 41*, 184–198.

Duffy, E. (1941). An explanation of "emotional" phenomena without the use of the concept of "emotion." *Journal of General Psychology, 25*, 282–293.

Duncker, K. (1945). On problem-solving. *Psychological Monographs, 58* (Whole No. 5).

Easterbrook, J. A. (1959). The effect of emotion on cue utilization and the organization of behavior. *Psychological Review, 66*, 183–201.

Estrada, C. A., Isen, A. M., & Young, M. J. (1997). Positive affect facilitates integration of information and decreases anchoring in reasoning among physicians. *Organizational Behavior and Human Decision Processes, 72*, 117–135.

Estrada, C., Young, M., & Isen, A. M. (1994). Positive affect influences creative problem solving and reported source of practice satisfaction in physicians. *Motivation and Emotion, 18,* 285–299.

Fiske, S. T., & Taylor, S. E. (1991). *Social cognition* (2nd ed.). Reading, MA: Addison-Wesley.

Forgas, J. P., & Bower, G. H. (1987). Mood effects on person-perception judgments. *Journal of Personality and Social Psychology, 53,* 53–60.

George, J. M., & Brief, A. P. (1996). Motivational agendas in the workplace: The effects of feelings on focus of attention and work motivation. In L. L. Cummings & B. M. Staw (Eds.), *Research in organizational behavior,* (Vol. 18, pp. 75–109). Greenwich, CT: JAI Press.

Greene, T.R., & Noice, H. (1988). Influence of positive affect upon creative thinking of problem solving in children. *Psychological Reports, 63,* 895–898.

Hilgard, E. R., & Bower, G. H. (1967). *Theories of learning,* (3rd ed.). New York: Appleton-Century-Crofts.

Hirt, E. R., Melton, R. J., McDonald, H. E., & Harackiewicz, J. M. (1996). Processing goals, task interest, and the mood-performance relationship: A mediational analysis. *Journal of Personality and Social Psychology, 71,* 245–261.

Isen, A. M. (1987). Positive affect, cognitive processes, and social behavior. In L. Berkowitz (Ed.), *Advances in experimental social psychology* (Vol. 20, pp. 203–253). San Diego, CA: Academic Press.

Isen, A. M. (1990). The influence of positive and negative affect on cognitive organization: Implications for development. In N. Stein, B. Leventhal, & T. Trabasso (Eds.), *Psychological and biological processes in the development of emotion* (pp. 75–94). Hillsdale, NJ: Erlbaum.

Isen, A. M. (1993). Positive affect and decision making. In M. Lewis & J. Haviland (Eds.), *Handbook of emotion* (pp. 261–277). New York: Guilford Press.

Isen, A. M., Ashby, F. G., and Waldron, E. (1997). The sweet smell of success. *Aromachology Review.*

Isen, A. M., & Baron, R. A. (1991). Positive affect in organizations. In L. L. Cummings & B. M. Staw (Eds.), *Research in organizational behavior* (Vol. 13, pp. 1–52). Greenwich, CT: JAI Press.

Isen, A. M., Berg, J. W., & Chen, M. (1991). *The influence of affect on a creative vs. a routine task.* Unpublished manuscript, Cornell University, Ithaca, NY.

Isen, A. M., & Daubman, K. A. (1984). The influence of affect on categorization. *Journal of Personality and Social Psychology, 47,* 1206–1217.

Isen, A. M., Daubman, K. A., & Nowicki, G. P. (1987). Positive affect facilitates creative problem solving. *Journal of Personality and Social Psychology, 52,* 1122–1131.

Isen, A. M., & Geva, N. (1987). The influence of positive affect on acceptable level of risk: The person with a large canoe has a large worry. *Organization Behavior and Human Decision Processes, 39,* 145–154.

Isen, A. M., Johnson, M. M. S., Mertz, E., & Robinson, G. F. (1985). The influence of positive affect on the unusualness of word associations. *Journal of Personality and Social Psychology, 48,* 1413–1426.

Isen, A. M., & Kahn, B. E. (1992, July). *The effect of positive and negative framing on the influence of positive affect on variety seeking.* Paper presented at the annual meeting of the Marketing Science Association, London, England.

Isen, A. M., Niedenthal, P., & Cantor, N. (1992). The influence of positive affect on social categorization. *Motivation and Emotion, 16,* 65–78.

Isen, A. M., Nygren, T. E., & Ashby, F. G. (1988). The influence of positive affect on the subjective utility of gains and losses: It's just not worth the risk. *Journal of Personality and Social Psychology, 55,* 710–717.

Isen, A. M., & Patrick, R. (1983). The influence of positive feelings on risk taking: When the chips are down. *Organizational Behavior and Human Performance, 31,* 194–202.

Isen, A. M., Rosenzweig, A. S., & Young, M. J. (1991). The influence of positive affect on clinical problem solving. *Medical Decision Making, 11,* 221–227.

Isen, A. M., & Shalker, T. (1982). The effect of mood state on evaluation of positive, neutral, and negative stimuli: When you "accentuate the positive," do you "eliminate the negative?" *Social Psychology Quarterly, 48,* 58–63.

Isen, A. M., Shalker, T., Clark, M., & Karp, L. (1978). Affect, accessibility of material in memory, and behavior: A cognitive loop? *Journal of Personality and Social Psychology, 36,* 1–12.

Isen, A. M., & Williams, K. (1988). *The influence of positive affect on children's creativity in play.* Unpublished manuscript, Cornell University, Ithaca, NY.

Johnson, E., & Tversky, A. (1982). Affect generalization and the perception of risk. *Journal of Personality and Social Psychology, 45,* 20–31.

Kahn, B., & Isen, A. M. (1993). The influence of positive affect on variety-seeking among safe, enjoyable products. *Journal of Consumer Research, 20,* 257–270.

Koestler, A. (1964). *The act of creation.* New York: Macmillan.

Kraiger, K., Billings, R. S., & Isen, A. M. (1989). The influence of positive affective states on task perception and satisfaction. *Organizational Behavior and Human Decision Processes, 44,* 12–25.

Lacey, J. I. (1967). Somatic response patterning and stress: Some revisions of activation theory. In M. H. Appley & R. Trumball (Eds.), *Psychological stress: Issues in research* (pp. 14–44). New York: Appleton-Century-Crofts.

Lacey, J. I. (1975). Psychophysiology of the autonomic nervous system. In J. R. Nazarrow (Ed.), *Master lectures in physiological psychology.* [cassette recording] Washington, DC: American Psychological Association.

Lacey, J. I., Kagan, J., Lacey, B., & Moss, H. A. (1963). The visceral level: Situational detemints and behavioral correlates of autonomic response patterns. In P. H. Knapp (Ed.), *Expressions of the emotions in man.* Madison, CT: International Universities Press.

LeDoux, J. E. (1996). *The emotional brain: The mysterious underpinnings of emotional life.* New York: Simon & Schuster.

Lewinsohn, S., & Mano, H. (1993). Multiattribute choice and affect: The influence of naturally occurring and manipulated moods on choice processes. *Journal of Behavioral Decision Making, 6,* 33–51.

Mackie, D. M., & Worth, L. (1991). Feeling good but not thinking straight: The impact of positive mood on persuasion. In J. P. Forgas (Ed.), *Emotion and social judgment* (pp. 201–220). Oxford, England: Pergamon.

Mandler, G. (1984). *Mind and body: Psychology of emotion and stress.* New York: W. W. Norton.

Mano, H. (1992). Judgments under distress: Assessing the role of unpleasantness and arousal in judgment formation. *Organizational Behavior and Human Decision Processes, 52,* 216–245.

Mano, H. (1998). Affect and persuasion: The influence of pleasantness and arousal on attitude formation and message elaboration. *Psychology & Marketing.*

Martin, L. L., Ward, D. W., Achee, J. W., & Wyer, R. S., Jr. (1993). Mood as input: People have to interpret the motivational implications of their moods. *Journal of Personality and Social Psychology, 64,* 317–326.

Matlin, M. W., & Zajonc, R. B. (1968). Social facilitation of word associations. *Journal of Personality and Social Psychology, 10,* 455–460.

Mednick, M. T., Mednick, S. A., & Mednick, E. V. (1964). Incubation of creative performance and specific associative priming. *Journal of Abnormal and Social Psychology, 69,* 84–88.

Mednick, S. A. (1962). The associative basis of the creative process. *Psychological Review, 69,* 220–232.

Murray, N., Sujan, H., Hirt, E. R., & Sujan, M. (1990). The influence of mood on categorization: A cognitive flexibility interpretation. *Journal of Personality and Social Psychology, 59,* 411–425.

Neiss, R. (1990). Ending arousal's reign of error: A reply to Anderson. *Psychological Bulletin, 107,* 1010–1050.

Pruitt, D.G. (1983). Strategic choice in negotiation. *American Behavioral Scientist, 27,* 167–194.

Rosch, E. (1975). Cognitive representations of semantic categories. *Journal of Experimental Psychology: General, 104* 192–233.

Russ, S. (1993). *Affect and creativity:* The role of affect and play in the creative process. Hillsdale, NJ: Erlbaum.

Schwarz, N., & Bless, H. (1991). Happy and mindless, but sad and smart? The impact of affective states on analytic reasoning. In J. P. Forgas (Ed.), *Emotion and social judgment* (p. 55–71). Oxford, England: Pergamon.

Showers, C., & Cantor, N. (1985). Social cognition: A look at motivated strategies. *Annual Review of Psychology, 36,* 275–305.

Smith, S. M., & Shaffer, D. R. (1991). The effects of good moods on systematic processing: "Willing but not able, or able but not willing?" *Motivation and Emotion, 15,* 243–279.

Staw, B. M., & Barsade, S. G. (1993). Affect and managerial performance: A test of the sadder-but-wiser vs. happier-and smarter hypotheses. *Administrative Science Quarterly, 38,* 304–331.

Staw, B. M., Sutton, R. I., & Pelled, L. H. (1994). Employee positive emotion and favorable outcomes at the workplace. *Organizational Science, 5,* 51–71.

Sternberg, R. (1988). *The triarchic mind: A new theory of human intelligence.* New York: Viking.

Taylor, S. E., & Aspinwall, L. G. (1996). Mediating and moderating processes in psychosocial stress: Appraisal, coping, resistance and vulnerability. In H. B. Kaplan (Ed.), *Psychosocial stress: Perspectives on structure, theory, life-course, and methods* (pp. 71–110). San Diego, CA: Academic Press.

Tversky, A., & Gati, I. (1978). Studies of similarity. In E. Rosch & B. B. Lloyd (Eds.), *Cognition and categorization* (pp. 79–98). Hillsdale, NJ: Erlbaum.

Venables, P. H. (1984). Arousal: An examination of its status as a concept. In M. G. H. Coles, J. R. Jennings, & J. A. Stern (Eds.), *Psychophysiological perspectives: Festschrift for Beatrice and John Lacey* (pp. 134–142). New York: Van Nostrand Reinhold.

Wertheimer, M. (1945). *Productive thinking.* New York: Harper & Row.

Yerkes, R. M., & Dodson, J. D. (1908). The relationship of strength of stimulus to rapidity of habit formation. *Journal of comparative and Neurological Psychology, 18,* 459–482.

Zajonc, R. B. (1965). Social facilitation. *Science, 149,* 269–274.

2

Mood and Creativity Research: The View From a Conceptual Organizing Perspective

Suzanne Vosburg
University of Bergen, Norway

Geir Kaufmann
Norwegian School of Management, Norway

The research on mood and creativity is scattered, and it is therefore difficult to form a coherent view of the findings and their theoretical meaning. In this chapter, we introduce a conceptual framework that could serve as a means to classify and systematically review existing studies in the field and pinpoint areas that need to be further examined. First, we need to clarify the nature of the pivotal concepts of this research domain.

WHAT IS MEANT BY "CREATIVITY"?

Novelty of ideas is generally seen as the hallmark of creative thinking. However, novelty is not sufficient, because an idea can be novel simply because it makes no sense or is idiosyncratic. Creative ideas or products not only are novel, but also have a certain value or meaning, either for the creator or the culture, in the sense of being useful, appropriate, or valuable (Boden, 1991; Kaufmann, 1988; Newell, Shaw, & Simon, 1979). Thus, it has become customary to define creativity as the process that leads to ideas that are both novel and useful, appropriate, or valuable (e.g., Amabile, 1983; Eysenck, 1994; MacKinnon, 1978; Stein, 1974; Sternberg & Lubart, 1995; Weisberg, 1988).

Kaufmann (1993) took this idea a step further, suggesting that the second part of the concept of creativity, variously described as usefulness, appropriateness, or value, can be subsumed under the general concept of *validity*. He described the term as including such areas as the basic meaningfulness of an idea (conceptual validity), the internal consistency of a theoretical model (theoretical validity), the esthetic value of artistic products (expressive validity), the function of a device (instrumental validity), and a novel social practice (social validity).

However, the twin concepts of novelty and validity are hardly exhaustive as defining criteria for creativity. As Kaufmann (1993) pointed out, this definition of creativity is not sufficiently distinct from standard definitions of intelligence. This is seen in the fairly representative definition of the concept of intelligence suggested by Gregory (1981), who singled out novelty and successfulness as hallmarks of intelligent behavior. The concept of successful novelty is clearly seen to be almost synonymous with standard definitions of creativity.

Newell, Shaw, & Simon (1979) hinted at a possible solution to this problem when they argued that it is necessary to qualify the novelty in question by adding the feature of a *modification or rejection of previously accepted ideas*. Kaufmann (1993) elaborated on this qualification, arguing that adding this feature to the criteria of novelty and validity provides a solution to the problem of discriminating between the concepts of creativity and intelligence in a way that captures the unique aspects of creativity.

A similar argument was put forward by Boden (1991), who distinguished between *first-time novelty* and *radical novelty*. Radical novelty was described as "thinking the impossible," which comes about by making a radical departure from a standard outlook on a problem. The radical departure consists of challenging the basic rules of a particular conceptual space, as exemplified by Schoenberg's reorganization of the standard musical space of tonality. The definition of creativity that forms the point of departure for the present treatment thus contains three basic features: *novelty, unconventionality* (or anticonventionality), and *validity*.

SORTING MOOD CONCEPTS

Emotion, mood, and affect appear to be overlapping concepts, and researchers have not reached an agreement on the distinguishing characteristics and functions of each construct (e.g., see Ekman & Davidson, 1994). However, there are some similar trends across different suggestions for conceptual clarification.

Mood Morris (1989) distinguished between mood as "figure" and as "ground." As ground, mood is the backdrop against which a person experiences and evaluates events; as figure, mood comes into the forefront of attention, which may result in an attempt to explain why a particular mood is present and, if it is negative, an attempt to "repair" or replace the current mood state. Moods are seen to be pervasive and global and to have the capability to influence a broad range of thought processes and behavior (M. S. Clark & Isen, 1982; Isen, 1984; Morris, 1989, 1992).

Feeling States A potential confusion lies in the use of the term *feeling states*. Feeling states are induced by pleasant or unpleasant experience, are pervasive, and can influence thoughts. In other words, they are the same as moods (M. S. Clark & Isen, 1982).

Emotion Emotions are generally thought of as being more intense and short-lived than moods (Watson & Clark, 1994); more likely to interrupt behavior and demand attention (Simon, 1982); and more directly experienced, that is, attributable (Morris, 1989); and as having positive or negative valence (Clore, 1994). Emotions are thought to represent a response to a subjective experience (Watson & Clark, 1994) and have a defined onset and decline (Morris, 1989; Oatley & Jenkins, 1992). They can be elicited by evaluating events that concern a person's important needs or goals (Frijda, 1993).

Affect Affect has been conceptualized as an overarching category of which emotion and mood are subsets (e.g., Russ, 1993; Simon, 1982). In the view of Watson and Clark (1984, 1994) and Tellegen (1985), affect is a disposition to experience certain emotions or feeling states. Positive Affect is the extent to which a person experiences a level of pleasure, whereas Negative Affect is the degree to which one is prone to experience distress. Besides the valence dimension, researchers have distinguished between a state and a trait dimension of both emotion and mood (e.g., Izard, 1991; Tellegen, 1985; Watson & Clark, 1994).

According to Kaufmann (1998), a way of solving the conceptual intricacies involved in distinguishing between emotion, feeling, affect, and mood is to view these concepts in *pairs* that can be characterized along two dimensions: background versus foreground expressions and general disposition versus specific manifestation.

In this scheme, *emotion–feeling* is one pair, wherein emotion is a general disposition such as fear, aggression, jealousy, happiness, etc., and a feeling is the overt, specific expression of this general state or disposition. *Mood–affect* is the other pair, wherein mood is a background state, and affect is the corresponding overt manifestation of it. In the same way we can talk about emotions being manifested in overt feelings, we can say that moods are manifested in overt affects. Thus, positive mood may be manifested in the affective state of elation and negative mood, in the overt state of depression. By definition, then, mood is a background state not consciously articulated by the individual.

Methodological Design	Core	Adjunct	Peripheral
Controlled	• Greene & Noice, 1988 • Isen, et al., 1987 (Studies 1 and 2) • Jausovec, 1989 • Kaufmann & Vosburg, 1997 (Study 2)	• Abele, 1992 • Estrada et al., 1994 • Greene & Noice, 1988 • Isen, et al., 1987 (Studies 3 and 4) • Kaufmann & Vosburg (in preparation) • Melton, 1995	• Isen & Daubman, 1984 • Isen et al., 1985 • Melton, 1995 • Mitchell & Madigan, 1984 • Murray et al., 1990
Quasi-Experimental	• Andreasen, 1987 • Andreasen & Cantor, 1974 • Andreasen & Powers, 1975 • Jamison, 1989 • Kaufmann & Vosburg, 1997 Study #1 • Ludwig, 1994 • Rothenberg, 1983 • Rothenberg & Burkhardt, 1984 • Weisberg, 1994	• Andreasen & Powers, 1974 • Bowden, 1994 • Vosburg, in press	
Correlational	• Eisenmann, 1990 • Richards & Kinney, 1990 • Richards et al., 1992 • Richards et al., 1988	• Mraz & Runco, 1994 • Schuldberg, 1990	• Staw & Barsade, 1993
Naturalistic	• Bower, 1989 • Frosch, 1987 • Jamison, 1993 • Rothenberg, 1990 • Schildkraut Hirschfeld, 1990		

Figure 1

A FRAMEWORK FOR MOOD AND CREATIVITY RESEARCH

The organizing, conceptual framework we propose is designed around two basic dimensions: The horizontal axis of the model classifies the *type of creativity process* examined in a particular investigation, and the vertical axis is the *methodological design* employed. Figure 1 presents this framework as an attempt to synthesize the mood and creativity research literature.

Type of Creativity Process

In the first dimension, *core processes* refers to processes that contain all three elements in the definition of creativity proposed earlier: novelty, unconventionality (or anticonventionality), and validity. *Adjunct processes* refers to processes that are important parts of the creative process but do not sample all three elements. *Peripheral processes* refers to processes that may sort under different areas of inquiry but are clearly linked to and relevant to understanding creativity. We describe these classifications in more detail later.

Methodological Design

The vertical axis is organized in hierarchical order according to the level of experimental control implemented. The top end of this axis is the controlled experiment, where mood is manipulated as an independent variable and effects on the dependent variable are examined. There are several difficulties inherent in this method. Individual differences as well as the difficulty of inducing sufficient and equal levels of positive and negative mood, make mood induction a complex undertaking. Conversely, the strength in experimental designs is the experimental manipulation, which allows for results that are thoroughly comparable and more easily interpretable.

The lower end of the axis is the naturalistic approach, that is, studies aimed at examining a phenomenon in its natural state under ecologically valid conditions. A typical example of the naturalistic approach is the case study. For our purposes, we limit the case studies to those that document the moods or mood disorders of past or present creators (however, most of these studies are concerned with past creators).

Between these two extremes are quasi-experimental studies, which compare matched groups with contrasting characteristics, and correlational studies, which primarily compare (or correlate) groups of instrumental measures and draw inferences about relationships within the data. Quasi-experimental designs allow for meaningful comparisons between groups for whom an experimental manipulation may not be possible or appropriate. However, the weaknesses of the two designs are similar: Without an experimental manipulation or randomization (in the case of quasi-experimental design), causal effects of the observed relationships may be difficult to interpret.

Tasks and Processes

Creative Problem-Solving Tasks   Creative problem-solving tasks are operationalizations of the creative process.

Measures of Core Processes   Insight problems require a radical restructuring of the conventional way of looking at the problem and a novel solution that is appropriate according to the solution requirements. Thus, we argue that insight problems constitute a miniature model of creative thinking (for a similar view, see Sternberg & Davidson, 1982, 1995). In our scheme, insight tasks qualify as measures of core processes.

Measures of Adjunct Processes   In contrast, divergent-thinking problems require the production of many different original ideas. These tasks model only the process of idea generation and are geared to the novelty aspect of creativity, which we see as an adjunct-process measure.

Finally, remote associates are founded on an associative theory of creativity (Mednick, 1962). A typical example of remote association is the Remote Associates Test (RAT; Mednick, 1962), which measures the ability to find the associative link that will connect three stimulus words. (For example, the words *blue, mouse,* and *moon* are given, and the response is *cheese).* Such associative combinations may be important ingredients of creative thinking, but as Boden (1991) succinctly argued, this mechanism per se does not distinguish between combinations of ideas that are valid, or promise to be valid, and those that are outlandish and have no validity.

Measures of Peripheral Processes Some processes are linked to the creative process peripherally, because they index creative ability indirectly but also sort more generally under other cognitive functions. An example is categorization. Certainly, categorization may be important to creative thinking, but it is not uniquely and intrinsically linked to creativity, as are the core processes defined above. It is possible to link categorization tasks to creativity because the studies here are concerned with original groupings evoked by a presented rule.

Other tasks included in this category are means–end problem-solving tasks, which are rather general tasks of problem solving. However, they are designed in such a way that they call for successful use of the kind of heuristics (e.g., analogies) that often figure prominently in the process of creative thinking. Thus, we place studies of more general cognitive processes in this dimension only if they explicitly draw connections to creativity.

Criteria for Inclusion of Studies in the Review

Studies were subjected to selective inclusion and exclusion criteria in order to retain the most targeted and appropriate studies. Only investigations focused specifically on mood and the creativity processes defined above—core, adjunct or peripheral processes—were included. We excluded some of the other mood literature, including research on mood and memory (Blaney, 1986; G. Bower, 1981), mood and persuasion (Abele & Hermer, 1993; Bless, Bohner, Schwarz, & Strack, 1990; Mackie & Worth, 1989; Schwarz, Bless, & Bohner, 1991; Worth & Mackie, 1987), mood and impression formation (Abele & Petzold, 1994; Martin, Ward, Achee, & Wyer, 1993), mood and information-processing (Brown & Taylor, 1986; Schwarz & Clore, 1983, 1988), mood and social behavior (Bodenhausen, Kramer, & Süsser, 1994; Isen, Clark, & Schwartz, 1976; Isen & Levin, 1972; Isen, Niedenthal, & Cantor, 1992; Isen, Shalker, Clark, & Karp, 1978; Isen & Simmonds, 1978), mood and task perception (Kraiger, Billings, & Isen, 1989), mood and negotiation (Carnevale & Isen, 1986), mood and variety-seeking behavior (Kahn & Isen, 1993), anxiety and creativity (Matthews, 1986a), and arousal and creativity (Matthews, 1986b; Toplyn & Maguire, 1991), even if issues and findings might indirectly be related to the core issues of mood and creativity.

Further, we included only studies that defined mood in the strict conceptual sense and excluded studies of other affective experience, such as emotion (Ekman & Davidson 1994; Izard, 1991) and affect (L. A. Clark, Watson, & Mineka, 1994; Diener & Iran-Nejad, 1986; Watson, 1988; Watson, Clark, & Carey, 1988; Watson, Clark, McIntyre, & Hamaker, 1992; Watson & Walker, 1996).

Clearly, the mood and creativity literature could be classified in different ways. Our present aim is to provide a theory-neutral, comprehensive, yet domain-specific classification of the literature that provides a good overview of the present state of the research and indicates direction for future investigation.

REVIEW OF THE RESEARCH ON MOOD AND CREATIVITY

Controlled on Core Process Studies

Core processes in a controlled setting are specifically insight problems, according to our definition. Greene and Noice (1988) and Isen, Daubman, and Nowicki (1987, Studies 1 and 2) found that positive mood facilitated creative problem solving on Duncker's (1945) candle task. Isen et al. induced positive and neutral moods (using film segments) in Study 1; and induced positive mood (by film and a small gift), negative mood (by film), and arousal (by exercise) in Study 2. They presented the task in physical object form (as opposed to written form). Greene and Noice induced positive mood by a small gift or compliment and presented the task in object form. Both studies showed that positive mood facilitated the solution of Duncker's candle task.

Two other studies produced contradictory results. Jausovec (1989) induced positive, negative, and neutral moods by film segments. He presented base information and problem-solving tasks in written form, with the aim of examining the influence of mood on analogical transfer of information from base form to the problem-solving tasks. From his results, a general conclusion that positive mood facilitates creative problem solving could not be drawn, because he found that positive mood did not facilitate analogical transfer with respect to Duncker's radiation task—an insight problem much like the one Isen et al. used. Kaufmann and Vosburg (1997, Study 2) examined the effects of positive, negative, and neutral mood, induced by film, on the solution of two insight problems presented in writing to participants. In stark contrast to Isen et al., they found that positive mood was detrimental to performance on insight tasks. In their study, the *negative* mood induction group solved the insight problems with the greatest ease, followed by the neutral, and then the control group; positive-mood participants had the most difficulty solving the problems. Task performance was recorded by both error rates and solution latencies.

This particular quadrant seems to house the most contradictory results of the model. Kaufmann and Vosburg (1997) and Vosburg (1998) suggested that distinguishing between satisficing and optimizing criteria for solution (Robbins, 1993; Simon, 1977); could explain these seeming differences. Satisficing entails accepting the first solution that meets a subjective task fulfillment criterion. Optimizing means maximizing the outcome of problem solving by searching for the best possible solution.

Insight problems are an example of a strict optimizing requirement, because there is only one ideal solution according to the solution requirements. Kaufmann and Vosburg (1997) argued that positive mood promotes a satisficing strategy, whereas negative mood facilitates an optimizing strategy that is expedient in meeting the strict solution criteria required in these tasks.

This idea offers a possible solution to the discrepancy between Kaufmann and Vosburg's (1997) and Isen et al.'s (1987) findings, which are the most directly comparable experiments. Isen et al. had participants manipulate physical objects, whereas Kaufmann and Vosburg administered paper-and-pencil tasks. Solution feedback from physical objects can show that the solution attempt is not adequate and at the same time instigate further search. Participants in a positive mood may be more optimistic and less vulnerable to failure, so the search for an adequate solution continues until the solution is found. Kaufmann and Vosburg's tasks provided no outside feedback, so participants could stop prematurely before reaching an adequate solution. It was suggested that when participants are left to set their own subjective solution criterion, positive-mood participants set a lower criterion for solution acceptance and are prone to accept lower quality solutions without searching further for better ones. However, this explanation needs to be tested in independent experiments. An obvious possibility would be to compare the effects of mood on performance under feedback versus no-feedback conditions. Another interesting possibility consists in varying the instructions for solution requirements for the same insight problem (i.e., "Think of as many solutions as you can for this problem" vs. "Think of the one best solution").

Controlled Adjunct Process Studies

Ideational Fluency Tasks In two studies, Abele (1992) induced mood by using autobiographical recall and measured its effect on ideational fluency in two types of divergent-thinking tasks: "Unusual Uses" and "Fictitious Situations." She reported the main effect that positive mood facilitated performance measured as fluency on divergent thinking tasks. She also found an interaction between mood and task type: Performance on tasks that elicited positive ideas (high instrumental interest) was facilitated by positive mood in controls, but performance on tasks that evoked negative responses (low instrumental interest) was superior in the control group. The negative-mood group performed better than the control group on tasks that evoked positive or neutral responses but worse than controls on tasks that required negative responses.

In a similarly designed study, Kaufmann and Vosburg (1998) induced positive and negative mood with film segments and examined task performance in divergent-thinking tasks presented in written format. They found that positive mood facilitated early production of ideas, but the effect tapered off drastically, rendering negative mood facilitative of superior idea generation in later idea production. This finding is in keeping with the satisficing/optimizing model described by Kaufmann and Vosburg (1997). In early idea production there are less constraints, allowing generation under an "anything goes" model; as time progresses, more constraints may become apparent, and under these constraints negative mood may better facilitate more targeted idea production.

Mood and Making Remote Associates Many researchers have reported that RAT performance seems to be facilitated by positive mood (Estrada, Isen, & Young, 1994; Isen et al., 1987). Estrada et al. (1994) induced positive mood in physicians by giving a small gift of candy or reading statements about humanistic sources of practice satisfaction and explored the effects of mood on RAT performance and practice satisfaction. They found that positive mood (induced by candy) led to superior scores on the creativity test. Isen et al. (1987) induced positive mood by presenting a small bag of candy in Study 3 and via films in Study 4 and found that positive mood facilitated RAT performance. They attributed this finding to the tendency of positive mood to influence cognitive organization by affecting the pattern and degree of relatedness that people see between different cognitive elements, thereby enabling superior associational capabilities. It should be noted, however, that Melton (1995) induced mood by cartoons or a comedy tape and did not find that positive mood led to superior performance on the RAT.

A possible means to explain these contradictory findings would be to vary the solution requirements of the RAT. This could be accomplished by using items that involve superficial processing (an easier level of difficulty) versus items that require deeper associative links (more difficult items). Because positive mood is often associated with more superficial or shallow processing, it would be expected to facilitate RAT performance when a surface solution is required. Positive mood is not conducive to narrow and deeper processing, so it might be expected that if these were the solution requirements for certain items, task performance would not be facilitated by positive mood.

In sum, the adjunct-process studies support the hypothesis that positive mood facilitates creative problem solving. All show positive mood associated with superior performance on each task operationalizing the adjunct process.

Controlled Peripheral Process Studies

Categorization Tasks Isen and Daubman (1984) induced mood by giving a gift or showing a film segment and asked participants to rate items on a 10-point scale in terms of whether they belonged to a particular category. In a subsequent study, they asked participants to sort colored chips into as many or as few categories as they desired. They found that positive mood led to more inclusion: Participants grouped more unusual exemplars as members of given categories and created fewer categories that included a large number of chips. Isen, Johnson, Mertz, and Robinson (1985) induced moods in participants by having them read valenced words or by showing a film. They reported that positive mood led to giving more positive and unusual associations to neutral words. Murray, Sujan, Hirt, and Sujan (1990) reported that positive mood, induced by the Velten procedure (reading self-referent statements designed to induce positive or negative moods), led to generating more similarities and differences between television shows; that is, it resulted in more categorization flexibility.

Means–Ends Tasks Mitchell and Madigan (1984) examined the effects of mood on interpersonal problem-solving ability. Mood was induced by the Velten procedure, and the task required providing the ending to a presented story. The investigators found that participants in the positive-mood condition generated more words and more relevant means to solutions than did those in the negative- or neutral-mood condition. Because this task is similar to a divergent thinking task, Mitchell and Madigan thought this finding showed support for the theory that positive mood facilitates adjunct-process performance.

Relevant to the interpretation of mood effects on creative problem solving tasks is the study reported by Melton (1995), in which a distinction was made between task components of generation and evaluation. Melton argued that these components may be differentially related to mood effects: Positive mood tends to facilitate generation but not evaluation. He examined the effects of positive and neutral moods on syllogism performance and showed that participants in a positive mood did not solve syllogisms as well as participants in a neutral mood. He attributed this finding to the idea that participants in positive moods expend less effort on task, which supports the satisficing account for the discrepant insight task findings reported above.

Quasi-Experimental Core-Process Studies

The connection between quasi-experimental core-process studies and mood and creativity studies may not be obvious. Like naturalistic studies, this set of quasi-experimental studies investigated creative persons; however, explicit comparisons were made between assigned groups. Many of the participants in these studies suffered from some type of affective disorder, which can be thought of as one extreme end of a mood continuum (Morris, 1992), the other end of which is slightly positive or slightly negative mood, and therefore the studies are included in the mood and creativity field.

Andreasen and Canter (1974) compared 15 successful writers from the University of Iowa Writers' Workshop and 15 controls outside the creative arts, from whom they gathered history of psychiatric symptoms and family history.

They reported that a large percentage of the writers (and their first-degree relatives) experienced a greater incidence of psychiatric disorder, most commonly affective disorder, than did controls and their relatives. Furthermore, they reported a tendency for writers to suffer primarily from a depressive type of affective disorder. Andreasen and Powers (1975) compared performance on an object-sorting test between creative writers and manic and schizophrenic patients. They concluded with caution that writers' thought processes resembled those in the manic phase of bipolar disorder; however, they carefully specified that the writers' overinclusion of objects was qualitatively different from the manic patients'. In response to Andreasen and Canter's study, Rothenberg and Burkhardt (1984) compared writers' word association response rates with those of psychiatric inpatients (depressive and schizophrenic). They reasoned that if writers had a tendency to be depressed, they would have slower latency rates to stimulus words. This hypothesis was not supported by their data and was therefore at odds with the trend of a greater incidence of depression in writers reported by Andreasen and Canter. Rothenberg (1983) also found that individuals identified by high-level creative performance (Nobel laureates) gave the most rapid opposite responses to stimuli (an indication of Janusian thinking, which is simultaneously conceptualizing opposite terms or concepts) compared with psychiatric patients and high- and low-creativity students. The patient group responded with the slowest latencies, again indicating a distinction between creative and psychopathological thought.

A more recent group of studies produced similar findings. Andreasen (1987) studied another group of writers from the Iowa Writers' Workshop, a matched comparison group, and first-degree relatives. She conducted structured interviews with the writers and the control group. Jamison (1989), too, carried out a series of interviews with a group of eminent British writers and artists, including poets, playwrights, novelists, and artists (biographers served as a comparison group). Lastly, Ludwig (1994) studied a group of women writers, based on interviews and completed questionnaires.

In each study, the selected sample had a disproportionate degree of mental illness, usually some type of affective disorder. Andreasen specifically noted that in her sample of writers there was a close association between mental illness and creativity. The majority of Jamison's participants said that intense moods and feeling states were integral or very important to their work.

Rothenberg (1990) has been consistently definitive in stating that creative thought processes are healthy ones and comparisons of the processes that occur in creative thinking and those that take place in affective disorders should be made carefully, if at all.

In Kaufmann and Vosburg's (1997) quasi-experimental Study 1, in which people who differed on positive- and negative-mood measures were compared on the basis of their task performance—the same procedure they used in their

Study 2, described in detail in the Controlled Core Process Studies section—there were results similar to those in Study 2: Positive mood was detrimental to insight problem performance. This is in line with their reported experimental manipulations.

Weisberg (1994) provided a different way to study creativity. He examined the career and productivity of the composer Robert Schumann with the goal of determining whether Schumann produced high-quality work in the years when he was hypomanic and highly productive. Weisberg used music guides to design an "archival measure of quality" which included two facets: Absolute equality for a given year was a measure of the number of recordings made of the pieces Schumann composed in that year, and relative quality was the average number of recordings available for each year's compositions. His finding suggested that the proportion of high-quality works remained constant over Schumann's life, implying that when the composer was more productive (in a hypomanic state), he was not more creative.

The concern that their sample sizes are small and participants were selected from a very unique group of individuals could be raised about most of these studies (with the exception of Kaufmann & Vosburg, 1997, Study 1). On the other hand, because these studies represent fundamental components of creative thinking, the findings can be be generalized.

Quasi-Experimental Adjunct-Process Studies

Replicating the general finding in the controlled experiments of adjunct-processes, Vosburg (1998) found the same pattern (as previously mentioned in this dimension) of positive mood rendering superior performance and negative mood leading to worse performance in terms of ideational fluency measured with divergent-thinking tasks. Furthermore, with these tasks, an equally large but diametrically opposite effect of positive and negative mood was found. Positive mood improved ideational fluency, while negative mood decreased it, establishing further support for positive mood's facilitating adjunct process.

Comparing manic and schizophrenic patients with normal controls, Andreasen and Powers (1974) administered a test of overinclusion and found that mania tended to be associated with more overinclusiveness than schizophrenia. From these findings, they drew a connection between affective disorder and overinclusive thinking, a hypothesis that was expanded by Andreasen and Powers (1975).

Correlational Core-Process Studies

Richards and her colleagues have made large contributions to the area of correlational core-process studies and made significant progress in demystifying the relationship between creativity and mental illness. Instead of moving in the direction from creativity to disorder, they figuratively "traced backward" to identify how disorders may or may not be related to creativity in the general population as determined by the Lifetime Creativity Scales (Richards, Kinney, Benet, & Merzel, 1988). Everyday creativity appeared to be enhanced in a milder form of bipolar illness; that is, there may be a creative advantage in certain mood disorders. Richards and Kinney (1990) asked people with bipolar disorder to fill out questionnaires eliciting background demographics and diagnoses and asked them to rate at what mood they felt the most creative (along with other characteristics) and how they felt when they were most creative. The results showed that participants with a bipolar disorder of Type I, II, or III found a mildly elevated mood, rather than an extremely elevated mood, to be conducive to creativity. Richards, Kinney, Daniels, and Linkins (1992) found job creativity to be higher in persons with bipolar disorder with milder mood elevations than in those with more severe forms.

These studies help clarify the relationship between creativity, mental health, and mental illness. The question is no longer whether the optimal environment for creativity is mental health or mental illness, but rather, if mental or affective illness is involved, what circumstances link illness course or treatment to productivity and creativity. Richards et al. (1988) and Jamison (1993) have shown that there may be a creative advantage in having a disorder that involves fluctuating senses of energy, confidence, well-being, fluency of thoughts and productivity.

Correlational Adjunct-Process Studies

Both of the correlational adjunct-process studies explored the relationships between creativity and other kinds of mental experiences, from suicidal ideation to an inclination toward subclinical psychopathological tendencies or experiences. Schuldberg (1990) administered paper-and-pencil tests designed to explore the subclinical features of psychopathology and everyday levels of creativity. Scales measuring subclinical negative symptoms (lack of emotional responding and movement retardation) were negatively related to creative functioning, whereas scales measuring subclinical positive symptoms (hallucinations or delusions) were positively related.

In a similarly designed study, Mraz and Runco (1994) administered scales that measured suicide ideation, hopelessness, and stress, as well as two categories of real world divergent thinking tasks: Problem solving and problem generation tasks. They found that suicide ideation was positively associated with problem generation fluency and negatively associated with problem solving flexibility, suggesting that the participants who showed strong negative mood tendencies were able to generate many problems but not able to generate adaptive solutions.

In contrast to the clinical populations investigated in the correlational core-process studies, both correlational studies of adjunct processes focused on normal populations and subclinical symptoms. At least two conclusions can be drawn from their results. First, creativity appears to follow a normal distribution, and is not an all-or-none phenomenon, and it may be studied in small samples drawn from the normal population rather than investigations of extreme groups. Second, particular subclinical features of psychopathology involving an affective component appear to be associated with problem-solving abilities.

Correlational Peripheral-Process Studies

Staw and Barsade (1993) compared the "sadder-but-wiser" hypothesis (i.e., that those with depressive tendencies have a more realistic outlook) to the "happier-and-smarter" hypothesis (that those who have a positive outlook do not suffer from an optimism bias) in a managerial decision-making simulation. They found that people who tended to have a positive disposition tended to make better decisions and were rated more favorably by their peers and supervisors. They attributed this finding to the idea that positive people may be more productive, especially with interpersonal relations and decision making. Although this study confirms general characteristics associated with positive mood, it could be argued that the conclusion is limited, because no measure of negative affect was included.

Naturalistic Core-Process Studies

Naturalistic studies are observational studies of real-world creativity. In our classification, we include studies of how people manage their affective disorders, along with their creative lives. Jamison (1993), for example, documented manic–depressive illness and aspects of it that can lead to greater artistic imagination and productivity. She argued for the association between manic–depressive illness and creativity in the arts by reviewing current thinking and research about the illness and then documented the lives, productivity and illnesses of many major writers, artists and thinkers. H. Bower (1989) documented Beethoven's depressive illness, while Frosch (1987) studied affective illness in musical composition by documenting many musical composers' lives. Schildkraut and Hirschfeld (1990) documented the role melancholy and depression played in the artist Joan Miro's life.

A THEORY OF MOOD EFFECTS ON CREATIVE PROBLEM SOLVING

The research findings presented in this chapter are highly discrepant and do not seem to lead to any kind of straightforward link between mood and creativity, as has been claimed by some researchers (e.g., see Isen et al., 1987). In fact, examples of mood effects in all directions have been reported: A positive effect of positive mood, a negative effect of positive mood, a positive effect of negative mood, and a negative effect of negative mood. We do not believe this is a matter of improper research with poorly conceptualized designs. Such results may seem

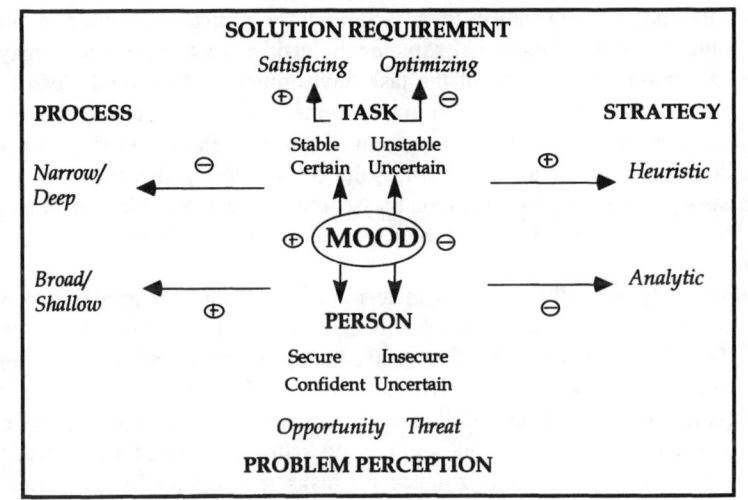

MOOD AND CREATIVITY RESEARCH: A CONCEPTUAL ORGANIZING MODEL

```
                        TASK CONSTRAINTS
        ┌─────────────────────────────────────────────────┐
        │            SOLUTION REQUIREMENT                 │
        │           Satisficing    Optimizing             │
   T    │    PROCESS     ⊕ ↑ TASK ↑ ⊖     STRATEGY       │  T
   A    │                 Stable  Unstable                │  A
   S    │    Narrow/   ⊖  Certain Uncertain   ⊕           │  S
   K    │    Deep     ←──────    ↑            ──→ Heuristic│ K
        │                                                  │
   C    │                ⊕ ( MOOD ) ⊖                      │  C
   O    │                                                  │  O
   N    │    Broad/                           ──→ Analytic │  N
   S    │    Shallow  ←──────  ↓ ↓            ⊖           │  S
   T    │              ⊕       PERSON                      │  T
   R    │                                                  │  R
   A    │              Secure    Insecure                  │  A
   I    │              Confident Uncertain                 │  I
   N    │                                                  │  N
   T    │              Opportunity   Threat                │  T
   S    │              PROBLEM PERCEPTION                  │  S
        └─────────────────────────────────────────────────┘
                        TASK CONSTRAINTS
```

Figure 2

in less disarray if they are incorporated within a larger organizational structure, as demonstrated in Figure 1. However, grouping studies by their defining characteristics is not sufficient to provide a path through the discrepancies. A more inclusive model to account for the different effects of mood on creative problem solving is needed.

Kaufmann (1998) suggested that mood influences problem solving in four general dimensions: *problem perception*, or how the problem is represented to the individual in general terms; *solution requirements*, or the criteria for an adequate solution to the problem; *process*, or what type of processing of problem information is best to deal with the problem at hand; and *strategy*, or what kind of general method of solving the problem is required. Figure 2 illustrates the relationships between mood and these four dimensions. To summarize the interrelationships, problem perception is important in the study of problem solving. A problem can be perceived as an opportunity or threat. How the problem is perceived (whether as an opportunity or as a threat) depends on the personality characteristics (whether the person is secure or insecure, confident or uncertain) and the mood (positive or negative) of the individual perceiving the problem. Positive mood may be conducive to perceiving the problem as an opportunity, whereas negative mood should increase the likelihood of perceiving the problem as a threat.

As can be seen, solution requirement consists of the satisficing/optimizing model for solution criteria, described earlier in this chapter. Positive mood could facilitate performance in a task where satisficing criteria is present (choosing the first solution that satisfies the task requirement), whereas negative mood could facilitate performance in a task under optimizing solution contraints (choosing the best solution that satisfies the task requirement). Mood may also affect a person's perception of the task environment, which could lead him or her to favor one or the other solution requirement. That is, a person in a negative mood may perceive the task environment as unstable and therefore work within a stricter criterion for an acceptable solution, rendering the one best answer, whereas a person in a positive mood may perceive the task environment as stable and therefore more easily accept the first solution that satisfied the requirements of the task.

Process type is distinguished in terms of level and breadth of processing (Anderson, 1990). Positive mood has been shown to facilitate broad processing (e.g., Isen & Daubman, 1984; Isen et al., 1985) and may lead to a less cautious approach to the task than negative mood (Clore, Schwarz, & Conway, 1994), promoting more superficial or shallow processing. Negative mood may lead to more constricted (or narrow) but deeper processing. It follows that positive mood would be conducive to performance on tasks that require the generation of many and varied ideas, whereas negative mood may inhibit this kind of task performance. In contrast, negative mood could facilitate performance on tasks that require one correct solution, whereas positive mood could be detrimental.

The last dimension incorporated in this model is strategy. Choice of strategy may be determined by the individual's general assessment of the structure of the task and confidence in his or her ability to solve the problem. It follows that positive mood would increase the likelihood that a person will use heuristic, shortcut strategies, whereas negative mood should lead to more cautious, analytic, and systematic methods of dealing with the task at hand. We would like to add, however, that the availability of feedback on solution attempts may significantly change the postulated pattern, and people in whom a positive mood has been induced, when continuously informed of their success at the task, may be more flexible in shifting strategies than negative-mood participants.

A border indicating task constraints surrounds figure 2 in order to take into account the possible effects of task requirements and the restraints this could place on the effect of the mood. What kind of restraint this is and how it operates remains to be determined.

In this chapter, we have presented a conceptual organizing model as a basis for classifying the mood and creativity research and a model intended to develop a more elaborate theoretical account of the research. Both constructs may be seen as a start toward forming a coherent and meaningful pattern within the apparent disarray of seemingly contradictory findings in the mood and creativity field.

CONCLUSION

The mood and creativity research has been scattered. This seeming lack of structure has been due to the relatively new (or renewed) interest taken in the field, which has resulted in disparate studies. This is reflected in the various research questions that have incorporated the full scope of research designs, ranging from the strict experimental design through the case study. Moreover, the operational definitions of creativity have differed considerably, further impeding meaningful interpretations of available research findings. Thus, there is a clear need for conceptual frameworks that can serve to integrate existing research and provide direction for future studies.

In this chapter, we have presented a conceptual organizing model as a basis for classifying the mood and creativity research by type of design and type of task employed. We hope that this chapter will contribute to a taxonomy of current and past work and provide an initial focus from which other research agendas may be generated. A conceptual framework such as ours may be fruitful as a heuristic organizer of research. However, if findings in the field are not linked to a theoretical process model, such as the one suggested by Kaufmann (1998), meaningful interpretations of the effects of mood on creativity may be difficult to draw.

REFERENCES

Abele, A. (1992). Positive and negative mood influences on creativity: Evidence for asymmetrical effects. *Polish Psychological Bulletin, 23,* 203–221.
Abele, A., & Hermer, P. (1993). Mood influences on health-related judgments: Appraisal of own health versus appraisal of unhealthy behaviors. *European Journal of Social Psychology, 23,* 613–625.
Abele, A., & Petzold, P. (1994). How does mood operate in an impression formation task? An information integration approach. *European Journal of Social Psychology, 24,* 173–187.
Amabile, T. M. (1983).The social psychology of creativity: A componential conceptualization. *Journal of Personality and Social Psychology, 45,* 357–376.
Anderson, J. R. (1990). *Cognitive psychology and its implications.* New York: W. H. Freeman.
Andreasen, N. C. (1987). Creativity and mental illness: Prevalence rates in writers and their first-degree relatives. *American Journal of Psychiatry, 144,* 1288–1292.
Andreasen, N. J. C., & Canter, A. (1974). The creative writer: Psychiatric symptoms and family history. *Comprehensive Psychiatry, 15,* 123–131.
Andreasen, N. J. C., & Powers, P. S. (1974). Overinclusive thinking in mania and schizophrenia. *British Journal of Psychiatry, 125,* 452–456.
Andreasen, N. J. C., & Powers, P. S. (1975). Creativity and psychosis. *Archives of General Psychiatry, 32,* 70–73.
Blaney, P. H. (1986). Affect and memory: A review. *Psychological Bulletin, 99,* 229–246.
Bless, H., Bohner, G., Schwarz, N., & Strack, F. (1990). Mood and persuasion: A cognitive response analysis. *Personality and Social Psychology Bulletin, 16,* 331–345.
Boden, M. A. (1991). *The creative mind: Myths and mechanisms.* New York: Basic Books.
Bodenhausen, G. V., Kramer, G. P., & Süsser, K. (1994). Happiness and stereotypic thinking in social judgment. *Journal of Personality and Social Psychology, 66,* 621–632.
Bower, G. (1981). Mood and memory. *American Psychologist, 36,* 129–148.
Bower, H. (1989). Beethoven's creative illness. *Australian and New Zealand Journal of Psychiatry, 23,* 111–116.
Brown, J. D., & Taylor, S. E. (1986). Affect and the processing of personal information: Evidence for mood-activated self schema. *Journal of Experimental Social Psychology, 22,* 436–452.

Carnevale, P. J. D., & Isen, A. M. (1986). The influence of positive affect and visual access on the discovery of integrative solutions in bilateral negotiation. *Organizational Behavior and Human Decision Processes, 37,* 1–13.

Clark, L. A., Watson, D., & Mineka, S. (1994). Temperament, personality, and the mood and anxiety disorders. *Journal of Abnormal Psychology, 103,* 103–116.

Clark, M. S., & Isen, A. M. (1982). Toward understanding the relationship between feeling states and social behavior. In A. H. Hastorf & A. M. Isen (Eds.), *Cognitive social psychology* (pp. 73–108). New York: Elsevier/North-Holland.

Clore, G. L. (1994). Why emotions require cognition. In P. Ekman & R. J. Davidson (Eds.), *The nature of emotion: Fundamental questions* (pp. 181–191). New York: Oxford University Press.

Clore, G. L., Schwarz, N., & Conway, M. (1994). Affective causes and consequences of social information processing. In T. K. Srull & R. S. Wyer (Ed.), *Handbook of social cognition: Vol. 1. Basic processes* (2nd ed., pp. 323–417). Hillsdale, NJ: Erlbaum.

Diener, E., & Iran-Nejad, A. (1986). The relationship between various types of affect. *Journal of Personality and Social Psychology, 50*(5), 1031–1038.

Duncker, K. (1945). On problem solving. *Psychological Monographs, 58 (Whole No. 270).*

Ekman, P., & Davidson, R. J. (Eds.). (1994). *The nature of emotion: Fundamental questions.* New York: Oxford University Press.

Estrada, C. A., Isen, A. M., & Young, M. J. (1994). Positive affect improves creative problem solving and influences reported source of practice satisfaction in physicians. *Motivation and Emotion, 18*(4), 285–299.

Eysenck, H. J. (1994). The measurement of creativity. In M. A. Boden (Ed.), *Dimensions of creativity* (pp. 199–242). Cambridge, MA: MIT Press.

Frijda, N. H. (1993). The place of appraisal in emotion. *Cognition and Emotion, 7,* 357–387.

Frosch, W. A. (1987). Moods, madness, and music. I. Major affective disease and musical creativity. *Comprehensive Psychiatry, 28,* 315–322.

Gregory, R. (1981). *Mind in science.* Middlesex, England: Penguin Books.

Greene, T. R., & Noice, H. (1988). Influence of positive affect upon creative thinking and problem solving in children. *Psychological Reports, 63,* 895–898.

Isen, A. M. (1984). Toward understanding the role of affect in cognition. In R. Wyer & T. Srull (Eds.), *Handbook of social cognition* (Vol. 3, pp. 179–236). Hillsdale, NJ: Erlbaum.

Isen, A. M., Clark, M., & Schwartz, M. F. (1976). Duration of effect of good mood on helping: "Footprints on the sands of time." *Journal of Personality and Social Psychology, 34,* 385–393.

Isen, A. M., & Daubman, K. A. (1984). The influence of affect on categorization. *Journal of Personality and social Psychology, 47,* 1206–1217.

Isen, A. M., Daubman, K. A., & Nowicki, G. P. (1987). Positive affect facilitates creative problem solving. *Journal of Personality and Social Psychology, 52,* 1122–1131.

Isen, A. M., Johnson, M. M. S., Mertz, E., & Robinson, G. F. (1985). The influence of positive affect on the unusualness of word associations. *Journal of Personality and Social Psychology, 48,* 1413–1426.

Isen, A. M., & Levin, P. F. (1972). Effect of feeling good on helping: Cookies and kindness. *Journal of Personality and Social Psychology, 21,* 384–388.

Isen, A. M., Niedenthal, P. M., & Cantor, N. (1992). An influence of positive affect on social categorization. *Motivation and Emotion, 16,* 65–78.

Isen, A. M., Shalker, T. E., Clark, M., & Karp, L. (1978). Affect, accessibility of material in memory, and behavior: A cognitive loop? *Journal of Personality and Social Psychology, 36,* 1–12.

Isen, A. M., & Simmonds, S. F. (1978). The effect of feeling good on a helping task that is incompatible with good mood. *Social Psychology, 41,* 346–349.

Izard, C. E. (1991). *The psychology of emotions.* New York: Plenum Press.

Jamison, K. R. (1989). Mood disorders and patterns of creativity in British writers and artists. *Psychiatry, 52* (May), 125–134.

Jamison, K. R. (1993). *Touched with fire: Manic depressive illness and the artistic temperament.* New York: Free Press.

Jausovec, N. (1989). Affect in analogical transfer. *Creativity Research Journal, 2,* 255-266.
Kahn, B. E., & Isen, A. M. (1993). The influence of positive affect on variety seeking among safe, enjoyable products. *Journal of Consumer Research, 20,* 257-270.
Kaufmann, G. (1993). The content and logical structure of creativity concepts: An inquiry into the conceptual foundations of creativity research. In S. G. Isaksen, M. C. Murdock, R. L. Firestien, & D. J. Treffinger (Eds.), *Understanding and recognizing creativity: The emergence of a discipline* (pp. 141-157). Norwood, NJ: Ablex.
Kaufmann, G. (1988). Problem solving and creativity. In G. Kaufmann & K. Grønhaug (Eds.), *Innovation: A cross-disciplinary perspective* (pp. 87-137). Oslo: Norwegian University Press.
Kaufmann, G. (1998). *The mood-and-creativity puzzle: Toward a theory of mood effects on problem solving.* Manuscript submitted for publication.
Kaufmann, G., & Vosburg, S. K. (1997). "Paradoxical" mood effects on creative problem solving. *Cognition and Emotion, 11,* 151-170.
Kaufmann, G., & Vosburg, S. (1998). *Mood effects on divergent thinking.* (Unpublished manuscript).
Kraiger, K., Billings, R. S., & Isen, A. M. (1989). The influence of positive affective states on task perceptions and satisfaction. *Organizational Behavior and Human Decision Making, 44,* 12-25.
Ludwig, A. M. (1994). Mental illness and creative activity in female writers. *American Journal of Psychiatry, 151,* 1650-1656.
Mackie, D. M., & Worth, L. T. (1989). Processing deficits and the mediation of positive affect in persuasion. *Journal of Personality and Social Psychology, 57,* 27-40.
MacKinnon, D. W. (1978). *In search of human effectiveness.* Buffalo, NY: Creative Education Foundation/Bearly Limited.
Martin, L. L., Ward, D. W., Achee, J. W., & Wyer, R. S. (1993). Mood as input: People have to interpret the motivational implications of their moods. *Journal of Personality and Social Psychology, 64,* 317-326.
Matthews, G. (1986a). The effects of anxiety of intellectual performance: When and why are they found? *Journal of Research in Personality, 20,* 385-401.
Matthews, G. (1986b). The interactive effects of extraversion and arousal on performance: Are creativity tests anomalous? *Personality and Individual Differences, 7,* 751-761.
Mednick, S. A. (1962). The associative basis of the creative process. *Psychological Review, 69,* 220-232.
Melton, R. J. (1995). The role of positive affect in syllogism performance. *Personality and Social Psychology Bulletin, 21,* 788-794.
Mitchell, J. E., & Madigan, R. J. (1984). The effects of induced elation and depression on interpersonal problem solving. *Cognitive Therapy and Research, 8,* 277-285.
Morris, W. N. (1989). *Mood: The frame of mind.* New York: Springer-Verlag.
Morris, W. N. (1992). A functional analysis of the role of mood in affective systems. In M. S. Clark (Ed.) Emotion. *Review of personality and social psychology,* 13. (pp. 256-293). Beverly Hills, CA: Sage.
Mraz, W., & Runco, M. A. (1994). Suicide ideation and creative problem solving. *Suicide and Life-Threatening Behavior, 24,* 38-47.
Murray, N., Sujan, H., Hirt, E. R., & Sujan, M. (1990). The influence of mood on categorization: A cognitive flexibility interpretation. *Journal of Personality and Social Psychology, 59,* 411-425.
Newell, A., Shaw, J. C., & Simon, H. A. (1979). The processes of creative thinking. In H. A. Simon (Ed.), *Models of thought* (Vol. 1, pp. 144-174). New Haven, CT: Yale University Press.
Oatley, K., & Jenkins, J. M. (1992). Human emotions: Function and dysfunction. *Annual Review of Psychology, 43,* 55-85.
Richards, R., & Kinney, D. K. (1990). Mood swings and creativity. *Creativity Research Journal 3,* 202-217.
Richards, R., Kinney, D. K., Daniels, H., & Linkins, K. W. (1992). Everyday creativity and bipolar and unipolar affective disorder: Preliminary study of personal and family history. *European Psychiatry, 7,* 49-52.

Richards, R., Kinney, D. K., Benet, M., & Merzel, A. P. C. (1988). Assessing everyday creativity: Characteristics of the lifetime creativity scales and validation with three large samples. *Journal of Personality and Social Psychology, 54,* 476–485.

Robbins, S. P. (1993). *Organizational behavior.* Englewood Cliffs, NJ: Prentice-Hall.

Rothenberg, A. (1983). Psychopathology and creative cognition. *Archives of General Psychiatry, 40,* 937–942.

Rothenberg, A. (1990). *Creativity & madness: New findings and old stereotypes.* Baltimore, MD: Johns Hopkins University Press.

Rothenberg, A., & Burkhardt, P. E. (1984). Difference in response time of creative persons and patients with depressive and schizophrenic disorders. *Psychological Reports, 54,* 711–717.

Russ, S. W. (1993). *Affect and creativity: The role of affect and play in the creative process.* Hillsdale, NJ: Erlbaum.

Schildkraut, J. J., & Hirshfeld, A. J. (1995). Mind and mood in modern art I: Miro and "Melancolie." *Creativity Research Journal, 8,* 139–156.

Schuldberg, D. (1990). Schizotypal and hypomanic traits, creativity, and psychological health. *Creativity Research Journal, 3,* 218–230.

Schwarz, N., Bless, H., & Bohner, G. (1991). Mood and persuasion: Affective states influence the processing of persuasive communications. *Advances in Experimental Social Psychology, 24,* 161–199.

Schwarz, N., & Clore, G. L. (1988). How do I feel about it? The informative function of affective states. In J. Forgas & K. Fiedler (Eds.), *Affect, cognition and social behavior* (pp. 44–62). Toronto: Hogrefe.

Schwarz, N., & Clore, G. L. (1983). Mood, misattribution, and judgments of well-being: Informative and directive functions of affective states. *Journal of Personality and Social Psychology, 45,* 513–523.

Simon, H. A. (1977). *The new science of management decision.* Englewood Cliffs, NJ: Prentice-Hall.

Simon, H. A. (1982). Comments. In S. T. Fiske & M. S. Clark (Eds.), *Affect and cognition: The Seventeenth Annual Carnegie Symposium on Cognition* (pp. 333–342). Hillsdale, NJ: Erlbaum.

Staw, B. M., & Barsade, S. G. (1993). Affect and managerial performance: A test of the sadder-but-wiser vs. happier-and-smarter hypotheses. *Administrative Science Quarterly, 38,* 304–331.

Stein, M. I. (1974). *Stimulating creativity* (Vol. 1). San Diego, CA: Academic Press.

Sternberg, R. J., & Davidson, J. E. (1982, June). The mind of the puzzler. *Psychology Today, 16,* 37–44.

Sternberg, R. J., & Davidson, J. E. (Eds.). (1995). *The nature of insight.* Cambridge, MA: Bradford.

Sternberg, R. J., & Lubart, T. I. (1995). *Defying the crowd: Cultivating creativity in a culture of conformity.* New York: Free Press.

Tellegen, A. (1985). Structures of mood and personality and their relevance to assessing anxiety, with an emphasis on self-report. In J. D. Maser & A. H. Tuma (Ed.), *Anxiety and the anxiety disorders* (pp. 681–706). Hillsdale, NJ: Erlbaum.

Toplyn, G., & Maguire, W. (1991). The differential effect of noise on creative task performance. *Creativity Research Journal, 4,* 337–347.

Vosburg, S. K. (1998). The effects of positive and negative mood on divergent thinking performance. *Creativity Research Journal, 11*(2), 165–172.

Watson, D. (1988). Intraindividual and interindividual analyses of positive and negative affect: Their relation to health complaints, perceived stress, and daily activities. *Journal of Personality and Social Psychology, 54,* 1020–1030.

Watson, D., & Clark, L. A. (1984). Negative affectivity: The disposition to experience aversive emotional states. *Psychological Bulletin, 96,* 465–490.

Watson, D., & Clark, L. A. (1994). Emotions, moods, traits and temperaments: Conceptual distinctions and empirical findings. In P. Ekman & R. J. Davidson (Eds.), *The nature of emotion: Fundamental questions* (pp. 89–93). New York: Oxford University Press.

Watson, D., Clark, L. A., & Carey, G. (1988). Positive and negative affectivity and their relation to anxiety and depressive disorders. *Journal of Abnormal Psychology, 97,* 346–353.

Watson, D., Clark, L. A., McIntyre, C. W., & Hamaker, S. (1992). Affect, personality, and social activity. *Journal of Personality and Social Psychology, 63,* 1011–1025.

Watson, D., & Walker, L. M. (1996). The long-term stability and predictive validity of trait measures of affect. *Journal of Personality and Social Psychology, 70,* 567–577.

Weisberg, R. W. (1988). Problem solving and creativity. In R. J. Sternberg (Ed.), *The nature of creativity* (pp. 148–176). Cambridge, England: Cambridge University Press.

Weisberg, R. W. (1994). Genius and madness? A quasi-experimental test of the hypothesis that manic-depression increases creativity. *Psychological Science, 5,* 361–367.

Worth, L. T., & Mackie, D. M. (1987). Cognitive mediation of positive affect in persuasion. *Social Cognition, 5,* 76–94.

3

The Emotional Resonance Model of Creativity: Theoretical and Practical Extensions

Isaac Getz
Paris Graduate School of Management (Groupe ESCP)

Todd I. Lubart
Université René Descartes, Paris

> Association depends in a much greater degree on the recurrence of states of feeling than on trains of ideas. (Samuel Taylor Coleridge, in Richards, 1950, p. 168)

Coleridge's reflection on the genesis of his work joins those of many other artists to indicate that emotions were a key to their creativity (Lubart & Getz, 1997). Yet, creativity has been traditionally studied from a cognitive perspective (cf. Lubart, 1994). Recently, researchers have begun to explore how emotion is related to creativity (Getz & Laroche, 1996; Russ, 1993; Shaw & Runco, 1994).

There are several ways in which the relationship between emotion and creativity may be conceived. First, as a conative variable, emotion can motivate

---

The research presented in this chapter was conducted in part when Isaac Getz was a visiting research scholar with the University of Massachusetts. It was supported by a research grant from the Chambre de Commerce et d'Industrie de Paris (CCIP). We thank Lisette Garrido and Linda Jarvin for their assistance with the empirical studies. We acknowledge the use of some material in this chapter from Lubart, T. I. & Getz, I. (1997). Emotion, Metaphor, and the Creative Process; *Creativity Research Journal, 10,* 285–301, published by Lawrence Erlbaum Associates.

creativity. For example, expressing emotions about personal experiences is an inherent drive acknowledged by many creators (see Freud, 1908/1959). In a related way, creative work is often viewed (e.g., in the humanistic perspective on creativity) as a means of expressing one's idiosyncratic emotions and affective response to the world.

Second, as a contextual variable, emotion (mood) may place the individual in a heightened mental state that influences creativity. For example, it has been found that people put in a mildly positive state interpret stimuli in novel ways or generate novel solutions to a problem (Isen, 1987, 1996). Other emotional states, such as negative or strongly positive ones, seem to exercise a more complex pattern of influences on creativity (Kaufmann, 1996). The theoretical account of this pattern is a subject of ongoing debate (Isen, 1996; Kaufmann, 1996).

Third, as a functional variable, emotion may stimulate specific concepts. Coleridge and many other eminent creators suggested that emotions may provide an associative bridge between cognitively remote concepts representing objects, persons, or events in memory. In a related vein, Russ (1993) suggested that access to affect-laden thoughts or primary process material may contribute to divergent thinking and free association.

Finally, the emotion–creativity relationship does not need to be conceived only in terms of emotions' effect on creativity. Emotions may accompany or be a consequence of creative work (Feist, 1994, Chapter 6 in this book). Furthermore, in the dynamic multistep creative process, the emotion resulting from one step may spark or mediate a following one. Researchers such as Feist (1994) and Oatley (1992) have examined this dynamic relationship of emotion and creativity.

In this chapter, we focus on the functional relationship between emotion and creativity. We describe briefly our emotional resonance model (ERM), which specifies how idiosyncratic emotions contribute to the access and association of cognitively remote concepts in memory. We then consider metaphor, one way to instantiate the associative basis of creativity. In the remainder of the chapter, we propose two extensions of our model: a theoretical extension that attempts to account for some of emotion's contextual influences on creativity and a practical extension consisting of a theory-based method for creativity improvement, an important area suffering from an abundance of atheoretical methods.

THE EMOTIONAL RESONANCE MODEL FOR GENERATING ASSOCIATIONS

There are three main components of the ERM: (a) endocepts that represent idiosyncratic experientially acquired emotions attached to concepts or images in memory; (b) an automatic resonance mechanism that propagates a current endocept's emotional profile through memory and activates other endocepts; and

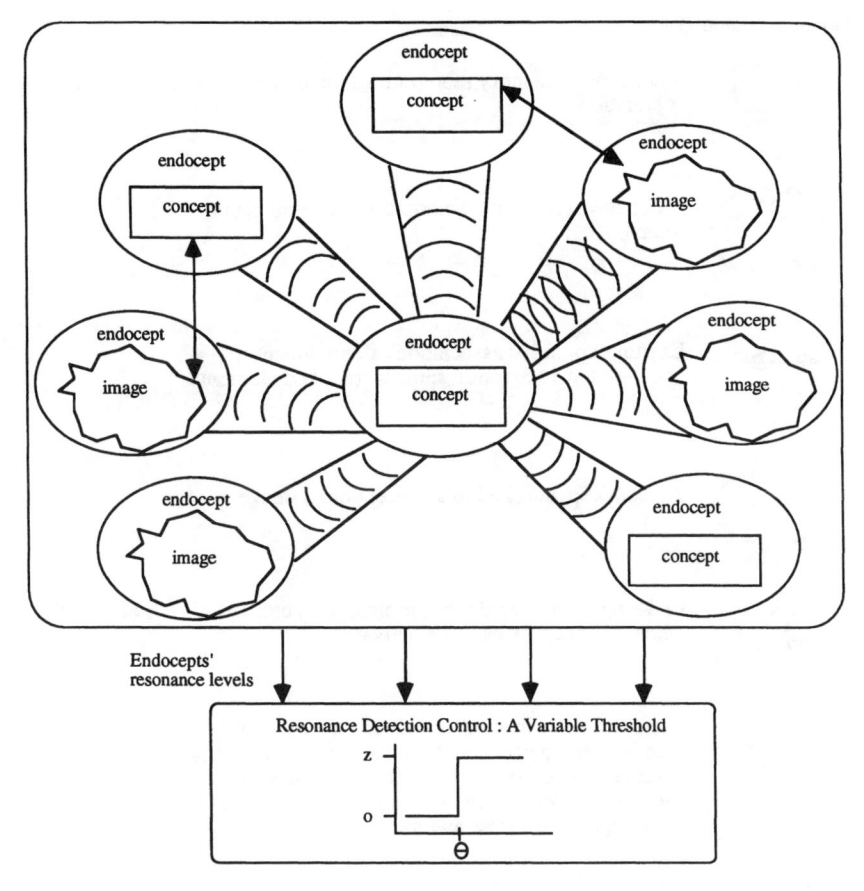

Figure 1. The emotional resonance model of concept association (Lubart & Getz, 1997)

(c) a resonance detection threshold that determines whether a resonance-activated endocept (and its concept or image) enters working memory. These components are illustrated in Figure 1 and briefly described now (a more detailed description may be found in Lubart and Getz, 1997).

Endocepts in Memory

Following several psychological theorists, we view emotions as constructions organized by biological, social, and psychological factors (Averill, 1992; Malatesta, 1988; for a review of approaches to emotions, see Ekman & Davidson, 1994; Fiske & Taylor, 1991). We focus on the emotions, sometimes termed "affective experiences" or "feelings," that are organized primarily by psychological factors; they are idiosyncratic and experientially acquired and cannot be easily described in terms of socially determined emotional categories (e.g., anger

Figure 1. Legend

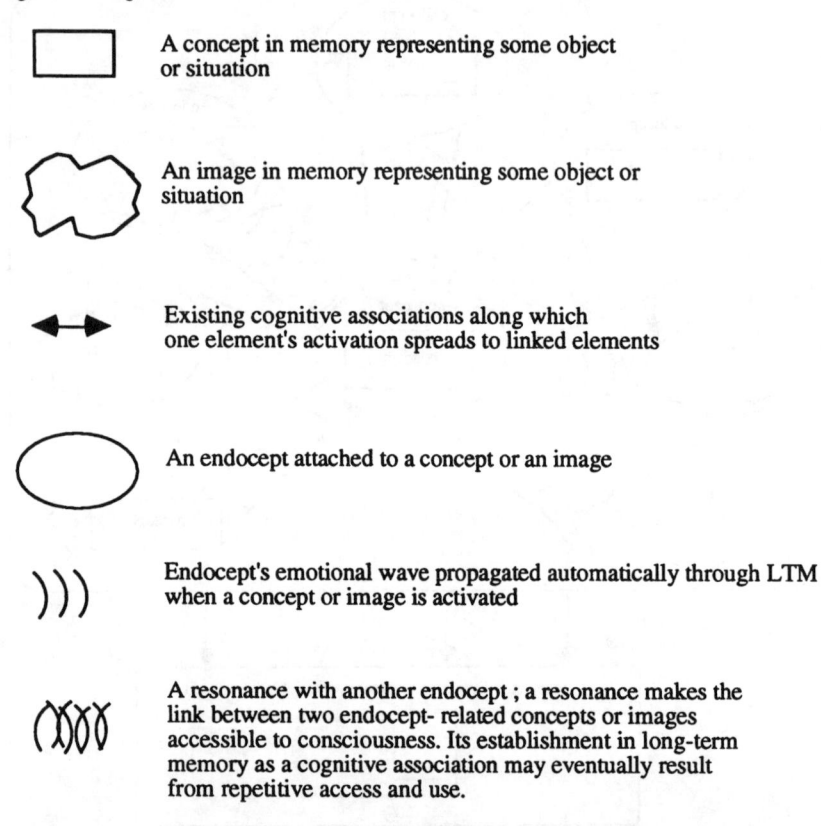

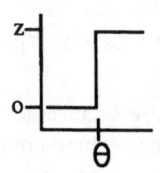

▭	A concept in memory representing some object or situation
⬡	An image in memory representing some object or situation
◄──►	Existing cognitive associations along which one element's activation spreads to linked elements
◯	An endocept attached to a concept or an image
)))	Endocept's emotional wave propagated automatically through LTM when a concept or image is activated
(XXX)	A resonance with another endocept ; a resonance makes the link between two endocept- related concepts or images accessible to consciousness. Its establishment in long-term memory as a cognitive association may eventually result from repetitive access and use.
[step function z/θ]	If the resonance passes an individually-set threshold θ then the similarity of the proximate concept or image is detected (z) by the individual and a link between two concepts or images is established in working memory.

or love). Arieti (1976) and Averill and Nunley (1992) referred to these emotions as "endocepts," a term we adopt to designate these emotions' memory representations.

We suggest that because of their experiential basis, endocepts are attached in memory to concepts or images representing objects, persons, or events. This suggestion is supported by the research on emotional priming of concepts (e.g., Bartlett, 1932; Paivio, 1978; Zajonc, 1980) and on automatic affective-evaluative priming of concepts (e.g., Bargh, Chaiken, Govender, & Pratto, 1992; Fazio, Sanbon matsu, Powell, & Kardes, 1986). For example, Paivio studied reaction times of pleasantness judgments for words and images referring to objects; he found that pleasantness information is closely linked to objects' representation in memory and that this information can be activated through pictures and, less directly, names of objects.

The suggestion that endocepts are attached in memory to concepts is further supported by several multicomponential views of memory integrating emotion (Epstein, 1994; Oatley & Johnson-Laird, 1987; Ortony, 1991). For example, Ortony, focusing on a person representation, suggests that along with fact-based (John has power) and trait-based (John is ambitious) components, there is an affective-experiential component consisting of a record of emotional experiences with a specific person (John was sad at our last meeting).

As in a traditional information-processing view of memory systems, we assume concepts to be partially interconnected and thus to be able to activate each other along the established links (see Figure 1). This, however, is not the only way to link concepts in memory.

An Automatic Resonance Mechanism

We suggest that endocepts attached to concepts may resonate with each other, providing an alternative way to link concepts in memory. Specifically, an endocept activated by an attached concept (itself activated by external stimuli or internal thought) propagates its emotional profile as a "wave" throughout the memory system. At this point, if some other endocept's emotional profile matches sufficiently the propagated profile, the two endocepts begin resonating in memory.

This emotional resonance suggestion is consistent with diverse theoretical proposals that emotions attached to concepts or images may interact, resonate, or reverberate in memory (e.g., Berggren, 1962, 1963; Isen, 1987; Miall, 1987; Spiro, Crismore, & Turner, 1982), as well as with proposals of global propagation and spreading of emotions (Damasio, 1994; Lang, 1994; Oatley & Johnson-Laird, 1987). For example, Isen (1987) proposed that if the affective tones of two concepts are shared, the concepts might be perceived as more related than they would otherwise. It should be noted that the suggested emotional propagation is distinct from both the above-mentioned spreading activation along established cognitive links and the Freudian psychodynamic transfer/displacement of affective memory traces along established associative links.

However, just because a link is resonating does not mean it will be noticed and accessed consciously by an individual. In order to be detected, the resonance needs to pass an individually set detection threshold.

Resonance Detection Threshold

In our model, whether or not the resonating link is detected depends on the interplay between (a) the individual's threshold value for bringing the link into working memory and (b) the resonating power of the linked endocept. For example, an individual with a high resonance detection threshold (i.e., an emotionally "deaf" individual) may have as much difficulty detecting a link with a strongly resonating endocept as an individual with a low threshold may have noticing a weakly resonating endocept. This suggestion of a resonance detection threshold is consistent with Poincaré's (1921) proposal that an emotional sensibility acts as a seive allowing only aesthetically pleasing ideas to enter consciousness and Miall's (1987) suggestion that some concepts may be activated by the currently activated concept's affect at a subthreshold level of excitement.

The resonance detection threshold value is one of several sources of individual differences specified in our model. Discussion of these individual difference parameters in the next section completes the presentation of our model.

Sources of Individual Differences in the Emotional Resonance Model

Individual differences in generating associations can arise from each aspect of our model. First, individuals may differ in their acquired knowledge and experiences and thus, in terms of our model, in the richness and content of their concept- and image-based memory. Second, individuals with the same experience may differ with regard to their propensity to dwell on it (Tellegen, 1982) or to respond emotionally to it in complex and idiosyncratic ways (Averill, 1994; Lane, Quinlan, Schwartz, Walker, & Zeitlin, 1990). In terms of our model, these individuals differ with regard to the multiaspectual and idiosyncratic nature of their endocepts. We wish to emphasize that endocepts are not copies of original emotional responses, but an elaboration in complex ways of these (possibly covert) responses in memory. In fact, one of the traits of creative people is their emotional independence, that is, their tendency to be reserved, withdrawn, or introverted (Ochse, 1990). Finally, individuals may differ with regard to their ability to attend to their internally felt emotions (Averill, 1994; Salovey, Mayer, Goldman, Turvey, & Palfai, 1995); in terms of our model, these individuals differ with regard to the level of their emotional resonance detection threshold.

Together, these differences indicate the conditions under which individuals will be most effective in generating emotion-based associations for creativity. Specifically, individuals with a significant personal experience on which they have dwelt and for which they have acquired complex and idiosyncratic emotions, and who, furthermore, are highly attentive to their emotional processes, will be the most effective in generating emotion-based associations for creativity. Though these "ideal" conditions may be met by only a small fraction of individuals (e.g., eminent creators), understanding them may illuminate the conditions necessary for ordinary individuals to achieve creativity.

Besides individual differences stemming from the ERM, there are other differences related to the specific means by which an association is expressed. As we discuss in the next section, in order to contribute to creativity, an emotionally generated association needs to be expressed in a specific form and medium.

CREATIVE METAPHOR: A WAY TO EXPRESS EMOTION-BASED ASSOCIATIONS

An emotion-based association can be expressed in a variety of ways, such as visualization, aphorisms, narratives, and metaphors, each implying a different degree of association's elaboration and later interpretation (Ahsen, 1982; Bruner, 1986; Epstein, 1994; Finke, Ward, & Smith, 1992; Jennings, 1991). Here we focus on metaphors considered to allow the elaboration, organization, and expression of emotion-laden experiences (but only when an individual avoids conventional, "frozen" metaphors; Ortony, 1975; cf. Lakoff & Johnson, 1980). Though parts of the processing have been studied, the overall psychological mechanism for generating metaphors for creativity remains a mystery (Clevenger & Edwards, 1988; Hoffman & Kemper, 1987; Miall, 1987).

We argue that generating metaphors for creativity may be conceived as a recurrent process composed of two phases: (a) noticing a source domain that may be used to generate a novel metaphor relevant to a target phenomenon or domain, and (b) mapping out and appreciating the metaphor for appropriateness. Research on metaphor generation typically has focused on the second phase of this process, providing participants with a target domain (e.g., a presidential candidate) and one of several source domains (e.g., animals; Clevenger & Edwards, 1988; Katz, 1989). Various mapping and appreciation cognitive mechanisms have been proposed (e.g., Gentner, 1988; Indurkhya, 1992; Tourangeau & Rips, 1991). Such an emphasis may be compared to early research on chess that placed the burden of chess move generation on the calculation phase, downplaying the fundamental phase of "seeing" or "feeling" a specific pattern of pieces in a chess position to which a calculation has to be applied (see Getz, 1996; Gobet & Simon, 1996).

Focusing on the first and fundamental phase of metaphor generation, we suggest that individualized, experientially acquired emotion is a key to noticing a very distant domain. We suggest further that the psychological process underlying this phase is the automatic emotional resonance described in our model. The emotional resonance leads to an association between a target phenomenon and an emotionally proximate but cognitively distant concept/domain. If detected and put in the working memory, this association becomes a subject for the second phase of cognitive processing and finally is expressed as a metaphor (if the second phase is skipped, an aphorism, instead of a metaphor, results).

Similar to automatic pattern recognition explaining move generation insights in expert chess players, automatic detection of a specific semantic domain via emotional resonance may be the only way to explain the metaphor generation insights reported by eminent creators (Lubart & Getz, 1997). This understanding provided by our model may be used to produce a theoretical account for the relation of mood and creativity as well as a practical way to improve creativity in non-eminent individuals. We discuss these theoretical and practical extensions of our model below.

ACCOUNTING FOR MOOD INFLUENCES ON CREATIVITY

Two theoretical extensions of the ERM have been proposed: one accounting for the positive relation of the Jungian intuitive style and creativity and the other accounting for the role of emotions in the production of artistic work (Lubart & Getz, 1997). Here we want to address another important issue for creativity: accounting for some of the effects of mood on creativity.

In Western culture, emotions and mood have been traditionally assigned a disruptive role with regard to rational thinking. Consistently, the earlier treatments of the effect of mood emphasized that negative mood interrupts cognitive processes. For example, fear may halt the execution of a plan. Similar interruptive effects may be observed with regard to the creative process. Beginning in the 1970s, there was a growing interest in the effect of positive mood. Some studies found that strong positive mood may be disruptive. More interestingly, Isen and her colleagues found that mild positive mood may be facilitative for diverse cognitive and creative tasks. For example, Isen, Daubman, and Nowicki (1987) found that after they were induced into a mild positive state, people performed better than controls on Duncker's candle task. Recently, Kaufmann (1996) integrated Isen et al.'s results with his own and others' findings in the following pattern of mood effects on creativity: (a) Positive mood has a facilitative effect on broader categorization, performance of a remote-associates task, divergent thinking, and solution of insight problems and complex problems; (b) negative mood has a facilitative effect on finding the problem, making unbiased judgments, and solving insight problems; (c) positive mood has a detrimental effect on searching for information, making unbiased judgments, and solving insight problems; and (d) negative mood has a detrimental effect on ideational fluency. These effects of mood on creative tasks, and in particular some puzzling mood effects on insight-focused creative tasks, are the subject of rich and ongoing theoretical debate.

Figure 1. Legend

There are several ways to account for the diverse findings, each emphasizing mood's interaction with conative, cognitive, or emotional aspects of creative performance. Considering conative aspects, mood may be viewed as regulating different motives and goals involved in the creative process (Simon, 1967). For example, a mild positive mood—as opposed to negative mood—does not lead an individual to switch to or consider another goal, thus reducing the extent of informational search. A person who is mildly happy while working on a new idea may tend to accept the first generated plan, thus halting the informational search.

Considering cognitive aspects, mood may be viewed as interacting with memory, organizing it in a different way, and making more material available (Isen, 1987). Mood may be also viewed as interacting with various properties of the creative problem-solving process, leading (depending on the properties) to either facilitative or detrimental effects on the creative performance (Kaufmann, 1996).

For example, when a task requires one ideal solution, positive mood may be detrimental because it promotes satisficing behavior.

Finally, one may consider emotional aspects of creative performance and how mood interacts with them. One such interaction was hypothesized by Isen (1987), who suggested that concepts that share a positive emotional tone may be perceived as close, thus facilitating their association in memory. In her hypothesis, mood is interacting with emotional aspects of memory. We suggest and develop at the level of psychological mechanisms how mood may interact with the emotion-based process of generating associations. Specifically, mood is interacting with the resonance detection component of the ERM: Positive mood lowers the individual's threshold level, increasing the likelihood that automatically resonating endocepts/concepts will be detected; inversely, negative mood raises the individual's threshold level, decreasing the likelihood that automatically resonating endocepts/concepts will be noticed. The rationale behind this operationalization is that happy people tend to accept easily every idea and, inversely, people who are upset tend to reject every idea.

The interaction of positive mood with the resonance detection component may account for positive mood's facilitating effects on creative tasks with an associative basis. Specifically, it may account for facilitating effects on such tasks as associating unusual words and certain parts of divergent thinking. Similarly, the interaction of negative mood with the resonance detection component may account for some detrimental effects of negative mood on creative tasks with an associative basis. Specifically, it may account for inhibiting effects on certain parts of ideational fluency. Our model's extension has more difficulty accounting for mood effects on creative tasks that have no clear associative basis. For example, insight problems, the solution of which often relies on discovering potential links between objects, are related but not identical to associative thinking. One way to account for mood effects on such psychologically complex tasks may be through an interaction of mood with all three—conative, cognitive, and emotional—components of creative performance.

Thus the ERM may foster a new understanding of the task-specific pattern of mood effects on creative thinking. Now we turn to another extension of the ERM—how to enhance creativity.

IMPROVING CREATIVITY IN ORDINARY PEOPLE

For at least four decades, improving creativity has been acknowledged to be an important individual, organizational, and social goal (Gordon, 1956; Sternberg & Lubart, 1995, 1996; see also humanistic psychologists such as Maslow and Rogers). Along with measurement and selection, creativity methods have been a traditional means for achieving this goal. Yet, these methods have not always performed as expected. The following brief discussion of existing creativity methods proposes the importance of theory for the reliability of creativity techniques.

Limitations of the Existing Methods

One way to organize creativity improvement methods is according to the creative (as opposed to the analytic) contents they offer for one or several steps of the problem-solving process. This process includes

1) Recognizing that a problem exists;
2) Identifying the nature of the problem;
3) Generating a strategy for solving the problem;
4) Allocating resources to problem solving;
5) Monitoring problem solving while it is occurring; and
6) Evaluating the quality of the problem solving.

For example, among the most traditional methods, brainstorming affects the search step through an increased number of generated ideas (step 3), whereas synectics (Gordon, 1961) and certain lateral thinking (DeBono, 1970) techniques affect problem identification (Step 2) through problem reconceptualization. The diversity of creativity improvement methods explains some of the positive improvement results reported in a dozen studies on creativity programs (e.g., Basadur, Graen, & Green, 1982; Couger, Higgins, & McIntrye, 1993; Parnes, 1987). For example, it explains why a combination of methods (or a combined method) has a higher chance to improve creativity than each method separately, an intuition supported experimentally by Ekvall and Parnes (1984). However, considering the interaction between the individual creative problem-solving process and the complex real-world environment reveals some basic limitations of the existing methods. These methods' creativity improvement results are typically obtained with some participants, some problems, and some settings but not with others. The techniques are unreliable, and the effectiveness of a method used with different people, problems, or settings is usually not predictable.

Besides the reliability limitation, the existing programs and methods also suffer from an emphasis on a facilitator (an expert who helps individuals apply the technique). Because creativity improvement programs typically do not train people how to facilitate, but simply how to use creativity methods, these methods may fail when used by a less experienced facilitator or by users themselves. We suggest that using a theoretical model that specifies the nature of the creative problem-solving process enables the existing methods' limitations to be overcome.

Specifically, a model's postulated creative process may be used to devise a method with concrete tools and procedures to be used in a facilitator-free fashion. In addition, a theoretical model may be used to specify a limited nonarbitrary set of participants, problems, and settings with which the proposed method will perform reliably. In the next section, we describe how our model can be extended in a practical, creativity improvement direction.

The Creativity Improvement Method Based on the Emotional Resonance Model

Our emotion-based model focuses on creative contents in the second step of the problem-solving process, that is, identifying the nature of the problem: It offers creative contents for this step by reconceptualizing a problem through an emotion-based potentially distant association or metaphor. This may lead to a new perspective on a problem, resulting in a new strategy for solving it (the third step of the problem-solving process). On the basis of the individual differences specified by our theoretical model, we can isolate the emotion-based processing points where people can fail to be creative. Potentially, this allows us to devise a complete creativity improvement method intervening at each of these various points. We begin by devising a method that intervenes at one point—activating an individual's idiosyncratic emotions (see Getz & Lubart, 1996). The following classroom demonstration illustrates a method based on our model.

Students were asked to redesign a traditional department store sales process. They began by using a grid to activate their experiential individualized emotions about this sales process and then used these emotions to generate potentially remote associates to a department store. In group discussions, students expressed the generated associations as metaphors and chose one that they deemed the most appropriate for reconceptualizing the problem. One group picked the Louvre Museum as an associate and formed the metaphor "Department store is the Louvre." After reconceptualizing the problem through the Louvre metaphor, the group elaborated a large array of solutions enabling the museum's visitors to circulate easily. The group completed the method by translating these diverse solutions back to the department store problem. For example, the group proposed that human or electronic guides be available to accompany shoppers throughout their visit of the department store and that sales counter personnel be removed. Throughout the method, students worked in an autonomous, facilitator-free manner, using the following tools and procedure.

The central tool is a grid that characterizes people's individualized emotions on the problem phenomenon and activates these emotions. The grid consists of 15 bipolar adjectives (based on Osgood's 1963, 1969, work), 5 corresponding to the evaluation factor of affective-connotative meaning (e.g., good–bad), 5 to the potency factor (e.g., strong–weak), and 5 to the activity factor (e.g., fast–slow). There is a 7-point rating scale for each bipolar set of adjectives. According to Averill (1975), Osgood (1969), and Russell (1980), semantic differentials may be used effectively to assess and characterize people's emotions on a phenomenon. We extended the use of this tool, suggesting that it also activates such emotions and further sets in motion their resonance throughout the memory system. We are in the process of gathering evidence for this hypothesis. Empirically, it is consistent with the available evidence on the (sometimes undesirable) effects that experimental instruments with affective items have on participants' emotions (e.g., Mark, Sinclair, & Wellens, 1991). Theoretically, it is consistent with Averill's (1994) and our view of individualized emotions as vague and multiaspectual.

The rationale behind the use of this tool is our assumption that many individuals respond emotionally in complex and idiosyncratic ways to mundane experiences but do not typically dwell on them. Thus, in order to activate their endocepts, something more than merely thinking about the experience may be needed. The grid is intended to "hit the strings" composing the emotional profile of an endocept, activating it and setting in motion its resonance.

The second key step of the procedure involves asking participants to list whatever problem associates come to mind. This forces them to attend to the associative links that have formed preattentively. The rationale behind the use of this step is our assumption that many individuals are not able to detect such a link spontaneously because of their high resonance detection threshold. It may happen, however, that even this step is not enough to force emotionally "deaf" individuals to attend to their emotional processes. In a preliminary study (Getz & Lubart, 1996), ordinary individuals who measured low on their attention to emotions (mostly science-oriented students) could not benefit from this procedure, whereas individuals who measured high on their attention to emotions (mostly literature-oriented students) could benefit from it.

Is there a procedural manipulation that could help emotionally "deaf," rationally thinking individuals to benefit from an emotional process for creativity? One such manipulation stemming from our model would involve charging emotionally (e.g., through visualization or personification) a phenomenon that is too abstract or conceptual and then using the grid. This step would force individuals to dwell on and respond emotionally to the phenomenon, perhaps for the first time. Simultaneously, this step could block their supposedly preferred rational–cognitive processing of the phenomenon's semantic information. A recent study (Jarvin, Getz, & Lubart, 1997) provides initial support for this proposal.

We compared the creative contents our method offers to the analytic contents offered by a cognitively driven close-analogy method in the above described classroom demonstration. Prior to the use of our emotion-based method, students were asked to suggest some spontaneous solutions to the department store problem. One student suggested using a supermarket as a close analogy. However, translating the supermarket sales process solutions back to the original department store problem offered analytic information, but no creative contents for the problem-solving process. For example, the supermarket analogy offered a solution strategy of modifying the sales process through self-service, a solution already used in some department stores.

To summarize, using a theory-based methodology allowed us to devise a creativity improvement method with carefully selected tools and procedures. We began by intervening in one point of the process, looking to specify experimentally participants and conditions with which our method would be reliable. The same methodology may be used to devise the tools and procedures to intervene in other points of the ERM-postulated creative process (e.g., in the emotional resonance detection). Overall, we have provided an example of how theory may be used to improve creativity in practical, everyday realms with ordinary individuals.

CONCLUSION

From a creativity perspective, the ERM may be seen as a specific, emotion-based mechanism for the incubation (unconscious generation of associations) and the illumination (conscious detection of a promising perspective) stages of the widely held four-stage, product-oriented view of the creative process (Hadamard, 1945; Wallas, 1926). Furthermore, when considered together with our suggested process of metaphor generation for creativity, the ERM may be seen as a specific mechanism for the alternative—Eastern and humanistic—views of creativity: the model accounts for the self-realization, self-expression, and enlightenment processes central to these personality- rather than product-oriented views of creativity (Lubart, 1990).

From a broader psychological perspective, the ERM can be seen as proposing a fundamental, functional role of emotion in cognition. Beyond creativity, our model can be generalized, developed, and tested in such aspects of cognition as remembering, interpretation of artistic work, intuition, transfer of attitudes, primary/secondary processes, and child development. As mentioned earlier, we have begun to extend our model in some of these directions. Furthermore, when considered in interaction with cognitive processes (as in metaphor generation), our model is consistent with several emotion-inclusive global theories of cognition (e.g., Epstein, 1994; Tucker, 1981) and offers a specific mechanism with which these theories may operate.

REFERENCES

Ahsen, A. (1982). Principles of imagery in art and literature. *Journal of Mental Imagery, 6,* 213–250.
Arieti, S. (1976). *Creativity: The magic synthesis.* New York: Basic Books.
Averill, J. R. (1975). A semantic atlas of emotional concepts. *JSAS Catalogue of Selected Documents in Psychology, 5* (330, Ms. No. 421).
Averill, J. R. (1992). The structural bases of emotional behavior: A metatheoretical analysis. In M. S. Clark (Ed.), *Emotion* (pp. 1–26).Newbury Park, CA: Sage.
Averill, J. R. (1994, July). *Emotional creativity inventory: Scale construction and validation.* Paper presented at the meetings of the International Society for Research on Emotion, Cambridge, England.
Averill, J. R., & Nunley, E. P. (1992). *Voyages of the heart: Living an emotionally creative life.* New York: Free Fress.
Bargh, J. A., Chaiken, S., Govender, R., & Pratto, F. (1992). The generality of the automatic activation effect. *Journal of Personality and Social Psychology, 62,* 893–912.
Bartlett, F. C. (1932). *Remembering: A study in experimental and social psychology.* Cambridge, England: Cambridge University Press.
Basadur, M., Graen, G. B., & Green, S. G. (1982). Training in creative problem solving: Effects on ideation and problem finding and solving in an industrial research organization. *Organizational Behavior and Human Performance, 30,* 41–71.

Berggren, D. (1962). The use and abuse of metaphor. (Part 1) *Review of Metaphysics, 62,* 237–258.
Berggren, D. (1963). The use and abuse of metaphor. (Part 2) *Review of Metaphysics, 63,* 450–472.
Bruner, J. S. (1986). *Actual minds, possible worlds.* Cambridge, MA: Harvard University Press.
Clevenger, T., Jr., & Edwards, R. (1988). Semantic distance as a predictor of metaphor selection. *Journal of Psycholinguistic Research, 17,* 211–226.
Couger, J. D., Higgins, L. F., & McIntyre, S. C. (1993). (Un)Structured creativity in information systems organizations. *MIS Quarterly, 17,* 375–397.
Damasio, A. R. (1994). *Descartes error: Emotion, reason, and the human brain.* New York: Putnam's Sons.
DeBono, E. (1970). *Lateral thinking.* New York: Harper & Row.
Ekman, P., & Davidson, R. J. (Eds.). (1994). *The nature of emotions.* New York: Oxford University Press.
Ekvall, G., & Parnes, S. J. (1984). *Creative problem solving methods in product development: A second experiment* (Report No. 2). Stockholm: FA Radet.
Epstein, S. (1994). Integration of the cognitive and the psychodynamic unconscious. *American Psychologist, 49,* 709–724.
Fazio, R. H., Sanbonmatsu, D. M., Powell, M. C., & Kardes, F. R. (1986). On the automatic activation of attitudes. *Journal of Personality and Social Psychology, 50,* 229–238.
Feist, G. J. (1994). The affective consequences of artistic and scientific problem solving. *Cognition and Emotion, 8,* 489–502.
Finke, R. A., Ward, T. B., & Smith, S. M. (1992). *Creative cognition: Theory, research, and applications.* Cambridge, MA: MIT Press.
Fiske, S. T., & Taylor, S. E. (1991). *Social cognition* (2nd ed.) New York: McGraw-Hill.
Freud, S. (1959). Creative writers and day-dreaming. In J. Stratchey (Ed.), *Standard edition of the complete psychological works of Sigmund Freud* (Vol. 9, pp. 143–153). London: Hogarth Press. (Original work published 1908).
Gentner, D. (1988). Metaphor as structure mapping: The relational shift. *Child Development, 59,* 47–59.
Getz, I. (1996). *L'expertise cognitive aux échecs.* [Cognitive Expertise in Chess] Paris: Presses Universitaires de France.
Getz, I., & Laroche, H. (1996). The role of emotions in organizational cognition and creativity: An overview. In *Transactions of the 2nd Symposium on Cognition and Creativity in Organizational Settings* (pp.2–5). Paris, France.
Getz, I, & Lubart, T. I., (1996, August). *The key role of emotion in practical cognition and creativity.* Paper presented at the 104th Annual Convention of the American Psychological Association, Toronto, Canada.
Gobet, F., & Simon, H. A. (1996). The roles of recognition processes and look-ahead search in time-constrained expert problem solving: Evidence from grand-master-level chess. *Psychological Science, 7,* 52–55.
Gordon, W. J. J. (1956, November). Operational approach to creativity. *Harvard Business Review,* pp. 41–51.
Gordon, W. J. J. (1961). *Synectics: The development of creative capacity.* New York: Harper & Row.
Hadamard, J. (1945). *An essay on the psychology of invention in the mathematical field.* Princeton, NJ: Princeton University Press.
Hoffman, R. R., & Kemper, S. (1987). What could reaction-time studies be telling us about metaphor comprehension? *Metaphor and Symbolic Activity, 2,* 149–186.
Indurkhya, B. (1992). *Metaphor and cognition.* Dordrecht, The Netherlands: Kluwer.
Isen, A. M. (1987). Positive affect, cognitive processes and social behavior. In L. Berkowitz (Ed.), *Advances in experimental social psychology.* (pp. 203–253). San Diego, CA: Academic Press.
Isen, A. M. (1996, June). The influence of positive affect on creative problem solving and related processes in organizations. In *Transactions of the 2nd Symposium on Cognition and Creativity in Organizational Settings,* (pp. 13–15). Paris, France.

Isen, A. M., Daubman, K., & Nowicki, G. (1987). Positive affect facilitates creative problem solving. *Journal of Personality and Social Psychology, 52,* 1122–1131.

Jarvin, L., Getz, I., & Lubart, T. I. (1997). Emotion, creativity, and individual differences: A preliminary study. In T. Tuhel, T. Mariuain, & G. Rouxel (Eds), *Psychologie et différences individuelles* [Psychology and Individual Difference] (pp. 207–210). Rennes, France: Presses Universitaires de Rennes.

Jennings, J. L. (1991). Aphorisms and the creative imagination: Lessons in creativity, method, and communication.

Katz, A. N. (1989). On choosing the vehicle of metaphors: Referential concreteness, semantic distances, and individual differences. *Journal of Memory and Language, 28,* 486–499.

Kaufmann, G. (1996, August). *Mood and creative problem solving.* Paper presented at the 104th Annual Convention of the American Psychological Association, Toronto, Canada.

Lakoff, G., & Johnson, M. (1980). *Metaphors we live by.* Chicago: Chicago University Press.

Lane, R. D., Quinlan, D. Q., Schwartz, G. E., Walker, P. A., & Zeitlin, S. B. (1990). The Levels of Emotional Awareness Scale: A cognitive-developmental measure of emotion. *Journal of Personality Assessment, 55,* 124–134.

Lang, P. J. (1994). The varieties of emotional experience: A meditation on James-Lange theory. *Psychological Review, 101,* 211–221.

Lubart, T. I. (1990). Creativity and cross-cultural variation. *International Journal of Psychology, 25,* 39–59.

Lubart, T. I. (1994). Creativity. In E. C. Carterette & M. P. Friedman (Series Eds.) & R. J. Sternberg (Vol. Ed.), *Handbook of perception and cognition: Thinking and problem solving* (pp. 289–332). San Diego, CA: Academic Press.

Lubart, T. I., & Getz, I. (1997). Emotion, metaphor, and creative process. *Creativity Research Journal, 10,* 285–301.

Malatesta, C. Z. (1988). The role of emotions in the development and organization of personality. In R. A. Thompson & R. A. Dienstbier (Eds.), *Nebraska symposium on motivation: Vol. 36. Socioemotional development* (pp. 1–56). Lincoln: University of Nebraska Press.

Mark, M. M., Sinclair, R. C., & Wellens, T. R. (1991). The effect of completing the Beck Depression Inventory on self-reported mood state: Contrast and assimilation. *Personality and Social Psychology Bulletin, 17,* 457–465.

Miall, D. S. (1987). Metaphor and affect: The problem of creative thought. *Metaphor and Symbolic Activity, 2,* 81–96.

Oatley, K. (1992). *Best laid schemes: The psychology of emotions.* Cambridge, England: Cambridge University Press.

Oatley, K., & Johnson-Laird, P. N. (1987). Towards cognitive theory of emotions. *Cognition and Emotion, 1,* 25–50.

Ochse, R. (1990). *Before the gates of excellence: The determinants of creative genius.* New York: Cambridge University Press.

Ortony, A. (1975). Why metaphors are necessary and not just nice. *Educational Theory, 25,* 45–53.

Ortony, A. (1991). Value and emotion. In W. Kessen, A. Ortony, & F. Craik (Eds.), *Memories, thoughts, and emotions: Essays in honor of George Mandler* (pp. 337–353). Hillsdale, NJ: Erlbaum.

Osgood, C. E. (1963). Language universals and psycholinguistics. In J. H. Greenberg (Ed.), *Universals of language* (pp. 299–328). Cambridge, MA: MIT Press.

Osgood, C.E. (1969). On the whys and wherefores of E, P, and A. *Journal of Personality and Social Psychology, 12,* 194–199.

Paivio, A. (1978). Mental comparisons involving abstract attributes. *Memory and Cognition, 3,* 199–208.

Parnes, S. J. (1987). The creative studies project. In S. G. Isaksen (Ed.), *Frontiers in creativity research* (pp. 156–188). Buffalo, NY: Bear Limited.

Poincaré, H. (1921). *The foundations of science.* New York: Science Press.

Richards, I. A. (1950). *Coleridge on imagination.* New York: Norton.
Russ, S. W. (1993). *Affect and creativity: The role of affect and play in the creative process.* Hillsdale, NJ: Erlbaum.
Russell, J. (1980). A circumplex model of affect. *Journal of Personality and Social Psychology, 45,* 1281–1288.
Salovey, P., Mayer, J. D., Goldman, S. L., Turvey, C., & Palfai, T. P. (1995). In J. Pennebaker (Ed.), *Emotion, disclosure, and health.* (pp. 125–154). Washington, DC: American Psychological Association.
Shaw, M. P., & Runco, M. A. (Eds.). (1994). *Creativity and affect.* Norwood, NJ: Ablex.
Simon, H. A. (1967). Motivational and emotional controls of cognition. *Psychological Review, 74,* 29–39.
Spiro, R., Crismore, A., & Turner, T. J. (1982). On the role of pervasive experiential coloration in memory. *Text, 2,* 253–262.
Sternberg, R. J., & Lubart, T. I. (1995). *Defying the crowd: Cultivating creativity in a culture of conformity.* New York: Free Press.
Sternberg, R. J., & Lubart, T. I. (1996). Investing in creativity. *American Psychologist, 51,* 677–688.
Tellegen, A. (1982). *Brief manual for the Multidimensional Personality Questionnaire.* Unpublished manuscript, Department of Psychology, University of Minnesota, Minneapolis.
Tourangeau, R., & Rips, L. (1991). Interpreting and evaluating metaphors. *Journal of Memory and Language, 30,* 452–472.
Tucker, D. M. (1981). Lateral brain function, emotion, and conceptualization. *Psychological Bulletin, 89,* 19–46.
Wallas, G. (1926). *The art of thought.* New York: Harcourt, Brace.
Zajonc, R.D. (1980). Feeling and thinking: Preferences need no inferences. *American Psychologist, 35,* 151–175.

4

Play, Affect, and Creativity: Theory and Research

Sandra W. Russ
Case Western Reserve University, Cleveland, Ohio

What does children's play have to do with the great creative masterpieces of our time? Can we really learn about the underlying creative processes that are involved in the writing of *Naked Lunch* or *Howl* or the discovery of the DNA helix by studying children's play? I think we can see the beginning of some of the cognitive and affective processes important in creativity in play. These processes are, of course, in the early stages of development. They are the precursors of the mature processes that are integrated into the knowledge base, life experiences, social context, and worldview of the creative adult tackling a problem or looking for a new synthesis. Adults are not recreating the play experience when they create. They are using processes that they used and developed when they played as children. By studying children's play, we can learn about the development of these processes, the role they play in creative work, how they do or do not facilitate creativity, and how they can be facilitated. Play is a window on the beginnings of the creative process.

AFFECT AND CREATIVITY

What is the role of affect in creativity? Other chapters in this book review the current state of theory and research in the field. In my own recent attempt at an integrated model of affect and creativity (Russ, 1993), I identified five affective processes important in creativity. These categories are based on the theoretical and research literature and are as follows:

Access to affect-laden thoughts—the ability to think about thoughts and images that contain emotional content. Primary process thinking and affective fantasies in daydreams and in play are examples of this category. Thoughts that involve emotional themes such as aggressive and sexual ideation illustrate this blending of affect and cognition.

Openness to affect states—the ability to experience the emotion itself. Comfort with intense emotion and the ability to experience a range of emotions and mood states characterize this openness.

Affective pleasure in challenge—enjoying the excitement and tension involved in identifying a problem and working on a task.

Affective pleasure in problem solving—taking deep pleasure in solving a problem or creating a product.

Cognitive integration and modulation of affective material—the cognitive regulation and control of emotional processes.

In my model of affect and creativity, I linked the affective processes to cognitive processes and personality traits found to be important in creativity (see Figure 1). There is a general consensus among creativity researchers about which cognitive processes (Guilford, 1950) and personality traits (Barron & Harrington, 1981) are important in creativity. The proposed links between affective processes and cognitive and personality processes are based on empirical evidence and the clinical literature. For example, primary process thinking has been found to relate to divergent thinking and the ability to shift sets (Russ, 1982, 1988), and mood induction has been found to facilitate breadth of associations (Isen, Daubman, & Nowicki, 1987). Different configurations of these processes occur in different creative individuals and different domains of creativity (Helson, 1996).

PLAY, AFFECT, AND CREATIVITY

Play is important in the development of many of the cognitive, affective, and personality processes involved in creativity. Cognitive processes such as divergent thinking and affective processes such as affect-laden fantasy occur in play, are expressed in play, and develop through play experiences. The link between play and creativity may exist because play facilitates a number of different processes important in creativity.

The type of play most important to the area of creativity is pretend play. Pretend play is play that involves pretending, the use of fantasy and make-believe, and the use of symbolism. Fein (1987) stated that pretend play is a symbolic behavior in which "one thing is playfully treated as if it were something else" (p. 282). She also stated that pretense is charged with feelings and emotional intensity. Affect is intertwined with pretend play. Fein viewed pretend play as a natural form of creativity.

The following discussion focuses on the affective processes in play and the link between affect in play and creativity. For reviews of the literature that

AFFECT AND CREATIVITY
A MODEL

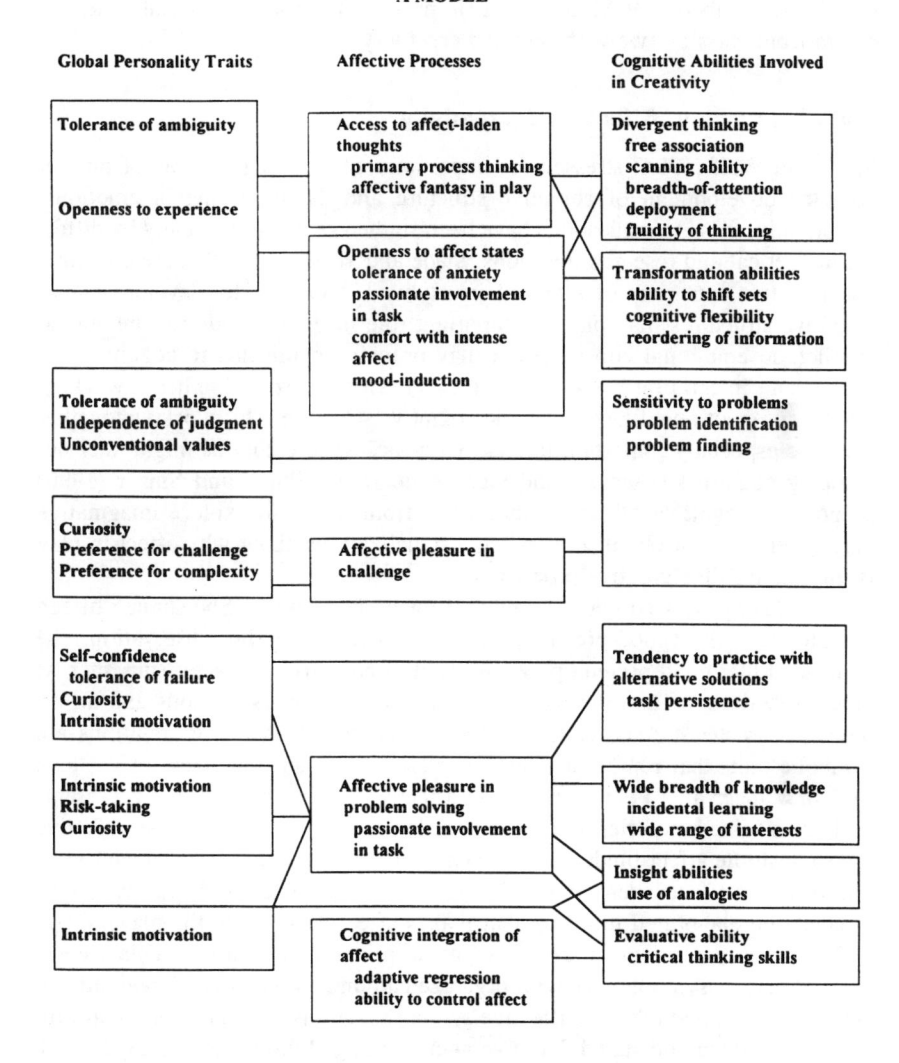

Global Personality Traits	Affective Processes	Cognitive Abilities Involved in Creativity

Tolerance of ambiguity
 	
Openness to experience
	Access to affect-laden thoughts
	  primary process thinking
	  affective fantasy in play
		Divergent thinking
		  free association
		  scanning ability
		  breadth-of-attention deployment
		  fluidity of thinking

	Openness to affect states
	  tolerance of anxiety
	  passionate involvement in task
	  comfort with intense affect
	  mood-induction
		Transformation abilities
		  ability to shift sets
		  cognitive flexibility
		  reordering of information

Tolerance of ambiguity
Independence of judgment
Unconventional values
		Sensitivity to problems
		  problem identification
		  problem finding

Curiosity Preference for challenge Preference for complexity	Affective pleasure in challenge	

Self-confidence
  tolerance of failure
Curiosity
Intrinsic motivation
		Tendency to practice with alternative solutions
		  task persistence

Intrinsic motivation
Risk-taking
Curiosity
	Affective pleasure in problem solving
	  passionate involvement in task
		Wide breadth of knowledge
		  incidental learning
		  wide range of interests

		Insight abilities use of analogies

Intrinsic motivation	Cognitive integration of affect
	  adaptive regression
	  ability to control affect
		Evaluative ability
		  critical thinking skills

    In this model of affect and creativity the major cognitive abilities which emerge as unique to and important in the creative process are linked to related specific affective processes and to global personality traits. In some case, the personality traits are behavioral reflections of the underlying affective process. One assumption of this model is that these specific affective processes and personality traits facilitate creative cognitive abilities.

Figure 1

discuss all types of creative processes and play, see D. L. Singer and Singer (1990), Vandenberg (1988), and Russ (in press). The material presented here is drawn from Russ's review of play and creativity.

Theories of Play, Affect, and Creativity

Slade and Wolf (1994) stressed the importance of studying the role of play in both the development of cognitive structure and the mastering of emotions. Historically, these two questions have been studied separately, usually by different theoretical and research traditions. Slade and Wolf argued that the cognitive and affective functions of play are intertwined. "Just as the development of cognitive structures may play an important role in the resolution of emotional conflict, so emotional consolidation may provide an impetus to cognitive advances and integration," they wrote (p. xv). This assertion implies a working together of emotional functioning and cognitive structure. This working together could be especially important in creativity—access to emotions might alter developing cognitive structure, and vice versa. D. L. Singer and Singer (1990) proposed a cognitive–affective framework from which to explore imaginative play. There are various theoretical conceptualizations about why affect in play is important in the creative process.

Fein (1987) viewed play as a natural form of creativity. She studied fifteen "master players" (good pretend players) and categorized her observation. She concluded that good pretend play consisted of cognitive characteristics such as object substitutions and the manipulation of object representations and an affective characteristic she called "affective relations." Affective relations are symbolic units that represent affective relationships, such as "fear of," "love of," or "anger at." Fein proposed an affective symbol system that represents real or imagined experience at a general level. She stated that these affective units constitute affect-binding representational templates that store salient information about affect-laden events. The units are "manipulated, interpreted, coordinated and elaborated in a way that makes affective sense to the players" (p. 292). These affective units are a key part of pretend play. In fact, Fein viewed pretend play as symbolic behavior organized around emotional and motivational issues. She implied that this affective symbol system is especially important for creative thinking and stated that divergent-thinking abilities such as daydreams, pretend play, or drawing can activate the affective symbol system. One of Fein's major conclusions was that creative processes cannot be studied independently of an affective symbol system, a system probably facilitated through pretend play.

Fein's conceptualization is consistent with the psychoanalytic concept of primary process and creativity, another major theoretical approach. Primary process thinking was first conceptualized by Freud (1915/1958) as an early, primitive system of thought that was drive laden and not subject to rules of logic or oriented to reality. Another way to view primary process thought is as affect-laden cognition. I have proposed that primary process is a subtype of affect in cognition (Russ, 1987, 1993, 1996). Primary process content is material around which a child experienced early intense feelings states (oral, anal, aggressive, etc.). It could be stored in the kind of affect symbol system proposed by Fein. According to psychoanalytic theory, primary process thinking facilitates creativity (Kris, 1952). Children and adults who have controlled access to primary process thinking should have a broader range of associations and be better divergent thinkers than individuals with less access to primary process. Freud's (1926/1959) formulation that repression of "dangerous" drive-laden content leads to a more general intellectual restriction predicts that individuals with less access to affect-laden cognitions have fewer associations in general. Thus, children who are more expressive of and open to affective content develop a richer, more complex store of affect-laden memories. This richer store of affect symbols and memories facilitates divergent-thinking and transformation abilities, because it provides a broader range of associations and a more flexible manipulation of images and ideas.

Primary process content is expressed in play. As Waelder (1933) said, play is a "leave of absence from reality" (p. 222) and is a place to let primary process thinking occur. Play can be important in the development of primary process thought.

Fein's (1987) theory and primary process theory are also consistent with Bower's (1981) conceptualization of affect and memory processes (see Russ, 1993). The work on mood and memory suggests that the search process for associations is broadened by the involvement of emotion. Russ (1993) proposed that if primary process is thought of as mood-relevant cognition, it could fit into a mood and memory theoretical framework. When stirred, primary process content triggers a broad associative network. Primary process content was stored into the memory system when emotion was present. Access to this primary process content activates emotion nodes and associations, broadening the search process. This conceptualization is also consistent with Getz and Lubart's emotional resonance model of creativity (see Chapter 3).

Vygotsky (1930/1967) also thought that play facilitated creativity. In a recent translation and integration of Vygotsky's work, Smolucha (1992) stated that Vygotsky viewed creativity as a developmental process facilitated through play. Vygotsky (1930/1967) stated "The child's play activity is not simply a recollection of past experience but a creative reworking that combines impressions and constructs forming new realities addressing the needs of the child" (p. 7). Through play, children develop combinatory imagination, that is, the ability to combine elements of experience into new situations and new behaviors. Combinatory imagination is part of artistic and scientific creativity. By adolescence, play evolves into fantasy and imagination, which combine with conceptual thinking. Imagination has two parts in the adolescent—objective and subjective. Subjective imagination includes emotion and serves the emotional life. Impulse and thinking are combined in the activity of creative thinking.

In my model of affect and creativity (Russ 1993), looking specifically at the affect categories, play is important in the expression and facilitation of all five affect processes. Both affect-laden fantasy and affect states are expressed in play. Children practice with the expression of a variety of feeling states and affective themes in fantasy. Also, the joy that most children experience when they become lost in pretend play may be similar to the flow (Csikszentmihalyi, 1990) experiences in creative work. The pleasure in play could also be similar to the intrinsic motivation so important in creativity (Amabile, 1990; Hennessey, Chapter 5 in this book). Taking pleasure in challenge and the tension necessary in the process of identifying and solving problems is also evident in play. Children do scare themselves as much as they can tolerate in pretend play. They also use play to work on and rework internal conflicts and situational traumas (Erikson, 1963). Finally, through play, the child learns to master feelings and develop cognitive structure that aids in the modulation and regulation of emotion (Freedheim & Russ, 1992).

Research Evidence of a Relationship Between Play and Creativity

A growing body of research has found a relationship between play and creativity. Most of the research has been correlational in nature. In a review of the literature, J. L. Singer and Singer (1976) concluded that the capacity for imaginative play is positively related to divergent thinking. D. L. Singer and Rummo (1973) found a relationship between play and divergent thinking in kindergarten children. Play was found to facilitate divergent thinking in preschool children by Dansky and Silverman (1973) and Dansky (1980). (See Russ, in press, for a thorough review of the research literature.)

Until recently, the research on play and creativity has focused on cognitive variables as the explanatory mechanisms underlying the relationship. The various theoretical explanations of affect in play and creativity are just beginning to be tested.

Lieberman's (1977) work supports a relationship between affect and divergent thinking. She focused on the variable playfulness, which included the affective components spontaneity and joy. She found that playful kindergarten children did better on divergent-thinking tasks than did nonplayful children. D. L. Singer and Singer (1990) reported that positive affect was related to imaginative play. J. L. Singer and Singer (1981) also found that preschoolers rated as high-imagination players showed significantly more themes of danger and power than did children with low imagination.

I was especially interested in investigating affective dimensions of play and creativity in my research program. To do so, I developed the Affect in Play Scale (APS) to meet the need for a standardized measure of affect in pretend play (Russ, 1987, 1993). Play sessions are individual puppet play involving two neutral-looking puppets, one boy and one girl, with three small blocks laid out on a table. The instructions are standardized and direct the children to play with the puppets any way they like for 5 min in a free-play period. The play task and instructions are unstructured enough that individual differences in the use of affect in pretend play emerge. The APS is appropriate for children from 6 to 10 years of age. The play session is videotaped so that coding can occur later.

The APS measures the amount and types of affective expression in children's pretend play. It also measures cognitive dimensions of the play, such as quality of fantasy and imagination. Conceptually, the APS taps three dimensions of affect in fantasy: affect states, or actual emotional experiencing through expression of feeling states; affect-laden thoughts, or affective content themes that include emotional content themes and primary process themes; and cognitive integration of affect. These three categories of affect are three of the five affective dimensions I proposed to be important in the creative process (Russ, 1993). This conceptualization of affect and creativity guided the development of the scale. In addition, I used Holt's (1977) scoring system for primary process on the Rorschach and J. L. Singer's (1973) play scales as models for the development of the scale. Details of the instructions and scoring system for the APS can be found elsewhere (Russ, 1993).

The major affect scores for the scale are frequency of affect units expressed, variety of affect categories expressed (there are 11 possible categories), and intensity of affect expression. There are also global ratings (on a 5-point scale) for comfort, quality of fantasy, and imagination. An affective integration score combines frequency and quality of fantasy.

Once the APS was constructed, pilot studies were carried out to ensure that the task was appropriate for young children and would result in adequate individual differences among normal school populations (Russ, Grossman-McKee, & Rutkin, 1984). By 1984, the basics of the task and scoring system were in place. Recent studies resulted in refinement of the scoring criteria and a shortening of the play period from 10 min to 5 min. Children who express a high frequency of affect in their play typically have the puppets playing competitive games, fighting with each other, having fun together, eating (oral content), and expressing affection.

Affect in Play Scale and Creativity

To date, my colleagues and I have carried out nine validity studies with the APS. In each study, we obtained interrater reliabilities on 15 or 20 participants. Interrate reliabilities have been good, usually in the .80s and .90s, using a variety of different raters. We also obtained split-half reliability for frequency of affective expression comparing the 2nd and 4th minutes with the 3rd and 5th minutes. We found a split-half reliability of .85, which is good (Russ, 1993; Russ & Peterson, 1990).

Two types of validating criteria have been used. One body of studies investigated affect in play and creativity. A second line of studies, not reviewed here, investigated play and coping/adjustment (Christiano & Russ, 1996; Russ, 1995).

The first study in the affect and creativity area (Russ & Grossman-McKee, 1990) investigated the relationships among the APS, divergent thinking, and primary process thinking on the Rorschach in 60 first- and second-grade children. As predicted, affective expression in play was significantly positively related to divergent thinking, as measured by the Alternate Uses Test (Wallach and Kogan, 1965). All major scores on the APS significantly correlated with divergent thinking, with correlations ranging from .23 ($p < .05$) between comfort and divergent thinking to .42 ($p < .001$) between frequency of affective expression and divergent thinking. All correlations remained significant when IQ was partialed out, because IQ had such low correlations with the APS. The lack of relationship between intelligence and any of the play scores is consistent with the theoretical model for the development of the scale and is similar to the results of J. L. Singer (1973). Also, there were no gender differences in the correlations between the APS and divergent thinking. This study also found a relationship between the amount of primary process thinking on the Rorschach and APS scores. Children who had more primary process responses on the Rorschach showed more primary process and more affect in their play and had higher fantasy scores than did children who showed less primary process on the Rorschach. This is an important finding, because it shows consistency in the construct of affective expression across two different situations.

The finding of a relationship between affect in play and divergent thinking (Russ & Grossman-McKee, 1990) was replicated by Russ and Peterson (1990) in a larger sample of 121 first- and second-grade children. Again, all the APS scores were significantly positively related to the Alternate Uses Test, independent of intelligence. Again, there were no gender differences in the correlations. This replication allows more confidence in the robustness of the finding of a relationship between affect in pretend play and creativity in young children. Children who have more access to emotion-laden fantasy and who can express emotion in play are more creative on divergent-thinking tasks.

An important question about the APS is whether it indeed measures two separate dimensions of play—an affective dimension and a cognitive dimension—or measures only an affect in fantasy dimension. The results of two factor analyses with the scale suggest that it measures two separate dimensions. In the Russ and Peterson (1990) study, a factor analysis of the total sample was carried out using the principal-component analysis with oblique rotation. An oblique solution yielded two separate factors as the best solution. The first and dominant dimension appeared to be cognitive. Imagination, organization, quality of fantasy, and comfort loaded on this dimension. The second factor appeared to be affective. Frequency of affective expression, variety of affect categories, and intensity of affect loaded on this factor. The factors, although separate, had a significant amount of shared variance ($r = .76$).

A recent study by D'Angelo (1995) replicated the finding of two factors, one cognitive and one affective, with a sample of 95 children in Grades 1–3. Another interesting finding by D'Angelo was a significant relationship between scores on the APS and responses in J. L. Singer's (1973) imaginative play predisposition interview. Good players in the APS reported that they prefer activities that require using imagination.

Stability of Dimensions of Play, Affect, and Creativity

A recent study (Russ, Robins, & Christiano, in press) followed-up the first and second graders in the Russ and Peterson study (1990) when they were in fifth and sixth grade. This was a longitudinal study that explored the ability of the APS to predict creativity over a 4-year period. Thirty-one children agreed to participate in the follow-up. The major finding was that quality of fantasy and imagination on the APS predicted divergent thinking over a 4-year period ($r = .34, p < .05$, and $r = .42, p < .01$, respectively). The correlations between variety of affect and divergent thinking was .25 but did not reach significance, possibly because of the small sample size.

Russ et al. (in press) also administered an adapted version of the play task to the older children (sixth and seventh graders), instructing them "to put on a play with the puppets." The task was scored using the scoring criteria for the APS. Raters were unaware of the earlier scores. Good stability was found in the dimensions being measured by the APS. For example, the correlation between the two frequency of affect scores was .33 ($p < .05$), that between the two variety of affect scores was .38 ($p < .05$), and that between the two frequency of positive affect scores was .51 ($p < .01$). Children who expressed more affect and better fantasy in play as first and second graders had more affect and better fantasy play in their play stories as sixth and seventh graders. In general, the sizes of the correlations are excellent for a period of 4 to 5 years and support the concept of enduring, stable constructs of affective expression in fantasy that are predictive of creative thinking over time. These findings also suggest an enduring quality to the affective and cognitive dimensions of the APS over a 5-year period.

These findings are consistent with those of Hutt and Bhavnani (1972), who found that creative inventiveness in preschool play related to later divergent thinking. Clark, Griffing, and Johnson (1989) also found a relationship between divergent thinking and play in preschoolers that was predictive of divergent thinking over a 3-year period.

In addition to testing the longitudinal stability of the play scale scores, Russ et al. (in press) tested the stability of the Alternate Uses Test scores over the 4 years. Both the fluency scores and the flexibility scores were significantly positively correlated over time ($r = .30, p < .05$; and $r = .46, p < .01$, respectively). It is noteworthy that the Alternate Uses Test was individually administered to the first and second graders but group administered when these children were older. Despite the introduction of other sources of variance, the correlations further attest to the stability of divergent-thinking abilities. My colleagues and

I hope to follow these children into adolescence to see if these processes remain stable.

POSITIVE AND NEGATIVE AFFECT IN CREATIVITY

What can play reveal about the role of positive and negative affect in creativity? After all, if play is fun, can any negative affect occur in play? To address this question, it helps to differentiate between affect states and affect-laden thoughts. In pretend play, much of what is expressed is affect-laden thoughts and fantasy. Affect states, the actual experiencing of a feeling state, may or may not accompany the affect-laden thought. For example, one puppet could be hitting the other puppet and saying "I hate you," which would be scored as intense aggressive affect fantasy. However, the child could be having fun and be in a positive mood state. Or, the child could be experiencing a mild degree of anger. If affect does accompany the fantasy, it can do so in varying degrees. In pretend play, the child is in charge of how much feeling is experienced. Especially with negative affect states, if the feelings become too uncomfortable, the child will change the theme or stop the play. Thus, the kind of negative affect experienced in pretend play is either mild in degree or in the form of a negative-affect theme or fantasy.

Mood Induction Research

No intervention study in the area of play and creativity has specifically manipulated affect in play and the effects on creativity. However, the research in the area of mood induction and creativity is relevant to the question of whether increasing affect in pretend play facilitates creative problem solving. Most of the research in the area of mood induction and creativity has been conducted with adults. The mood induction paradigm provides a way of altering affect states so that the effect on cognitive processes can be observed. In a series of studies, Isen found that induced positive affect facilitated creative thinking. Isen (1985) found that positive affect increased divergent associations to neutral words, and Isen et al. (1987) found that positive affect, induced by a comedy film, resulted in more creative problem solving than did control conditions. Induction of a negative mood state had no effect on creativity. Jausovec (1989) also found that induced positive affect facilitated performance on an analogical transfer task, thought to be important in creative thinking. He also found that negative mood induction had no effect. Both Isen et al. and Jausovec hypothesized that the negative mood induction method that was used (a Holocaust film) may have been too extreme. In a study by Adaman (1991), a milder form of negative mood induction that used sad music did facilitate divergent thinking in college students. Kaufman and Vosburg (1997) found that negative mood induction did facilitate performance on an insight task. The only published study with children found that induced positive affect in eighth-grade children facilitated creative problem solving (Green and Noice, 1988). It may be concluded that careful experimental work has shown that positive affect states facilitate transformation abilities, remote associations, and analogical transfer (see Chapters 1 and 2 for a review).

Pretend Play Research

The pretend play research also suggests that positive affect relates to and facilitates creative cognitive processes. Lieberman's (1977) finding that spontaneity and joy in play related to divergent thinking, D. L. Singer and Singer's (1990) finding that positive affect related to imaginative play, and Krasnor and Pepler's (1980) notion that intrinsic motivation (a pleasurable state) is part of pretend play are all consistent with the mood induction research findings.

Although, as reviewed earlier, a few studies have indicated a facilitative effect, by and large the mood induction research has not found much support for negative affect's facilitating creativity. However, in play research, negative play themes are related to creativity. Themes of danger and power occurred in high-imagination players (J. L. Singer & Singer, 1981), negative primary process themes related to creative thinking (Russ & Grossman-McKee, 1990), and frequency of affect consisting of both positive- and negative-affect themes in play related to divergent thinking (Russ, 1993; Russ & Grossman-McKee, 1990; Russ & Peterson, 1990). Theoretically, both positive and negative affect should facilitate creativity. Richards (1990), Russ (1993), and Feist (in press) have proposed a curvilinear relationship between affect and creativity. Positive and negative affect may facilitate creativity when they exist in low to moderate levels. At those levels, such as in well-controlled play, where the child is in charge of pacing the material, negative affect may trigger memories and associations important to the creative process. Because the child is in charge of the material in good pretend play, negative affect may not be so negative. Negative themes such as fear and aggression may not be accompanied by negative mood states. D. L. Singer and Singer (1990) stated that controlled expression of negative affect is reinforcing. Krasnor and Pepler (1980) thought that all pretend play involved mainly positive emotions. On the other hand, Morrison's (1988) idea of reworking old metaphors in play involves dealing with negative affect. Chuck Jones, the cartoonist, has stated that in the creative process, one must be open to and face down anxieties and fears (Goleman, Kaufman, & Ray, 1992). Joy arrives when the issue has been resolved, in the art. Vandenberg (1988) stated that play derives its thrill from the anxiety within it. Since safety is a prerequisite for play, threats and taboos can be explored.

The play situation is a place where children can develop modes of expression of both positive and negative affect. In this safe arena, children can call up a variety of pretend mood scales, memories and fantasies, and primary process themes. Negative affect can be expressed, worked through, and mastered. Children can practice with free associations and divergent thinking. Over time, this practice could alter cognitive structures, increase metaphors, foster a rich store of affect symbols (Fein, 1987), and result in increased divergent-thinking and transformation abilities.

Primary Process Thinking and Positive and Negative Affect

Psychoanalytic theory states that it is the conflict-laden, negative-affect themes that relate to and facilitate creativity. In Freud's (1926/1959) formulation, it is the repression of "dangerous" drive-laden content that leads to a more general restriction of cognition. Primary process content is mainly aggressive or libidinal (oral or sexual) content around which the child experiences conflict, and the child must work to master and integrate this material. An interesting theoretical question is whether primary process themes are negative-affect themes, or are a mix of both positive- and negative-affect themes around which the child experiences early intense feeling states. Learning to regulate these intense emotions and affect-laden thoughts and images is a major developmental task. These intense emotions include both negative (aggression) and positive (oral or affection) emotions.

Most of the studies in the primary process area used Holt's (1977) scoring system for primary process responses on the Rorschach. In the adult and child literature, the expression of well-integrated primary process thinking on the Rorschach consistently related to creativity in males, but usually not in females (for reviews, see Holt, 1977; Russ, 1993; Suler, 1980). In a series of studies that I carried out with children, I found that well-integrated primary process content on the Rorschach was positively related to flexibility in thinking as measured by Luchin's Water-Jar Test (Russ, 1982) and divergent thinking (Russ, 1988; Russ & Grossman-McKee, 1990), independent of intelligence. For the most part, these relationships were true for boys, not for girls. Two questions emerged from these studies:

Is it just the primary process affect-laden themes that relate to creativity, or do all affect-laden themes relate?
Why the sex differences? Would other types of affect themes relate to creativity in girls? Girls had expressed significantly less primary process content on the Rorschach than did boys (Russ, 1982).

Initially, I tried to answer these questions by scoring other types of affect themes on the Rorschach data. However, not enough nonprimary process themes occurred to allow a powerful statistical analysis. The Rorschach does not pull for a whole array of affect themes, at least not in children. I then developed the APS so that I could address these questions in the more natural medium of expression for children—pretend play.

In the Russ and Grossman-McKee (1990) study, the amount of primary process shown on the Rorschach related to all types of affect in play, not just

Table 1 Oblique Factor Structure of the Affect in Play Scale with Primary Process Affect for Total Sample

Play score	Cognitive	Affect — Primary Process	Affect — Nonprimary Process
Frequency of primary process	−.06	.92	−.09
Frequency of nonprimary process	−.01	−.10	.87
Variety of affect	16	.39	.48
Mean intensity	.32	.37	.13
Comfort	.67	.06	.11
Quality of fantasy	.75	.06	.10
Organization	.81	.00	−.03
Imagination	.75	−.01	.00

Note: N = 121.

primary process themes. Children who expressed more primary process on the Rorschach had more affective expression in general in their play. Frequency of total affect in play related to divergent thinking for boys ($r = .40$) and girls ($r = .44$). Primary process content related to divergent thinking for boys ($r = .38$) and girls ($r = .48$), and nonprimary process content did not predict creativity. Replication of this study with a second sample of 121 children again showed a relationship between affect in play and divergent thinking for both boys and girls (Russ & Peterson, 1990). However, in this study primary process and nonprimary process affect related equally to divergent thinking. Also, when affect content was examined in a different way and frequency scores were obtained for positive and negative affect, both positive- and negative-affect themes related to creativity.

Factor Analysis of the Affect in Play Scale

In order to get a better handle on what dimensions of affect are tapped by the APS, several factor analyses were carried out on the Russ and Peterson (1990) data set (Russ, 1993).

First, a principal-component analysis with oblique rotation of the seven major scores revealed two factors: a cognitive factor (organization of fantasy, imagination, quality of fantasy, and comfort) and an affective factor (frequency of affect, variety of affect categories, and intensity of affect).

Two principal-component analyses using the affect scores with an oblique solution were performed to examine the affect dimension. When the primary process and nonprimary process scores were used in place of the frequency of affect score, three factors were found. The first was a cognitive factor, the second was primary process affect, and the third was nonprimary process affect (Table 1). The second factor analysis, using the positive- and negative-affect scores, also revealed three factors: a cognitive factor, positive affect, and negative affect

Table 2 Oblique Factor Structure of the Affect in Play Scale with Positive and Negative Affect for Total Sample

		Affect	
Play score	Cognitive	Negative	Positive
Frequency of positive affect	−.02	−.12	.84
Frequency of negative affect	−.07	.93	−.07
Variety of affect	13	.42	.51
Mean intensity	.34	.41	.09
Comfort	.70	.15	−.02
Quality of fantasy	.73	.05	.1
Organization	.76	−.09	.06
Imagination	.73	−.02	−.00

Note: N = 121.

(Table 2). These results suggest that the hypothesized constructs have some conceptual validity.

Separate factor analysis using the oblique solution was then performed on the 11 affect content categories and, five different factors were found in the play (Table 3). The factors make sense theoretically. On the first factor, oral content and nurturance/affection combined. The second factor was composed of negative-affect themes of aggression, anxiety, sadness, and frustration. The third factor comprised happiness themes, with a low aggression loading. The fourth factor was low competition and high anxiety. The fifth factor was an association of sexual and anal content, which is understandable in that they are both unusual content themes in the play of young children. In this factor analysis of content categories, content clustered according to positive- and negative-affect themes, not primary process and non-primary process themes.

Table 3 Oblique Factor Structure of APS Content Categories in the Affect in Play Scale

	Factor				
Category	1	2	3	4	5
Oral	.806	−.022	.008	.081	.142
Sexual	−.024	−.044	.067	.061	.873
Competition	−.048	.349	.124	−.765	.165
Oral aggression	.841	.036	.015	−.042	−.003
Anal	.319	.073	−.12	−.185	.64
Aggression	.017	.548	−.649	.143	−.001
Happiness	.057	.136	.795	.063	−.024
Nurturance	.47	.195	.269	.392	.263
Anxiety	−.027	.463	.238	.536	.083
Sadness	−.025	.693	−.028	−.028	.02
Frustration	.08	.716	.05	−.226	−.048

The factor structure of the APS suggests that researchers need to go beyond differentiating between positive- and negative-affect or primary process and nonprimary process themes. There may be specific clusters of affect content categories that go together developmentally, are involved in different ways in the creative process, and work differently for girls than for boys. Different dimensions of positive and negative affect could differentially effect different types of cognitive processes (divergent thinking, metaphor construction, etc.) Also, this research on affect themes is looking at a different dimension of affect than is the research on mood states. For example, children differentiate how the puppets are feeling in the play from how they themselves are feeling (in an aggressive play condition in a recent experiment, 70% of the children reported feeling an affect state different from the puppets' state). As mentioned earlier, in play where the child is in charge of pacing the material, negative affect may not be so negative. Negative themes like aggression may not be accompanied by negative mood states.

In summary, the results of these studies support the hypotheses that both positive affect and negative affect in fantasy relate to creativity in children. My colleagues and I are just beginning to learn about the different types of affective processes involved in creativity, developmental trends, and gender differences.

PLAY, CREATIVITY, AND COPING IN CHILDREN

The research literature on creativity and coping in children is relevant to the general question of the relationship between creativity and adjustment. Although the area of creativity and adjustment has not been extensively investigated in children, there are several studies in the creativity and coping area that provide direction for future research.

Theoretically, children who are good at generating a variety of ideas and who can flexibly solve problems in creative endeavors should be able to apply these skills to everyday problem solving (Carson, Bittner, Cameron, Brown, and Meyer, 1994; Russ, 1988, 1993). This idea is also consistent with Richards' (1993) concept of everyday creativity. There is some empirical support for this hypothesis.

In several studies, my colleagues and I have found a relationship between divergent thinking and coping in children. I (Russ, 1988) found a strong relationship between the Alternate Uses Test and the Zeitlin Coping Inventory (teacher's ratings) for fifth-grade boys ($r = .58, p < .01$). In the Russ and Peterson (1990) study, divergent thinking related to the teacher's ratings of coping and self-report ratings of coping in first and second graders. In a longitudinal follow-up study of that sample, imagination and quality of fantasy in early play significantly predicted the number of different responses generated and the quality of coping responses on a self-report measure in fifth and sixth grade. In the fifth- and sixth-grade sample, divergent thinking significantly related to the quality of coping responses. (Russ et al., in press).

In all of our studies, my colleagues and I used the Alternate Uses Test. Carson et al. (1994) found similar results using the Torrance tests of divergent thinking. They found that figural (not verbal) divergent thinking in third to sixth graders was significantly related to the Zeitlin Coping Inventory and some other measures of coping. Resistance to premature closure was the best predictor of coping ability. Carson et al. concluded that "the extent to which children's coping skills and behavior could be positively influenced by augmenting their creative-thinking abilities is not only an intriguing empirical question but one that may have programmatic implications (i.e., practical significance) for children as well" (p. 154). The play, creativity, and adjustment area is a fruitful line of research for the future.

CONCLUSION

The converging research evidence that supports the links among play, affect, and creativity strongly suggests that researchers should continue investigating the play and creativity area. The following are suggested guidelines for future research.

There is a need for more longitudinal studies. Runco (1996) stressed the importance of understanding the development of creative processes. Longitudinal studies are needed but are difficult to plan and carry out. Attrition of participants is a problem. Nevertheless, researchers need to try and, at times, learn from the patterns of correlation in studies with small sample sizes. The field could also develop a support network for collecting longitudinal data.

The focus should be on the specific mechanisms and processes that underlie the play and creativity link. For example, how does having easy access to affect-laden fantasy facilitate divergent thinking? Does it facilitate divergent thinking only when emotional associations are important, or does it facilitate broad scanning ability in general?

More studies of the differential effects of different types of affect content on different types of creativity tasks are needed. Research suggests that positive and negative affect, and different content themes within those categories, may have different effects on various types of creative cognitive processes. Also, affect states and affect-laden fantasy may function quite differently from one another. The play and creativity paradigm may be more appropriate for studying affect-laden fantasy and creativity, and the mood-induction paradigm more appropriate for studying affect states and creativity (Russ, 1993).

Studies that investigate play and affect expression are also needed. How do researchers facilitate various types of affect expression in pretend play? Can it be done in one-shot studies, or does a series of play interventions over time need to be implemented?

Finally, studies of etiological factors involved in developing good play skills would have important practical implications for parents and for teachers.

The knowledge base of the play, affect, and creativity area has grown in the last 20 years. This growing knowledge base fits with the new theoretical models that are emerging in the affect and creativity area. Interaction between play scholars and affect and creativity researchers is crucial for a sophisticated understanding of the development of creative affective processes.

REFERENCES

Adaman, J. (1991). *The effects of induced mood on creativity.* Unpublished masters' thesis, University of Miami, Coral Gables, FL.

Amabile, T. (1990). Within you, without you: The social psychology of creativity and beyond. In M. Runco & R. Albert (Eds.), *Theories of creativity* (pp. 61–91). Newbury Park, CA: Sage.

Barron, F. & Harrington, D. (1981). Creativity, Intelligence, and Personality. In M. Rosenzweig & L. Porter (Eds.), *Annual Review of Psychology,* (Vol. 32, pp. 439–476). Palo Alto, CA. Annual Review.

Bower, G. (1981). Mood and memory. *American Psychologist, 36,* 129–148.

Carson, D., Bittner, M., Cameron, B., Brown, D., & Meyer, S. (1994). Creative thinking as a predictor of school-aged children's stress responses and coping abilities. *Creativity Research Journal, 7,* 145–158.

Christiano, B., & Russ, S. (1996). Play as a predictor of coping and distress in children during an invasive dental procedure. *Journal of Clinical Child Psychology, 25,* 130–138.

Clark, P., Griffing, P., & Johnson, L. (1989). Symbolic play and ideational fluency as aspects of the evolving divergent cognitive style in young children. *Early Child Development and Care, 51,* 77–88.

Csikszentmihalyi, M. (1990). *Flow: The psychology of optimal experience.* New York: Harper & Row.

D'Angelo, L. (1995). *Child's play: The relationship between the use of play and adjustment styles.* Unpublished doctoral dissertation, Case Western Reserve University, Cleveland, OH.

Dansky, J. (1980). Make-believe: A mediator of the relationship between play and associative fluency. *Child Development, 51,* 576–579.

Dansky, J., & Silverman, F. (1973). Effects of play on associative fluency in preschool-aged children. *Developmental Psychology, 9,* 38–43.

Erikson, E. (1963). *Childhood and society.* New York: Norton.

Fein, G. (1987). Pretend play: Creativity and consciousness. In P. Gorlitz & J. Wohlwill (Eds.), *Curiosity, imagination, and play* (pp. 281–304). Hillsdale, NJ: Erlbaum.

Feist, G. (1998). Affective states and traits in creativity: Evidence for non-linear relationships. In M. A. Runco (Ed.), *Handbook of creativity research* (Vol. 2). Cresskill, NJ: Hampton Press.

Freedheim, D., & Russ, S. (1992). Psychotherapy with children. In C. Walker & M. Roberts (Eds.), *Handbook of clinical child psychology* (2nd ed., pp. 765–781). New York: Wiley.

Freud, S. (1958). The unconscious. In J. Strachey (Ed. and Trans.), *The standard edition of the complete psychological works of Sigmund Freud* (Vol. 14, pp. 159–215). London: Hogarth Press. (Original work published 1915)

Freud, S. (1959). Inhibition, symptoms, and anxiety. In J. Strachey (Ed. and Trans.), *The standard edition of the complete psychological works of Sigmund Freud* (Vol. 20, pp. 87–172). London: Hogarth Press. (Original work published 1926)

Goleman, D., Kaufman, P., & Ray, M. (1992). *The creative spirit.* New York: Dutton.

Guilford, J. P. (1950). Creativity. *American Psychologist, 5,* 444–454.

Greene, T., & Noice, H. (1988). Influence of positive affect upon creative thinking and problem solving in children. *Psychological Reports, 63,* 895–898.

Helson, R. (1996). In search of the creative personality. *Creativity Research Journal, 4,* 295–306.

Holt, R. R. (1977). A method for assessing primary process manifestations and their control in Rorschach responses. In M. Rickers-Ovsiankina (Ed.), *Rorschach psychology* (pp. 375–420). New York: Kreiger.

Hutt, C., & Bhavnani, R. (1972). Predictions for play. *Nature, 237,* 171–172.

Isen, A. (1985). The asymmetry of happiness and sadness in effects on memory in normal college students. *Journal of Experimental Psychology: General, 114,* 388–391.

Isen, A., Daubman, K., & Nowicki, G. (1987). Positive affect facilitates creative problem solving. *Journal of Personality and Social Psychology, 52,* 1122–1131.

Jausovec, N. (1989). Affect in analogical transfer. *Creativity Research Journal, 2,* 255 266.

Kaufmann, G., & Vosburg, S. K. (1997). "Paradoxical" mood effects on creative problem solving. *Cognition and Emotion, 11,* 151–170.

Krasnor, L., & Pepler, D. (1980). The study of children's play: Some suggested future directions. *New Directions for Child Development, 9,* 85–94.

Kris, E. (1952). *Psychoanalytic exploration in art.* New York: International Universities Press.

Lieberman, J. N. (1977). *Playfulness: Its relationship to imagination and creativity.* San Diego, CA: Academic Press.

Morrison, D. (1988). The child's first ways of knowing. In D. Morrison (Ed.), *Organizing Early Experience: Imagination and Cognition in Childhood,* (pp. 3–14). Amityville: Baywood.

Richards, R. (1990). Everyday creativity, eminent creativity and health. Afterward for CRT issues in creativity and health. *Creativity Research Journal, 3,* 300–326.

Richards, R. (1993). Everyday creativity, eminent creativity, and psychopathology. *Psychological Inquiry, 4,* 212–217.

Runco, M. A. (1996). Creativity and development: Recommendations. In M. Runco (Ed.), *Creativity from childhood through adulthood: The developmental issues* (pp. 87–90). San Francisco: Jossey-Bass.

Russ, S. (1982). Sex differences in primary process thinking and flexibility in problem solving in children. *Journal of Personality Assessment, 45,* 569–577.

Russ, S. (1987). Assessment of cognitive affective interaction in children: Creativity, fantasy, and play research. In J. Butcher & C. Spielberger (Eds.), *Advances in personality assessment* (Vol. 6, pp. 141–155). Hillsdale, NJ: Erlbaum.

Russ, S. (1988). Primary process thinking on the Rorschach, divergent thinking, and coping in children. *Journal of Personality Assessment, 52,* 539–548.

Russ, S. (1993). *Affect and creativity: The role of affect and play in the creative process.* Hillsdale, NJ: Erlbaum.

Russ, S. (1995). Play psychotherapy research: State of the science. In T. Ollendick & R. Prinz (Eds.), *Advances in clinical child psychology* (Vol. 17, pp. 365–391). New York: Plenum.

Russ, S. (1996). Psychoanalytic theory and creativity: Cognition and affect revisited. In J. Masling & R. Borstein (Eds.), *Psychoanalytic perspectives on developmental psychology* (pp. 69–103). Washington, DC: American Psychological Association.

Russ, S. (1998). Play and creativity. In M. Runco (Ed.), *Creativity research handbook* (Vol. 3), Cresskill, NJ: Hampton Press.

Russ, S., & Grossman-McKee, A. (1990). Affective expression in children's fantasy play, primary process thinking on the Rorschach, and divergent thinking. *Journal of Personality Assessment, 54,* 756–771.

Russ, S., Grossman-McKee, A., & Rutkin, Z. (1984). [Affect in Play Scale: Pilot project]. Unpublished raw data.

Russ, S., & Peterson, N. (1990). *The Affect in Play Scale: Predicting creativity and coping in children.* Unpublished manuscript.

Russ, S., Robins, D., & Christiano, B. (1997). Pretend play: Longitudinal prediction of creativity and affect in fantasy in children. *Creativity Research Journal.*

Singer, D. L., & Rummo, J. (1973). Ideational creativity and behavioral style in kindergarten age children. *Developmental Psychology, 8,* 154–161.

Singer, D. L., & Singer, J. (1990). *The house of make-believe.* Cambridge, MA: Harvard University Press.
Singer, J. L. (1973). *Child's world of make-believe.* San Diego, CA: Academic Press.
Singer, J. L. (1976). *Daydreaming and fantasy.* London: Allen and Unwin.
Singer, J. L., & Singer, D. L. (1976). Imaginative play and pretending in early childhood: Some experimental approaches. In A. Davids (Ed.), *Child personality and psychopathology* (Vol. 3, pp. 69–112). New York: Wiley.
Singer, J. L., & Singer, D. L. (1981). *Television, imagination, and aggression.* Hillsdale, NJ: Erlbaum.
Slade, A., & Wolf, D. (1994). *Children at play.* New York: Oxford University Press.
Smolucha, F. (1992). A reconstruction of Vygotsky's theory of creativity. *Creativity Research Journal, 5,* 49–67.
Suler, J. (1980). Primary process thinking and creativity. *Psychological Bulletin, 88,* 144–165.
Vandenberg, B. (1988). The realities of play. In D. Morrison (Ed.), *Organizing early experience: Imagination and cognition in childhood* (pp. 198–209). Amityville: Baywood, NY.
Vygotsky, L. S. (1967). Vaobraszeniye I tvorchestvo v deskom voraste [Imagination and creativity in childhood]. Moscow: Prosvescheniye. (Original work published 1930)
Waelder, R. (1933). Psychoanalytic theory of play. *Psychoanalytic Quarterly, 2,* 208–224.
Wallach, M. & Kogan, N. (1965). *Modes of Thinking in Young Children: A Study of the Creativity–Intelligence Distinction.* New York: Holt, Rinehart, & Winston.

5

Intrinsic Motivation, Affect, and Creativity

Beth A. Hennessey
Wellesley College, Wellesley, Massachusetts

Is there a recipe for creativity? Have the necessary components been identified? Can just the right combinations be prescribed? A perusal of the chapters in this book would suggest that special talents, psychopathologies, a playful perspective, and feelings of tension and disequilibration all play an important role. To this list many social psychologists would add one more ingredient: intrinsic motivation. In this chapter, I explore the research on intrinsic motivation and propose a theoretical explanation for the impact of motivation on creativity that is based on an individual's affective response to the task at hand.

Rather than attempting to identify stable individual differences between people, social psychologists generally seek to understand the "average" person and hope to establish and identify commonalities in behavior. In other words, creativity theorists and researchers trained in this approach are relatively unconcerned with within-group variability. Instead, they investigate between-groups differences brought on by situational variables—social and environmental conditions that can positively or negatively affect the creativity of most individuals.

One of the first theorists to advance formally a social psychology of creativity was Teresa Amabile (1983a). The formulation on which her work and the work of her colleagues is based states that there is a direct relation between the motivational orientation a person brings to a task and the creativity of the person's performance on that task. And it is the environment, or at least certain aspects of the environment, that in large part determines that motivational orientation. In essence, people have been found to be most creative when they feel motivated primarily by the interest, enjoyment, satisfaction, and challenge of the work itself—not by external pressures. This relation between creativity and motivation is the *intrinsic-motivation principle of creativity:* The intrinsically motivated state is conducive to creativity, while the extrinsically motivated state is detrimental (Amabile, 1983a, 1983b, 1996; Hennessey & Amabile, 1988b).

In the past 20 years, numerous empirical studies have provided evidence to support this view. (For more complete reviews of the relevant research in this area, see Hennessey & Amabile, 1988; Cameron & Pierce, 1994.) Pioneers in this research effort were Lepper, Greene, and Nisbett, who in 1973 investigated the effect of expected reward on children's motivation and artistic performance. These researchers found that for preschoolers who initially displayed a high level of intrinsic interest in drawing with magic markers, working for an expected "Good Player Award" decreased their interest in the task. Compared with a group who received an unexpected reward and a control (no reward) group, the children who had made their drawings in order to receive a Good Player Award spent significantly less time using the markers during subsequent free-play periods, and this decrement in interest persisted for at least a week after the initial experimental session. Furthermore, the globally assessed quality of the drawings produced under expected-reward conditions was lower than that of the drawings produced by the unexpected-reward and control groups.

Taking a similar approach, Greene and Lepper (1974) and Kernoodle-Loveland and Olley (1979) also offered rewards to preschoolers. Again, children working under the reward conditions produced drawings of lower quality than did their nonrewarded counterparts; a reduction in intrinsic interest in the drawing task was also replicated. Using a different experimental task, Garbarino (1975) found that fifth- and sixth-grade girls who received a reward for tutoring younger children conducted sessions that were characterized as high-pressure, businesslike, hostile, and tense. Nonrewarded tutors, on the other hand, were observed to be both warm and relaxed and highly efficient. Pittman, Emery, and Boggiano (1982) also observed important differences in the behavior of rewarded and nonrewarded persons. Children who were offered a reward for their participation showed a strong subsequent preference for simpler versions of a game, whereas nonrewarded children chose more complex versions. And Shapira (1976) reported that participants who expected payment for success chose to work on relatively easy puzzles, whereas those who expected no payment preferred much more challenging puzzles.

A number of more recent studies have focused on the effect of reward on the *creative* aspects of people's performance. One early investigation of this type was conducted by Kruglanski, Friedman, and Zeevi (1971). High school students were given two open-ended creativity tasks. Product originality was assessed, and there emerged a statistically significant superiority for nonrewarded students. In addition, differences were found between the reward and no-reward groups on two intrinsic-interest measures: students' expressed enjoyment of the activities and their willingness to volunteer for further participation.

Another investigation of the effect of expected reward on participants' creativity of performance was conducted by Amabile (1982). In this case, the experimental task involved artistic creativity and the reward was introduced in a competitive setting. Girls ages 7–11 years made paper collages during one of two parties. Girls in the experimental group competed for prizes, whereas those in the control group expected that the prizes would be raffled off. Artist-judges later rated each collage, and the control group was judged significantly higher than the experimental group on collage creativity.

Each of these investigations points to the same conclusions as do the original findings of Lepper et al. (1973). For participants who initially display a high level of interest in a task, working for an expected reward decreases their motivation and undermines the creativity and globally assessed quality of their performance.

Imposing restrictions on how a task must be completed has also proven detrimental to intrinsic motivation and creativity. In an investigation conducted with nursery school students, Amabile and Gitomer (1984) found that children who had been allowed to select the materials they would use to make a collage produced products that were rated as significantly more creative than those made by children whose materials had been selected for them. In addition, observations made 2 weeks after this initial experimental session revealed that children in the open-selection condition spent somewhat more time with collage materials during free play than did children in the no-choice condition.

In a number of other investigations, the role of choice has also proven significant. Folger, Rosenfield, and Hays (1978) found that for people who had freely chosen to participate in a study, the promise of reward significantly undermined intrinsic interest. Under conditions of no choice, however, rewarded participants actually showed increased levels of interest. Finally, in a related series of studies (Amabile, Hennessey, & Grossman, 1986; Studies 2 and 3), the presence or absence of choice was crossed with the presence or absence of reward. As predicted, creativity was undermined only in participants who freely chose to participate in the experiment and completed a target task in order to receive a promised reward. For people who did not perceive the decision to complete the task as under their control, no such deleterious effects of expected reward were observed.

In addition to rewards, the expectation of evaluation can have a significant negative impact on people's interest and task performance. One early investigation (Amabile, 1979) revealed that women who expected that the collages they were making would be evaluated showed less creativity and task interest than did nonconstraint controls. Two subsequent studies, one a replication with artistic creativity (Amabile, Goldfarb, & Brackfield, 1990, Study 2) and the other a replication with verbal activity (Amabile et al., 1982, Study 1), yielded parallel results.

The message is clear. What these and many other investigations like them reveal is that the motivation necessary for creative performance cannot be engendered from without. Intrinsic interest cannot be taught, and it cannot be coerced.

Intrinsic interest must come from *within* the individual. This delicate and often fleeting motivational state springs from a passion and excitement about a task and is particularly susceptible to the undermining effects of extrinsic constraints.

PROPOSED MECHANISMS OF DECREASED MOTIVATION WITH REWARD EXPECTATION

If we accept the research evidence that extrinsic motivation is detrimental to creativity, it makes sense that a competitive atmosphere or an impending evaluation would undermine creativity of performance. But what is it that makes the expectation of a reward damaging? One group of theorists (e.g., Reiss & Sushinsky, 1975) has suggested that people may be so distracted by the anticipation of reward during initial task engagement that their enjoyment of the activity is hampered. According to this explanation, people's later lack of interest in an activity occurs because their intrinsic enjoyment has been directly blocked by the "competing response" of reward anticipation.

Although the competing-response hypothesis is not without intuitive appeal, it cannot account for people's behavior under all circumstances. For example, Amabile et al. (1986) conducted a study in which the incentive offered to children was not a tangible gift to be delivered after task completion. Instead, the reward was an attractive activity—playing with a Polaroid camera—that the children were allowed to engage in *before* completing the target storytelling task. Children assigned to the reward condition signed a contract and promised to tell a story later in order first to have a chance to use the camera. Children in the no-reward condition were simply allowed to use the camera and then were presented with the target task; there was no contingency established between the two. Results indicated that, overall, children in the no-reward condition told more creative stories than did children in the reward condition. This main effect of reward was, in fact, statistically significant, even though the children had already enjoyed the reward before the experimental activity began, and it was unlikely that any reward-related competing responses were operating.

If competing responses cannot always be blamed for the negative impact of environmental constraints such as expected reward on task motivation and creativity, what other explanations might be offered? One possibility is that the imposition of extrinsic constraints presents a bit of a dilemma. Whether people are attempting to explain their own behavior or discover the reasons behind someone else's activity, they are faced with the question of whether internal or external factors are primarily responsible for it. When both internal and external forces are present, that is, when extrinsic incentives such as reward have been paired with a task that is itself interesting or enjoyable, it is as if there are too many possible justifications for the behavior. Is she engaging in that activity because she enjoys it, or is she in it simply for the reward? Am I completing this assignment because it is fun, or am I motivated primarily by the fact that it will be graded?

INTRINSIC MOTIVATION, AFFECT, AND CREATIVITY

Termed the "overjustification effect" by social psychologists, people's reasoning in such situations is most often explained by the "discounting principle" (Kelley, 1973; Kruglanski, 1975). When adults and older children are presented with stories that give several adequate reasons for a hypothetical character's behavior, they consistently downplay possible internal motivation and attribute behavior to external causes such as rewards, commands, obligations, and threats (DiVitto & McArthur, 1978; Morgan, 1981; Smith, 1975). Similarly, in situations where there are multiple plausible causes for their own actions, adults and older children typically favor an extrinsic explanation. They discount the possibility that they are intrinsically motivated, and their creativity suffers.

The fact that very young children also experience decreased interest in an activity after being rewarded seems to indicate that they, too, are engaging in this process. Yet although their outward behavior nicely parallels that evidenced by adults, children under the age of 7 or 8 have consistently been shown to lack the cognitive capabilities necessary for weighing multiple sufficient causes and discounting (e.g., Shultz, Butkowsky, Pearce, & Shanfield, 1975; Smith, 1975). In fact, some studies have indicated that many young children use an additive algorithm and interpret the expectation of reward as an *augmentation* of intrinsic interest (e.g., DiVitto & McArthur, 1978; Morgan, 1981).

A great deal of research attention has focused on the apparent discrepancy between young children's inability to discount and the fact that their behavior mirrors that of adults and older children experiencing overjustification. Two plausible explanations for this phenomenon have been offered. The first is that the testing procedures used to evaluate discounting ability may be too abstract and may require memory and verbal skills that are too demanding for younger children. In other words, current assessment methods may be underestimating the abilities of young participants. This position is not without empirical support. Researchers who have sought to simplify the testing process have had some success in increasing the amount of discounting evidenced by preschoolers (see Kassin & Gibbons, 1981; Kassin, Gibbons, & Lowe, 1980; Newman & Ruble, 1992; Peterson & Gelfand, 1984; Shultz & Butkowsky, 1977). However, even the most developmentally appropriate procedures have failed to reveal any consistent discounting ability among children under the age of 7.

Even with the use of carefully revised testing procedures, researchers have been unable to demonstrate that children under the age of 6 or 7 understand the ulterior motives behind the offer of reward (e.g., Cohen, Gelfand, & Hartmann, 1981; Karniol & Ross, 1976; Kassin & Ellis, 1988; Newman & Ruble, 1992, Study 2). Although they may evidence discounting ability when presented with vignettes involving commands, they frequently appear to regard the presence of a reward as evidence that an activity is attractive (Karniol & Ross, 1979; Newman & Ruble, 1992, Study 1). In response to these findings, Karniol and Ross (1979) questioned whether the manipulative intent behind the offer of reward is obvious to young children. It would seem that such an understanding would be basic to the discounting process, but this issue has received little research attention.

THE WORK–PLAY STUDY

In a recent study of young children's understanding of the reward process a colleague and I simplified our testing procedures as much as possible (Hennessey & Berger, 1993). Unlike previous researchers, we did not require that our participants make inferences about the preferences of hypothetical characters for activities and toys. Instead, we reasoned that young children might be more apt to demonstrate discounting ability if they were presented with situations in which they could actively engage. Toward this end, we asked our young participants to decide *themselves* which of two characters deserved a reward.

Two major hypotheses guided this investigation. First, we predicted that preschoolers, although unable to discount, would be able to distinguish between work and play activities. Further, we expected that children would be more likely to reward a character engaging in work rather than play, because rewards are typically paired with undesirable chores. This study improved on earlier methodologies in that fewer cognitive demands were placed on the participants. Rather than asking children to speculate about the reactions and interests of hypothetical characters who were not seen and had or had not been promised some incentive, the children in this investigation actually delivered a reward to either a working or a playing doll.

After being tested for discounting using a standard interview procedure (i.e., DiVitto & McArthur, 1978; Smith, 1975), our participants, who ranged in age from 3 to 6 years, were presented with 10 illustrated story pairs, each contrasting two activities that needed to be done. (Importantly, pretesting had determined that preschoolers consistently perceived one of the tasks in each pair as "fun" and the other as "not so fun.") After deciding which of two paper dolls (matched with the gender of the participant) was to perform each of the activities, the children were instructed to give a sticker (e.g., ice cream cone or toy) to the doll who they believed most deserved a reward. Next, they were asked which of the two dolls really liked what he or she was doing. Finally, the experimenter commented, "One of these dolls was working and one was playing. Point to the doll that was working. Point to the doll that was playing."

As expected, the majority of children evidenced little, if any, discounting ability. Of the 27 children tested, 4 scored as discounters, 10 as transitional, and 13 as nondiscounters (i.e., they showed an additive, rather than a discounting, process). There were no significant effects of age or sex on this (or any other) dependent measure. Analyses did reveal that our young participants had, in fact, developed scripts for work and play. Across the 10 story pairs, those activities that in pretesting had been identified as "not so fun" were consistently labeled as work. In addition, when asked which of the dolls really liked what he or she was doing, children were more likely to choose the doll they believed to be

INTRINSIC MOTIVATION, AFFECT, AND CREATIVITY

playing than to choose the doll they had labeled as working. Although performance on this measure was not flawless, children chose the "player" significantly more often than they did the "worker" in 6 of the 10 scenarios presented.

Although the children were able to distinguish between work and play tasks, they were no more likely to reward the doll who was working than they were the doll who was playing. The majority of the children performed no better than chance on each of the 10 story pairs presented. Apparently, they had not yet developed an understanding that rewards are typically paired with undesirable activities. Importantly, this failure to make a connection between the promise of reward and the attractiveness of a task did not appear to stem from an inability to speculate accurately about how the dolls felt about the activities they were performing. When asked which of the two dolls really liked what he or she was doing, children were far more likely to nominate the doll they believed to be playing.

Why is the interest of preschool-aged children undermined by the expectation of reward? Our results clearly indicate that the young children participating in this investigation were not yet able to recognize the manipulative intent behind the offer of reward. Given the fact that this highly structured testing situation failed to reveal such a level of understanding, it is unlikely that the actual promise of a reward in a real-life situation would trigger in these children the cognitions necessary for the discounting process to take place.

AN ALTERNATIVE AFFECTIVE EXPLANATION

For years, researchers such as myself have been intent on proving that young children are, in fact, capable of discounting. We have spent endless hours tweaking our testing procedures and modifying our protocols, and yet we still have little understanding of why extrinsic constraints negatively affect the motivation and creativity of children. I believe it is time that researchers take a different approach and search for an explanation for the undermining of intrinsic interest based on something other than an attributional framework. The impact of a promised reward (or other extrinsic constraint) on young children may well be mediated by something other than a discounting mechanism.

One viable alternative explanation is that the reduction of intrinsic interest in young children occurs when they learn that rewards are associated with activities that need to be done, that is, with activities that are not enjoyable and often even aversive. The undermining of intrinsic interest may result from a negative emotional or affective response to the offer of a reward, rather than from a thoughtful analysis. Children may learn through experience to react negatively to a task as work when their behavior is controlled by socially imposed factors (e.g., rewards), and they may react positively to a task as play when there are no constraints imposed. Simply put, they may learn that when rewards are present, work is at hand. And work is not fun, so they feel worse from the outset about rewarded tasks. Negative affect resulting from socially learned stereotypes or scripts of work (see Morgan, 1981; Ransen, 1980) may be what leads to decrements in intrinsic interest.

Only a few investigations have directly tested this proposition (see Hennessey & Berger, 1993), yet there is good evidence that even very young children develop scripted knowledge about the differences between work and play. In one investigation (Amabile et al., 1986, Study 1), my colleagues and I found that elementary school students (ages 5–10) who had been promised a reward for their participation were more likely to label a storytelling task as work, whereas children who had not been promised a reward were more likely to label the same task as play. Tucker (1980), in fact, identified distinct stages in the developmental sequence of acquiring work and play concepts. Children as young as age 3 were shown to label activities consistently as falling into one or the other category, and by age 5 or 6, they had acquired simple representational sets (scripts) about activities they identified as work or play.

In keeping with these findings, King (1982) noted that kindergartners' definitions of play are based on social criteria such as whether an activity is voluntarily chosen, is self-directed, and allows one an uninterrupted time span. Regarding the definition of work, King suggests that social criteria again play an important role and that kindergartners tend to define all required activity as work. Research carried out by Cunningham and Wiegel (1992) also confirms that preschoolers presented with a sorting task will consistently label activities that occur in a mandatory context as work.

THE IMMUNIZATION STUDIES: INDIRECT EVIDENCE TO SUPPORT THE AFFECTIVE WORK–PLAY HYPOTHESIS

If children learn to react negatively to a task as work when their behavior is controlled by socially imposed factors (e.g., rewards, evaluation, or competition) and if it is this negative affect resulting from socially learned stereotypes (scripts) of work that leads to decrements in intrinsic interest, how might researchers gain evidence to support these hypothesized connections? One option is to test whether a direct manipulation of children's perceptions of an activity as work or play significantly alters their interest in and creativity on that task. This is what happened in a recent series of investigations designed to train children to maintain an intrinsic focus even when extrinsic factors were present.

In the first of these studies (Hennessey, Amabile, & Martinage, 1989, Study 1), my colleagues and I set out to determine whether special training sessions designed to address directly motivational orientation could "immunize" or bolster children against the usually deleterious effects of reward on intrinsic motivation and creative aspects of performance. Elementary school students (ages 7–11) were randomly assigned to intrinsic-motivation-focus or control groups and met with an experimenter over 2 consecutive days for the purpose of viewing videos and engaging in directed discussion. The tapes shown to students in the intrinsic-motivation-focus condition depicted two 11-year-olds talking with an adult about various aspects of their school work. Scripts for this condition were constructed to help children focus on the intrinsically interesting, fun, and playful aspects of a task. Ways to make even the most routine assignment exciting were suggested, and participants were helped to distance themselves from socially imposed extrinsic constraints, such as rewards. Tapes shown to students in the control condition featured the same two young actors talking about some of their favorite things, including foods, music groups, movies, and seasons.

After this training procedure, all students met individually with a second adult for testing. Half the children in each of the training conditions were told that they could take two pictures with an instant camera if they promised to tell a story to the experimenter later. For children in the no-reward conditions, the picture taking was presented simply as the first in a series of "things to do."

In this 2 × 2 factorial design, presentation of reward was crossed with type of training received. We expected that only the children who had been specifically instructed in ways to overcome the usual deleterious effects of extrinsic constraints would maintain baseline levels of intrinsic motivation and creativity in situations of expected reward (i.e., they would be immunized against the effects of extrinsic constraints). The data from our first investigation not only confirmed these expectations, but gave us reason to believe that our intervention had much more of an impact than we had expected. We found that the offer of reward actually augmented the creativity of the trained group, and this effect was quite robust. In fact, the creativity of children who received intrinsic-motivation training and expected a reward was significantly higher than that of any other group.

This surprising finding led us to hypothesize that perhaps our assumption that the presence of extrinsic factors always detracts from intrinsic motivation was flawed. Although it is true that most existing intrinsic-motivation research has been based on a model that states that as extrinsic motivation increases, intrinsic motivation decreases (cf. Lepper & Greene, 1978), perhaps under certain specific conditions internal and external factors combine in additive fashion to augment intrinsic interest. Perhaps under certain conditions persons can be led to view extrinsic motivators in a positive, rather than negative, light.

This reformulation of the original overjustification model has in fact been suggested previously. Deci and Ryan (1985) pointed out that the individual's interpretation of a constraint plays a crucial role in determining the effect the constraint has on motivation or performance. In our initial discussion of these immunization study results, we conjectured that children who entered the creativity testing situation after having undergone intrinsic motivation training would have a much more salient awareness of their own intrinsic interest in school-type tasks. Thus, the reward may have served to heighten their already positive feelings about the tasks they were doing.

Two follow-up investigations of our intrinsic-motivation-focus techniques (Hennessey et al., 1989, Study 2; Hennessey & Zbikowski, 1993) were subsequently carried out. Each was designed as a conceptual replication of Study 1. The same experimental design was used, although the target creativity task in

Study 2 was a paper collage, and in Study 3 the control group viewed a tape about American Sign Language. In Study 2, it was again the children who had received immunization training and were expecting a reward who produced the most creative products. Yet, in this instance the effect was less dramatic. Statistical comparisons revealed that the creativity of the children who received training and expected a reward for their performance was significantly different from the creativity of only one of the other three groups.

Like those of Study 2, the results of the third investigation also mandate that researchers not be too quick to abandon their original notions about the universally negative effects of extrinsic constraints. Although children assigned to the intrinsic-motivation-focus/reward condition again produced the most creative products, their performance was significantly different only from that of the no-training-reward group. Together, the results of Studies 2 and 3 indicate that children who are exposed to intrinsic-motivation training and then offered a reward for their performance cannot be expected to demonstrate unusually high levels of creativity. They can, however, be expected to maintain baseline levels of intrinsic motivation and creativity under reward conditions.

What is it about our immunization procedures that allows children to maintain their creativity even when they expect a reward? It appears that children exposed to our training techniques learned to deemphasize the importance of reward. They were able to maintain a positive approach and bring to the experimental tasks a playfulness and a willingness to take risks that many researchers believe are crucial to creativity (Amabile, 1983a, 1996; Barron, 1968; Campbell, 1960; Crutchfield, 1962; Dansky & Silverman, 1975; Lieberman, 1965; Stein, 1974). In short, our training seems to help children to decouple negative affect from expected reward.

THE AFFECT/CREATIVITY LINK

In the past few years, the issue of how an individual responds on an affective level to a task has come to play an increasingly significant role in my own theorizing and that of many of my collaborators. This focus on affect did not happen all at once; neither was it intentional or particularly theory driven. Rather, the data themselves forced us to take this direction, as it became increasingly clear that the cognitive based attribution models on which our work was founded were no longer sufficient to explain many of our findings.

At first, our investigation (Hennessey & Berger, 1993) of children's conceptions of work and play, described earlier in this chapter, was driven by the need to come up with an alternative to the overjustification model. We knew that the youngest participants in our study were incapable of discounting, and we needed another explanation for why their motivation and creativity were being undermined by extrinsic constraints. As I have mentioned, negative affect engendered by socially learned stereotypes of work seemed to play a major role. In attempting to explain our intrinsic-motivation training results (Hennessey et al.,

1989; Hennessey & Zbikowski, 1993), we were also led to an affective explanation. The data we have gathered over the past few years have made it increasingly clear that affect plays a significant role in the creative process of young children.

Moreover, this role of affect may apply not just to preschoolers, but to people of all ages. No longer can researchers be satisfied with two separate explanations for the undermining of intrinsic motivation and creativity by extrinsic constraints. The overjustification model can be used to explain the behavior of older persons, who have been shown to be capable of discounting. But just because adults and school-aged children are able to engage in these cumbersome and complex cognitive machinations does not mean that they do so on a regular basis.

In fact, there is an extant literature that lends some support to this view. A number of studies conducted in the past decade have revealed that people show higher levels of associative fluency (believed to be an important component of the creative process) when they are in positive affective states. In a series of studies conducted by Isen (1987; Isen & Daubman, 1984; Isen, Johnson, Mertz, & Robinson, 1985), for example, persons who had been exposed to films designed to induce a happy mood made especially high numbers of unusual associations on subsequent verbal tasks. Yet the picture is not entirely clear. In a comprehensive discussion of social and environmental influences on creativity, Amabile (1996) disclosed that several attempts in her laboratory have failed to show any systematic effects of mood induction on creativity. In at least one instance (Tighe, 1992), adults who had seen a positive movie wrote stories that were rated as *less* creative than those produced by adults who had had a negative viewing experience.

How might these conflicting findings be explained? Although a great deal of research remains to be carried out, my belief is that the negative affect experienced by the participants who watched a film was different from the negative affect brought about by the promise of a reward or the expectation of an evaluation. In other words, it may not be negative affect *per se,* but the particular type of negative affect engendered by the imposition of extrinsic constraints that undermines intrinsic motivation and creativity of performance.

The fact that people exposed to a sad or upsetting film were able to maintain their creativity should come as no surprise. Consider the stereotypical starving artist. His last dollar has been spent on a tube of cerulean blue oil paint. The heat has been shut off for failure to pay the bills. It's cold and damp, and he hasn't eaten in almost two days. Yet the sky that covers the canvas before him is a creative masterpiece. How has he managed to maintain his creativity? The fact that his hands and feet are numb and he is hungry most probably has caused him to experience a great deal of negative effect, but this is not the kind of negative affect that undermines motivation. When the negative affect is not tied to the specific (creative) activity, it may have little influence on the individual's intrinsic motivation for the task at hand. His artistic performance has not suffered, because he is free of extrinsic constraints. There is no reward at stake.

His work is not being evaluated, and he need not compare his finished product with anyone else's.

CONCLUSION

Musings about hypothetical artists may be instructive, but they are not sufficient grounds for solid, scientific theory. What is needed now are carefully constructed investigations designed to examine directly this affective explanation for the undermining of intrinsic interest and creativity of performance. In planning this research program, it will be crucial to keep two guidelines in mind. First, although the negative effects of reward have in the past received the lion's share of attention, it will be essential to include investigations of a variety of extrinsic factors in future studies. Second, it will also be important to test this affective hypothesis across a wide range of people. Everyone from preschoolers to artists to R&D scientists should be expected to experience similar affective responses to extrinsic constraints.

If classrooms and work environments that optimize creativity are to become a reality, the first step must be to develop a comprehensive model of how social and environmental factors affect the motivation and performance of most individuals. Only when researchers understand both the positive and the negative consequences of promising a reward, imposing an evaluation, or setting up a situation of competition can they hope to foster the creativity of students and employees. Attention to the affective consequences of these factors may hold the key to such an understanding.

REFERENCES

Amabile, T. (1979). Effects of external evaluation on artistic creativity. *Journal of Personality and Social Psychology, 37*, 221–233.
Amabile, T. (1982). Children's artistic creativity: Detrimental effects of competition in a field setting. *Personality and Social Psychology Bulletin, 8*, 573–578.
Amabile, T. (1983a). *The social psychology of creativity.* New York: Springer-Verlag.
Amabile, T. (1983b). Social psychology of creativity: A componential conceptualization. *Journal of Personality and Social Psychology, 45*, 357–377.
Amabile, T. (1996). *Creativity in context.* Boulder, CO: Westview.
Amabile,T., & Gitomer, J. (1984). Children's artistic creativity: Effect of choice in task materials. *Personality and Social Psychology Bulletin, 10*, 209–215.
Amabile, T., Goldfarb, P., & Brackfield, S. (1990). Social influences on creativity: Evaluation, coaction, and surveillance. *Creativity Research Journal, 3*, 6–21.
Amabile, T., Hennessey,B., & Grossman, B. (1986). Social influences on creativity: The effects of contracted-for reward. *Journal of Personality and Social Psychology, 50*, 14–23.
Barron, F. (1968). *Creativity and personal freedom.* New York: Van Nostrand.
Cameron, J., & Pierce, W. (1994). Reinforcement, reward, and intrinsic motivation: A meta-analysis. *Review of Educational Research, 64*, 363–423.
Campbell, D. (1960). Blind variation and selective retention in creative thought as in other knowledge processes. *Psychological Review, 67*, 380–400.
Cohen, E., Gelfand, D., & Hartmann, D. (1981). Causal reasoning as a function of behavioral consequences. *Child Development, 52*, 514–522.

Crutchfield, R. (1962). Conformity and creative thinking. In H. Gruber, G. Terrell, & M. Wertheimer (Eds.), *Contemporary approaches to creative thinking* (pp. 120–140). New York: Atherton Press.

Cunningham, B., & Wiegel, J. (1992). Preschool work and play activities: Child and teacher perspectives. *Play and Culture, 5,* 92–99.

Dansky, J., & Silverman, I. (1975). Play: A general facilitator of fluency. *Developmental Psychology, 11,* 104.

Deci, E., & Ryan, R. (1985). *Intrinsic motivation and self-determination in human behavior.* New York: Plenum.

DiVitto, B., & McArthur, L. Z. (1978). Developmental differences in the use of distinctiveness, consensus, and consistency information for making causal attributions. *Developmental Psychology, 14,* 474–482.

Folger, R., Rosenfield, D., & Hays, R. (1978). Equity and intrinsic motivation: The role of choice. *Journal of Personality and Social Psychology, 36,* 557–564.

Garbarino, J. (1975). The impact of anticipated reward upon cross-age tutoring. *Journal of Personality and Social Psychology, 32,* 421–428.

Greene, D., & Lepper, M. (1974). Effects of extrinsic rewards on children's subsequent interest. *Child Development, 45,* 1141–1145.

Hennessey, B., & Amabile, T. (1988a).. Story-telling: A method for assessing children's creativity. *Journal of Creative Behavior, 22,* 235–246.

Hennessey, B., & Amabile, T. (1988b). The conditions of creativity. In R. J. Sternberg (Ed.), *The nature of creativity* (pp. 11–38). New York: Cambridge University Press.

Hennessey, B., Amabile, T., & Martinage, M. (1989). Immunizing children against the negative effects of reward. *Contemporary Educational Psychology, 14,* 212–227.

Hennessey, B., & Berger, A. (1993, March). *Children's conceptions of work and play: Exploring an alternative to discounting.* Poster presented at the meeting of the Society for Research in Child Development, New Orleans, LA.

Hennessey, B., & Zbikowski, S. (1993). Immunizing children against the negative effects of reward: A further examination of intrinsic motivation training techniques. *Creativity Research Journal, 6,* 297–307.

Isen, A. M. (1987). Positive affect, cognitive processes, and social behavior. In L. Berkowitz (Ed.), *Advances in experimental social psychology* (Vol. 20, 203–253). San Diego, CA: Academic Press.

Isen, A. M., & Daubman, K. A. (1984). The influence of affect on categorization. *Journal of Personality and Social Psychology, 47,* 1206–1217.

Isen, A. M., Johnson, M. M. S., Mertz, E., & Robinson, G. F. (1985). The influence of positive affect on the unusualness of word associations. *Journal of Personality and Social Psychology, 48,* 1413–1426.

Karniol, R., & Ross, M. (1976). The development of causal attributions in social perception. *Journal of Personality and Social Psychology, 34,* 455–464.

Karniol, R., & Ross, M. (1979). Children's use of a causal attribution schema and the inference of manipulative intentions. *Child Development, 50,* 463–468.

Kassin, S., & Ellis, S. (1988). On the acquisition of the discounting principle: An experimental test of a social-developmental model. *Child Development, 59,* 950–960.

Kassin, S., & Gibbons, F. (1981). Children's use of the discounting principle in their perceptions of exertion. *Child Development, 52,* 741–744.

Kassin, S., Gibbons, F., & Lowe, C. (1980). Children's use of the discounting principle: A perceptual approach. *Journal of Personality and Social Psychology, 39,* 719–728.

Kelley, H. (1973). The processes of causal attribution. *American Psychologist, 28,* 107–128.

Kernoodle-Loveland, K., & Olley, J. (1979). The effect of external reward on interest and quality of task performance in children of high and low intrinsic motivation. *Child Development, 50,* 1207–1210.

King, N. (1982). Children's conceptions of work and play. *Social Education, 46,* 110–113.
Kruglanski, A. (1975). The endogenous-exogenous partition in attribution theory. *Psychological Review, 82,* 387–406.
Kruglanski, A., Friedman, I., & Zeevi, G. (1971). The effects of extrinsic incentive on some qualitative aspects of task performance. *Journal of Personality, 39,* 606–617.
Lepper, M., & Greene, D. (Eds.). (1978). *The hidden costs of reward.* Hillsdale, NJ: Erlbaum.
Lepper, M., Greene, D., & Nisbett, R. (1973). Undermining children's intrinsic interest with extrinsic rewards: A test of the "overjustification" hypothesis. *Journal of Personality and Social Psychology, 28,* 129–137.
Lieberman, J. (1965). Playfulness and divergent thinking: An investigation of their relationship at the kindergarten level. *Journal of Genetic Psychology, 107,* 219–224.
Morgan, M. (1981). The overjustification effect: A developmental test of self-perception interpretations. *Journal of Personality and Social Psychology, 40,* 809–821.
Newman, L., & Ruble, D. (1992). Do young children use the discounting principle? *Journal of Experimental Social Psychology, 28,* 572–593.
Peterson, L., & Gelfand, D. (1984). Causal attributions of helping as a function of age and incentives. *Child Development, 55,* 504–511.
Pittman, T., Emery, J., & Boggiano, A. (1982). Intrinsic and extrinsic motivational orientations: Reward-induced changes in preference for complexity. *Journal of Personality and Social Psychology, 48,* 789–797.
Ransen, D. (1980). The mediation of reward-induced motivation decrements in early and middle childhood: A template matching approach. *Journal of Personality and Social Psychology, 35,* 49–55.
Reiss, S., & Sushinsky, L. (1975). Overjustification, competing responses, and the acquisition of intrinsic interest. *Journal of Personality and Social Psychology, 31,* 1116–1125.
Shapira, Z. (1976). Expectancy determinants of intrinsically motivated behavior. *Journal of Personality and Social Psychology, 39,* 1235–1244.
Shultz, T., & Butkowsky, I. (1977). Young children's use of the scheme for multiple sufficient causes in the attribution of real and hypothetical behavior. *Child Development, 48,* 464–469.
Shultz, T., Butkowsky, I., Pearce, J., & Shanfield, H. (1975). The development of schemes for the attribution of multiple psychological causes. *Developmental Psychology, 11,* 502–510.
Smith, M. (1975). Children's use of the multiple sufficient cause schema in social perception. *Journal of Personality and Social Psychology, 32,* 737–747.
Stein, M. (1974). *Stimulating creativity* (Vols 1 and 2). San Diego, CA: Academic Press.
Tighe, E. (1992). *The Motivational Influences of Mood on Creativity.* Ph.D. disscussion, Brandeis University.
Tucker, J. (1980). The concepts of and the attitudes toward work and play in children (Doctoral dissertation, University of Denver, 1979). *Dissertation Abstracts International, 40,* 3987B.

Part Two

Affect and Creative Expression

6

Affect in Artistic and Scientific Creativity

Gregory J. Feist
College of William and Mary, Williamsburg, Virginia

The artist's life is commonly viewed as an emotionally unstable, agony-filled, but creative life. Many people, including artists themselves, might even go so far as to assert that if artists are not tormented, morose, or at least distressed and unhappy, they cannot truly be creative or that if they were to go through therapy and "get better," that would be the end of their creativity. Their "creative juices" ostensibly are sustained by tragedy and turmoil. Or to put it bluntly: "Artists lick their wounds for nourishment not for healing" (Wayne, 1974, p. 107). Implicit in this view is the assumption that negative affect somehow acts as a cause of creativity or, at the very least, facilitates the creative process. These assumptions are in fact empirical questions, and one can ask, Does an artist really need to be miserable to be creative? Does an improved psychological state mean an end to creative productivity? Even if there is a relationship between negative affect and creativity, it is quite possible that the affect is a result, rather than a cause, of creative thought. In a related vein, there is the question of what impact psychotherapy generally has on a person's creative input. Does successfully going through therapy tend to increase or decrease creative achievement? Each of these questions can and ultimately must be addressed empirically if psychologists are to move beyond anecdotal lore. Moreover, these questions concern only negative affect, which is but half of the affect involved in the affect–creativity picture. An increasing body of literature demonstrates the importance of positive affect in the creative process, both as an antecedent (Estrada,

Isen, & Young, 1994; Isen, Daubman, & Nowicki, 1987) and as a consequent of creative insight (Feist, 1994; Gruber, 1995; Otto & Schmitz, 1993). Being in a positive mood appears to facilitate creative problem solving, and strong emotional reactions tend to follow creative insight.

In addition to the distinction between negative and positive affect, there is the critical role that career discipline plays in mediating the relationship between affect and creativity (Ludwig, 1995). Scientists, it is commonly believed, are quite the opposite of artists: hyperrational, logical, devoid of deep or frequent emotion. They avoid passion and emotion lest it cloud and bias their objectivity. And indeed, historically this assumption has resulted in scholars' bypassing the role affect plays in science and scientific creativity (Feist, 1994). Again, although a grain of truth may exist for such a stereotypic view of the scientific process, it may not be more than a grain and it may be as incomplete and stereotyped as the tormented artist syndrome.

In this chapter, I show where these perceptions are accurate and where they are misguided by reviewing theoretical and empirical work on affect in the artistic and scientific creative processes. The theoretical section is structured around three theoretical perspectives: psychoanalytic, developmental, and cognitive. The empirical section is structured around four topics: general findings, affective states and artistic creativity, affective traits and artistic creativity, and the aesthetic emotions and scientific creativity. In the final section of the chapter, I attempt to integrate the recent advances on affect and creativity, elucidate the gaps in knowledge, and suggest how these gaps might be filled.

THEORY ON AFFECT AND CREATIVITY

The theoretical attention devoted to affect and creativity can conveniently be classified into psychoanalytic, cognitive, cognitive–motivational, or integrative theories. In this section, Freud, Rank, and Kris represent the psychoanalytic perspective, Koestler and Lazarus the cognitive, Runco the cognitive–motivational, and Russ the integrative.

Freud's theory of defense mechanisms, in particular sublimation, is well known, so I discuss only its most basic propositions here. Freud's theory of creativity (1925/1958) was based on sublimation of unsatisfied impulse into constructive and creative expressions: "We can begin by saying that happy people never make phantasies, only unsatisfied ones. Unsatisfied wishes are the driving power behind phantasies" (p. 47). Freud went on to classify wishes into two groups—erotic or ambitious—but argued for the similarity and unity of these two wishes. Ultimately, Freud argued that creative activity is inherently repressed or unsatisfied sexual impulse.

Rank (1932/1964) disagreed with Freud's view that creative genius was motivated first and foremost by sexual impulse and argued that immortality stood at the origin of all creative achievement. The desire to cast one's artistic expressions and ultimately one's life in immortal forms is the fundamental motivation behind creation. Everyone fears death, and this fear of death is most pronounced in the artist's desire to leave behind creations for generations. In this way—and by having children—one can transcend death. Not only did Rank disagree with Freud's view of the central role of sexuality, but he even argued that it was "anti-sexuality" that lies behind creative expression. Creative expression is manifested in a controlling of life impulse and is in this sense "anti-sexual." In short, the emotion of fear is the motive for all creativity. Although Rank disagreed with Freud's basic premise, they were not far apart in one sense: both believed that emotion (dissatisfaction or fear) impelled the creative urge.

A more cognitive, yet still psychoanalytic, theory of creativity was offered by Kris (1952). He postulated that creative thinking involves the ability to regress to more primitive, proverbial, unconscious thought processes, and he called this *regression in the service of the ego*. Such regression, however, it adaptive and functional in that it allows one to connect heretofore disjointed ideas in a useful and potentially creative manner. To put it simply, the creative individual has the ability to regress but in the healthy and constructive service of the ego. Of all the psychoanalytic theories of creativity, Kris's stimulated the most empirical investigations. In the 1950s and 1960s, many researchers found support for the positive relationship between regressive and primary process thinking and creativity (Bush, 1969; Dudek, 1968; Gamble & Kellner, 1968; Gray, 1969; Hersch, 1962; Hilgard, 1962; Pine & Holt, 1960; Wild, 1965). For example, Pine and Holt (1960) reported that there was a significant positive correlation between adaptive regression shown on the Rorschach and Thematic Apperception Test and creativity as measured by Guilford's Unusual Uses and Consequences tests. Furthermore, some researchers (e.g., Hersch, 1962; Wild, 1965) found that creative artists, compared with noncreative persons and schizophrenic persons, were better able to move back and forth between mature and primitive thought processes. In his review of the literature on primary process thinking and creativity, Suler (1980) concluded; "The loose and at times illogical and fantastical ideation characteristic of formal primary process undoubtedly contributes to innovative thinking. . . . This capacity to master the cognitive complexity imposed by subjective states of drive and affect reflects the more general ability to cope with the complexities in thought inherent in any scientific or artistic creative process" (pp. 159–160).

Two theorists who were more purely cognitive in their orientation but who believed that cognition leads to affective responses are Koestler (1964) and Lazarus (1991). Koestler believed that creativity must involve the process of bisociation, or the sudden and unexpected bringing together of two heretofore disparate ideas. The suddenness and unexpectedness of the union of ideas is almost always experienced affectively as humor or happiness or excitement. Of course, with creative insight, such emotion and bisociation do not assure the correctness or adaptiveness of the idea. That must wait for logical, aesthetic, or empirical verification (depending on the domain of creativity). Recently, O'Quin and Derks (1996) pointed out the strengths and weaknesses in Koestler's argument by reviewing the theoretical and empirical literature on the topic.

The cognitive theorist of emotion, Lazarus (1991) did not explicitly discuss creativity, but elsewhere I have elaborated on how Lazarus's cognitive–relational theory of emotion could be applied to predict particular emotional antecedents and consequences of the creative process (Feist, 1994, in press). Lazarus argued that people experience an emotion whenever they appraise an event as relevant to their well-being (relevance), and the valence of the emotion is determined by its congruency with their goals and motives (goal congruency). Another key assumption of Lazarus's theory is the notion of "core relational theme." "A core relational theme is simply the central (hence core) relational harm or benefit in adaptational encounters that underlies each specific kind of emotion" (Lazarus, p. 121). For instance, the core relational theme for sadness is "irrevocable loss," while for anger it is "insult to me or mine."

Using Lazarus's concept of core relational themes, I have argued that anxiety would be a commonly experienced emotion before an insight (Feist, in press). The core relational theme for anxiety is "facing uncertain, existential threat," and to the extent that the problem is important to a person's well-being and existence and its outcome is uncertain, the person will experience some sort of threat. If an individual were convinced that he or she could solve the problem, anxiety would not be experienced. The problem would pose little existential threat. Next, there are two emotions that should occur during the insight stage (i.e., the few minutes during and immediately after the insight): relief and happiness. The core relational theme for relief involves having a goal-incongruent condition change for the better. Clearly, in creative problem solving not being able to solve the problem is goal incongruent. However, once it is solved, happiness should also be experienced during an insight—and maybe even right before—insofar that its core relational theme is "making reasonable progress toward the realization of our goals" (Lazarus, 1991, p. 267). Finally, after the insight has occurred (i.e., from hours to years later), a person should be likely to experience some degree of pride. Although pride is similar to happiness in that both are relevant and congruent to the person's goals, pride is distinguished from happiness to the extent that the person experiences the enhancement of his or her self-esteem and social esteem and to the extent that credit is to the person, rather than to someone or something else. The bigger and more difficult the problem, the more pride the individual should experience in solving it. For example, a chemist I interviewed had this to say:

> Well, there is a great deal of satisfaction out of seeing something work, and having the feeling that no one else has been able to do this. There is a certain ego satisfaction that goes with that. [For example, in graduate school] I stumbled upon a new compound, and I proudly took it to [my advisor] and he said, "That's nice, but you know there are 50,000 plus compounds discovered every year. What's so special about this one?" And I concluded that what was so special about it was that I was the one who discovered it.

The third theoretical perspective is the cognitive–motivational one. Runco (1994) recently put forth the argument that tension and negative affect are often essential antecedent conditions for creative thought. At the simplest level, tension can be something as straightforward as the cognitive dissonance created by not understanding something and being motivated to figure it out. That negative affect can spur creative expression is most clearly seen in cathartic expressions of grief after a loved one or important figure dies. Often people feel a need to write poetry or build a memorial. These are creative expressions of sadness, but they also are a constructive form of grieving. Tension most broadly defined can and sometimes does drive creative expression. More generally, Runco pointed to the growing body of literature that connects cultural and professional marginality, broken homes, and emotional dissatisfaction to the drive to solve problems creatively. More philosophically, this argument can be modeled dialectically as the tension between thesis and antithesis that leads to synthesis. Runco's line of argument originates in Barron's (1955, 1963) and MacKinnon's (1970) view that highly creative people seek out and even thrive in tension and disorder (cf. Sashin, 1993). MacKinnon called this the "divine discontent" of poets. The reader may also note the similarity between Runco's ideas and Freud's notion that unsatisfied wishes (dissatisfaction) underlie creativity. Finally, Kuhn (1977) also made a similar point with his concept of "essential tension" in science. Essential tension spurs scientific progress forward and consists of the dialectic between stable tradition (thesis) and the change of revolution (antithesis).

Finally, Russ (1993) recently integrated cognitive, motivational, and personality perspectives in her model of affect and creativity. She argued that the personality traits of tolerance of ambiguity and openness to experience lead to affect-laden thoughts, which lead to divergent thinking. In addition, she argued that intrinsic motivation, curiosity, and risk taking lead to taking affective pleasure in solving problems, which in turn leads to having a wide range of interests. Russ went on to make a cogent case for the more general antecedent role that the personality characteristics of openness, tolerance of ambiguity, preference for complexity, self-confidence, and risk taking play in a person's ability to tap into the deep, affective primary process modes of thought necessary for creative insight. What is most appealing about this theoretical model is the fact that whereas the causal paths and directionality may be speculative, the personality, affective, and cognitive processes in the model are based on consensual, robust empirical findings in the creativity literature.

RESEARCH ON AFFECT AND CREATIVITY

In addition to the theorists' contributions to affect and creativity, many researchers have begun to focus their energy on unraveling the relationship between the two processes. Although the focus of this section is on art and science, some general findings have recently emerged that elucidate the affect–creativity connection.

General Findings

Isen and her colleagues (Estrada et al., 1994; Isen & Daubman, 1984; Isen et al., 1987; Isen, Johnson, Mertz, & Robinson, 1985) have shown in a systematic set of studies that positive affective states lead people to be more inclusive in their categorization of stimuli and to give more unusual associations to neutral words compared with control participants. Isen et al. (1987); (see also Andreasen & Powers, 1974; Richards, 1994) explains this phenomenon primarily in terms of expanding one's cognitive search and integrating divergent concepts:

> Good feelings increase the tendency to combine material in new ways and to see relatedness between divergent stimuli. We hypothesize that this occurs because the large amount of cognitive material cued by the positive affective state results in defocused attention, and the more complex, cognitive context thus experienced by persons who are feeling happy allows them a greater number and range of interpretations. (p. 1130)

Influenced by the findings of Isen and her colleagues, Larson (1990) hypothesized that if positive feelings lead to a loosening of cognitive processes, boredom and anxiety, to the extent that they are associated with a narrowing of attention and a decrease in motivation (Mendelsohn, 1976), should lead to less creative thought (cf. Eysenck, 1993, 1995). In an experiment to test the constrictive effect of negative affect, Larson found that only boredom, not anxiety, was negatively related to creative output in high school students' term papers.

Isen and Larson each viewed affect as antecedent to creativity, but of course affect can also be a consequence of creativity (Feist, 1994). Otto and Schmitz (1993) investigated experimentally the effect that solving a creativity task has on positive affect. More specifically, they tested Fiedler's (1988) compatibility hypothesis, which holds that only when information style (creative vs. analytic) matches mood state (positive or neutral, respectively) will positive mood result. Therefore, they predicted that only participants who are solving creativity tasks and are already in a positive mood will maintain their positive mood. The hypothesis was supported: When information style (creativity) and mood state (positive) matched positive affect was maintained.

Affective States and Artistic Creativity

Heretofore no distinction has been made between affective states and affective traits. Yet the distinction is an important one. As discussed by Rosenberg, Ekman and Blumenthal (1998), affective experience has at least three temporal levels: emotion, mood, and trait. These three levels are on a continuum from shortest (emotion) to longest (trait). Affective states can be either antecedent or consequent to creative insight, whereas affective traits are primarily antecedent to it. In other words, short-term emotional states can immediately precede or immediately follow creative insight, but emotional traits such bipolar disorder or neurotic anxiety are much more likely to precede creative insight than to follow it.

That the artistic process can be an intensely affective experience seems obvious: There are many anecdotes attesting to the importance of emotion in artistic creativity. For instance, Duke Ellington apparently had an uncanny ability to tolerate tension and ambiguity and to put emotion and sensuality into musical form (Sashin, 1993). Fred Mitchell, a modern artist, described his feelings when he senses that a painting is coming together: "I feel a certain fusion of time and tenses and physicalities which seem to be present. . . . My life, such as it is, becomes a more meaningful thing to me. . . . I feel good about it. I feel confident. I feel very warm. I feel excited . . . I feel I am in possession of more of myself at these times" (quoted in Alexenberg 1981, p. 42). In addition to anecdotal evidence, there is some systematic and empirical research demonstrating the importance of affect and feeling in art (Bush, 1969; Gardner, 1973; MacKinnon, 1975; Suler, 1980).

Moreover, a commonly held view is that emotional states inherent to art and artistic creativity are more intense than those in science and scientific creativity (Bush, 1969; Csikszentmihalyi, 1978; Gardner, 1973; Suler, 1980). Although this may be true for the elaboration and verification stages of the creative process, it appears not to be true for the insight and discovery stages. I demonstrated this in a quasi-experimental design, assigning either an art or a science task to art and science students (Feist, 1994). The science task was a modification of the Science Test of Pine and Holt (1960): Half of the participants were told to imagine that they had discovered a species similar to humans, but with the sex organs of both males and females, and were asked to give possible scientific theories explaining such a species and suggest ways their theories could be tested. The other half of the participants, who were in the art task condition, were asked to look at a photograph by Ansel Adams ("Moonrise, Hernandez, New Mexico 1941") and write three modified Haiku poems of five lines each based on this photograph (cf. Amabile, 1983). All participants completed the Feeling and Thought Questionnaire (FTQ; Feist, 1991) three times (before, during, and after insight). The FTQ consists of a total of 37 emotion terms, such as *pleased, happy, excited, angry, sad,* and *anxious*. Participants rated the extent to which they experienced each emotion on a 7-point Likert scale from *not at all intense* (0) to *somewhat intense* (3) to *very intense* (6).

The emotion terms were classified into a positive or negative emotion scale based on loadings from a factor analysis with varimax rotation. It is important to note that the words were rated after the entire problem-solving process had occurred, not at three separate time periods during the problem-solving task. The primary hypothesis was that intensity of reported affect would be similar for the art and science students before and during the insight but that art students would report greater intensity of affect after the insight. No predictions were made concerning the valence (positive and negative) of the affect. As can be seen in Figure 1, the hypothesis was supported, but only for positive emotion. Art and science students experienced the same intensity of affect before and during the insight, and art students reported significantly more positive emotion

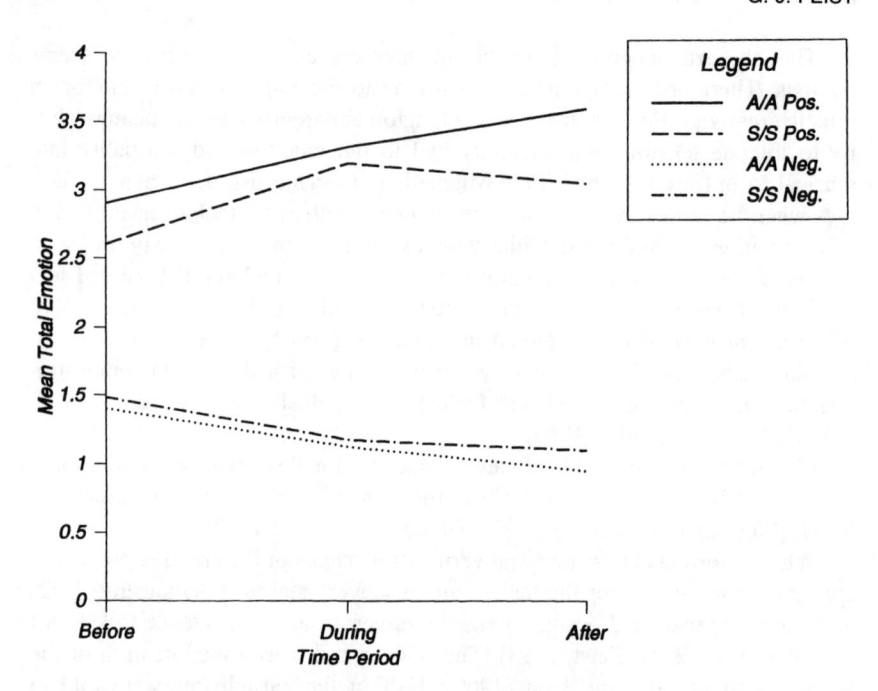

Figure 1 Positive and negative emotion before, during, and after the insight: Art students solving art tasks (A/A; $n = 26$) vs. science students solving science tasks (S/S; $n = 35$). Adapted from Feist (1994, *Cognition & Emotion, 8,* 489–502; Lawrence Erlbaum Associates) and reprinted with permission.

after the insight than did science students, $F(1, 60) = 4.07$, $p < .05$. The main effect, interaction, and simple comparisons for negative emotion were each nonsignificant.

Affective Traits and Artistic Creativity

Long-term affective dispositions as expressed in depression or manic–depressive illness have for a long time been implicated in the creative process. The pre-Socratics as well as Socrates, Plato, and Aristotle (see Jamison, 1993) each argued for the close connection between madness and creative insight. Indeed, the association between madness and genius has been pervasive both in the lay public and among researchers of the creative process for at least the last 100 years (see Lombroso, 1891/1976). However, only in the last 30 years has more systematic, empirical research been devoted to the topic, and the results appear to uphold the connection between mental illness and creativity only in artistic, not scientific, creativity (Andreasen & Glick, 1988; Andreasen & Powers, 1974; Barron, 1963; Jamison, 1993; Ludwig, 1992, 1995; Richards, 1994; Richards & Kinney, 1990). Furthermore, a consensual finding has emerged from this literature: The relationship between affective illness and artistic creativity is curvilinear, with the peak occurring at the mild levels of affective disturbance

(Andreasen & Glick, 1988; Barron, 1963; Feist, in press; Jamison, 1993; Matthews, 1986; Richards, 1994; Richards, Kinney, Lunde, Benet, & Merzel, 1988; Russ, 1993). Most of these studies, however, have not directly compared creativity in art with creativity in science.

One of the few studies that addressed the rates of affective disorder in the arts and sciences was conducted recently by Ludwig (1992, 1995). In a biographical study of 1,005 individuals in 18 different professions (including the creative arts and the sciences), Ludwig examined the relative rates of mental and affective illness across the professions. The main finding was that all forms of psychopathology (alcohol and drug abuse, psychosis, anxiety disorders, somatic problems, and suicide, among others) were more common in the artistic professions ($n = 555$) than in all other professions ($n = 450$). More specific to the art versus science comparison, mania was diagnosed in roughly 9% of the artists and in less than 3% of all other professions, while depression was diagnosed in approximately 40% of the artists and only 17% of the nonartists. Chi-square analyses revealed that both of these comparisons were statistically significant. Although Ludwig did not directly compare artists with scientists, from his published tables it could be calculated that the rate of mania was just over 1% and the rate of depression 17.5% for scientists (physical and social, $n = 112$), rates significantly lower than those for artists.

Such a difference in affective dispositions between artistic and scientific creativity is consistent with Gardner's (1973) observation: "Whereas the artist is interested in the subjective world, and is intent upon conveying his understanding and feeling for the world of human individuals or the 'living' aspects of objects, the scientist more typically investigates the world of the objective or treats individuals as objects" (p. 311). Suler (1980) also argued that scientists are more involved in objective, non-affect-charged secondary process thought than are artists (cf. Bush, 1969; Csikszentmihalyi, 1978; Feist, 1991, 1994). Using the Myers-Briggs Type Indicator, MacKinnon (1975) reported that, indeed, research scientists prefer thinking to feeling modes, whereas writers prefer feeling to thinking. In sum, there is little evidence for the connection between affective illness and creativity in science. The connection appears to be most pronounced in the arts.

The Aesthetic Emotions and Scientific Creativity

This is not to say that emotion plays no role in the scientific process. It does and this fact is most clearly seen in the aesthetics of scientific discovery. Just as is true with art, there is much historical and anecdotal evidence suggesting that strong aesthetic emotions are experienced by many scientists before and immediately after solving important scientific problems (Beveridge, 1957; Chandrasekhar, 1987; Curtin, 1982; Dyson, 1982; Einstein, 1934/1988; Gruber, 1995; Koestler, 1964; Lipscomb, 1982; Root-Bernstein, 1989; Yang, 1982). Einstein went so far as to say, "The most beautiful experience we can have is the mysterious. It is the fundamental emotion that stands at the cradle of true art and true science" (1934/1988, p. 9, translation mine). A few years later, the French mathematician Poincaré (1952) echoed Einstein's words:

> It may be surprising to see emotional sensibility involved *a propos* of mathematical demonstrations, which, it would seem, can only interest the intellect. This would be to forget the feeling of mathematical beauty, of the harmony of numbers and forms, of geometric elegance. This is a true esthetic feeling that all real mathematicians know, and it surely belongs to emotional sensibility. (p. 40)

Similarly, the great theoretical physicist, Paul Dirac, appeared to place beauty above truth when he said, "It is more important to have beauty in one's equations than to have them fit the experiments" (quoted by Yang, 1982, p. 36). Dirac did not believe that experimental results should be totally ignored; he simply meant that at the early stage of theoretical development, aesthetic solutions with intuitive appeal should not be thrown out because they do not fit current experimental findings. Indeed, such a strategy is congruent with the "confirm early–disconfirm late" heuristic that cognitive psychologists of science have recently described (Feist & Gorman, 1998; Mynatt, Doherty, & Tweney, 1977, 1978). "Confirm early" means that a bias toward confirming evidence is an adaptive strategy in the early stages of scientific problem solving. One can be too skeptical and too easily discard ideas that later prove to be correct. It is only after a few iterations of confirming the idea that a disconfirmation strategy becomes useful in attempting to falsify it. This is the idea behind "disconfirm late." But falsification should not prematurely edit potentially useful and original solutions. It is in this sense that Dirac's admonition to place aesthetics above evidence is best understood. Sometimes experimental technology is not up to the task of testing and falsifying truly original and beautiful ideas.

A component of beauty is the ability to experience awe and humility at the power and grandeur of nature. Nature is much more mysterious and powerful than humans' understanding of it will ever be, and the ability to be moved by its power is an essential element to being a scientist. Koestler (1964) called this "the oceanic feeling of wonder" (p. 258) and believed that artist, scientist, and jester each was moved and driven by it. The astronomer Carl Sagan (1996) recently wrote that the two necessary characteristics of being a scientist are the ability to experience awe and the ability to think skeptically. To be awe-struck by the magnitude and power of nature and thereby wanting to understand how nature works is both phylogenetically and ontogenetically the beginning of science. Without wonder, awe, and curiosity (each of which is affective), there is no science.

If beauty is a critical guiding force in scientific problem solving, a philosophical question must be asked: What is beauty? According to the philosopher Hartshorne (1982), beauty is experienced when two opposing bipolar dimensions are balanced: mere unity versus mere diversity and ultrasimplicity versus ultracomplexity. In short, beauty can be described as unified diversity, simple complexity, or both. Great scientific insights are profound experiences of beauty precisely because they unify diversity or bring simplicity to complexity. The desire to bring simplicity to complexity is a fundamental motivation behind all of science. The "parsimony urge," as it could be called, is most pronounced in physics and math, but it is also a goal of the biological and social sciences. Skinner (1953), among others, argued that a goal of all science is to discover general laws and principles of nature. A law or principle is nothing other than a conceptual heuristic that simplifies a diverse range of phenomena. Psychologically, the drive to experience beauty and to find simple principles for complex behavior is probably related to a greater drive to develop a codified and meaningful worldview and frame of orientation of life (Epstein, 1990; Fromm, 1973). In short, beauty, parsimony and the search for principles are essential to science, and each involves affective, motivational, and intuitive elements in addition to cognitive ones.

Yet aesthetics and being awestruck are not the only expressions of affect in science. Affect also is experienced more directly after the creative solution to a difficult scientific problem has been found (Chandrasekhar, 1987; Feist, 1994; Gruber, 1995; Koestler, 1964; Poincaré, 1952). Excitement, joy, and elation, along with frustration, anger, and depression are experienced throughout the scientific process. As mentioned earlier, Lazarus (1991) argued that people experience emotions whenever an event is meaningful and relevant to their well-being. Scientists who work months or years on a problem and finally solve it do have emotional reactions. For instance, Heisenberg had this to say about the moment he first came up with the idea of quantum mechanics:

> At first, I was deeply alarmed. I had the feeling that, through the surface of atomic phenomena, I was looking at a strangely beautiful interior, and felt almost giddy at the thought that I now had to probe this wealth of mathematical structure nature had so generously spread out before me. I was far too excited to sleep. (quoted in Chandrasekhar, 1987, p. 21)

Many other such historical instances could be amassed (e.g., Gruber, 1995; Koestler, 1964; Poincaré, 1952). The real question is not so much whether scientists experience emotion (they are human after all!), but what conditions elicit different kinds and intensities of emotion. If Lazarus's theory is valid, successful or unsuccessful problem solving has to be the context in which the most intense affect is experienced by scientists. The outcomes of problems and experimental results are most relevant and meaningful to a scientist's well-being and therefore should be the source of the most intense affect.

As yet, there is little empirical evidence regarding the kind and intensity of affect experienced in the process of doing science. The nature of affect as experienced by scientists as a result of their work in an area ripe for empirical exploration by psychologists of science (cf. Feist & Gorman, 1998). To put it simply, psychologists of science study scientific behavior. In addition to the developmental, cognitive, personality, and social influences on scientific behavior, emotion and motivation are central to a full understanding of scientific behavior. For example, what role does positive and negative affect play in facilitating, inhibiting, and motivating solutions to scientific problems? To what extent are beauty and awe motivators for scientists? Do the nature and intensity of affect experienced by scientists differ from the nature and intensity of affect experienced by people in other professions, especially the arts? These questions can and should be examined not only by psychologists of science, but by emotion and creativity researchers as well.

CONCLUSION

After a long period of neglect (Feist & Runco, 1993), the relationship between affect and creativity is finally being given the theoretical and empirical attention it deserves. Indeed, two books have appeared recently that are devoted exclusively to the topic (Russ, 1993; Shaw & Runco, 1994), and the current volume follows in that tradition. Affect is critical to the entire creative process: It influences as well as follows from the creative insight. Emotions also act as a primary reinforcer and motivator for creative behavior. A common theme throughout a diverse range of theories of creativity is the idea of affective processes as both a motivator and a consequence of creative insight. Sexual dissatisfaction, fear of death, and regression to primitive states highlight Freud's, Rank's, and Kris's theories, respectively. Even the cognitive theory of Koestler argues for the fundamental influence of emotion before, during, and after creative discovery. Lazarus's theory of emotion, although it does not explicitly focus on creativity, can easily be applied to predict which emotions should most likely occur before (anxiety), during (relief and happiness), and after (pride) insight. Runco's theory of the importance of tension as a motivator of creativity is similar to the ideas of Barron, MacKinnon, Freud, and Kuhn. Finally, Russ has integrated much of the findings from the last 30 years of empirical work on the creative process, person, and environment to create a comprehensive model of affect and creativity.

The empirical work on affect and creativity has demonstrated the important role that both positive and negative affective states play in creative solutions to problems. Positive emotion expands cognitive associations, while mild negative affect in the form of tension or dissatisfaction can actually motivate one toward creative problem solving. However, the relationship between creativity and negative affective states and traits (mania and depression) appears to be curvilinear (Andreasen & Glick, 1988; Feist, in press; Jamison, 1993; Matthews, 1986; Richards, 1994; Richards et al., 1988; Russ, 1993). Creative functioning peaks with mildly elevated negative affective states and traits. For instance, cyclothymia is a stronger predictor of creative activity than full-blown bipolar disorder (Andreasen & Glick, 1988; Jamison, 1993; Richards, 1994; Richards et al.,

1988). Furthermore, the difference between affective experience in art and science appears to exist primarily after, rather than before or during, creative insight (Feist, 1994). Indeed, it is clear from historical, anecdotal, and a smattering of empirical sources of evidence that the experiences of wonder, awe, and beauty as well as frustration and dissatisfaction are essential motivations behind all of science (Beveridge, 1957; Chandrasekhar, 1987; Curtin, 1982; Einstein, 1934/1988; Gruber, 1995; Koestler, 1964; Root-Bernstein, 1989). Finally, great scientific insights are often followed by intense affective reactions (Gruber, 1995; Koestler, 1964; Poincaré, 1952).

What does this mean for future research? What should the next step be in the study of affect and creativity? There are at least five major questions that need more empirical attention:

1. Under what conditions can negative affective states and traits facilitate creative thinking, and under what conditions can they inhibit it? In other words, what is the exact form of the curvilinear relationship between creativity and negative affective states and traits?
2. Which emotional processes play the most important role in scientific creativity, and under what conditions are they most likely to occur? This question can and should be addressed by at least three different groups of researchers: psychologists of science, creativity researchers, and emotion researchers.
3. Where are there commonalities and where are there differences in the affective processes that occur during artistic creativity as compared with scientific creativity?
4. Can various theories of emotion (e.g., Lazarus's) be generalized to the creative process and predict the types of emotional states that are likely to occur during different stages of creativity?
5. What are the developmental pathways that connect affective and creative development? How does the relationship between affect and creativity change with age? (Notice that I said nothing in this chapter about development. This is not only because the focus was not on development, but also because little work has been done on the topic.)

Given the recency with which the topic of affect and creativity and their interrelationship has garnered serious scholarly attention, it is rather impressive that researchers know as much as they do. Yet, with each answered question many new unanswered questions arise. That is the nature of science, and it is why the topic of affect and creativity should continue to fascinate, bedazzle, and even frustrate researchers for generations to come. But then again, fascination and frustration are necessary conditions for creative activity!

REFERENCES

Alexenberg, M. L. (1981). *The aesthetic experience in creative process.* Ramat Gan, Israel: Bar-Ilan University Press.

Amabile, T. (1993). *The Social Psychology of Creativity.* New York: Springer Verlag.
Andreasen, N. C., & Glick, I. D. (1988). Bipolar affective disorder and creativity: Implications and clinical management. *Comprehensive Psychiatry, 29,* 207–216.
Andreason, N. C., & Powers, P. (1974). Overinclusive thinking in mania and schizophrenia. *British Journal of Psychiatry, 125,* 452–456.
Barron, F. (1955). The disposition toward originality. *Journal of Abnormal and Social Psychology, 51,* 478–485.
Barron, F. (1963). *Creativity and psychological health.* New York: Van Nostrad.
Beveridge, W. I. B. (1957). *The art of scientific investigation* (3rd ed.). New York: Vintage.
Bush, M. (1969). Psychoanalysis and scientific creativity. *Journal of the American Psychoanalytic Association, 17,* 136–190.
Chandrasekhar, S. (1987). *Truth and beauty: Aesthetics and motivations in science.* Chicago: Chicago University Press.
Csikszentmihalyi, M. (1978). Phylogenetic and ontogenetic functions of artistic congition. In S. Madeja (Ed.), *The arts, cognition and basic skills (pp. 114–127).* St. Louis, MO: CERMEL.
Curtin, D. W. (1982). *The aesthetic dimension of science.* New York: Philosophical Library.
Dudek, S. Z. (1968). Regression and creativity. *Journal of Nervous and Mental Disease, 147,* 535–546.
Dyson, F. J. (1982). Manchester and Athens. In D. W. Curtin (Ed.), *The aesthetic dimension of science* (pp. 41–62). New York: Philosophical Library.
Einstein, A. (1988). *Mein Weltbild* (Original work published 1934) Frankfurt: Ullstein Materialien.
Epstein, S. (1990). Cognitive-experiential self theory. In L. A. Pervin (Ed.), *Handbook of personality: Theory and research* (pp. 165–192). New York: Guilford Press.
Estrada, C. A., Isen, A. M., & Young, M. J. (1994). Positive affect improves creative problem solving and influences reported source of practice satisfaction in physicians. *Motivation and Emotion, 18,* 285–299.
Eysenck, H. J. (1993). Creativity and personality. Suggestion for a theory. *Psychological Inquiry, 4,* 147–178.
Eysenck, H. J. (1995). *Genius: The natural history of creativity.* Cambridge, England: Cambridge University Press.
Feist, G. J. (1991). Synthetic and analytic thought: Similarities and differences among art and science students. *Creativity Research Journal, 4,* 145–155.
Feist, G. J. (1993). A structural model of scientific eminence. *Psychological Science, 4,* 366–371.
Feist, G. J. (1994). Affective consequences of insight in art and science students. *Cognition and Emotion, 8,* 489–502.
Feist, G. J. (1998). Affective states and traits in creativity: Evidence for non-linear relationships. In M. A. Runco (Ed.), *Handbook of creativity research* (Vol. 2) Cresskill, NJ: Hampton Press.
Feist, G. J., & Gorman, M. E. (1999). The psychology of science: Review and integration of a nascent discipline. *Review of General Psychology, 2,* 3–47.
Feist, G. J., & Runco, M. A. (1993). Trends in the creativity literature. An analysis of the research in the *Journal of Creative Behavior* (1967–1989). *Creativity Research Journal, 6,* 271–286.
Fiedler, K. (1988). Emotional mood, cognitive style, and behavior regulation. In K. Fiedler & J. Forgas (Eds.), *Affect, cognition, and social behavior* (pp. 100–119). Toronto: Hogrefe.
Freud, S. (1958). On creativity and the unconscious. ("Papers on Applied Psychoanalysis" [Vol. 4] *Collected Works of Sigmund Freud*) New York: Harper. (Original work published in 1925).
Fromm, E. (1973). *The anatomy of human destructiveness.* New York: Holt, Rinehart & Winston.
Gamble, K. R., & Kellner, H. (1968). Creative functioning and cognitive regression. *Journal of Personality and Social Psychology, 9,* 266–271.
Gardner, H. (1973). *The arts and human development.* New York: Wiley.
Gray, J. J. (1969). The effect of productivity on primary process and creativity. *Journal of Projective Techniques and Personality Assessment, 33,* 213–218.
Gruber, H. E. (1995). Insight and affect in the history of science. In R. J. Sternberg & J. E. Davidson (Eds.). *The nature of insight* (pp. 397–431). Cambridge, MA: MIT Press.

Hartshorne, C. (1982). Science as the search for the hidden beauty in the world. In D. W. Curtin (Ed.), *The aesthetic dimension of science* (pp. 85–106). New York: Philosophical Library.
Hersch, C. (1962). The cognitive functioning of the creative person: A developmental analysis. *Journal of Projective Techniques, 26,* 193–200.
Hilgard, E. R. (1962). Impulsive versus realistic thinking. An examination of the distinction between primary and secondary processes in thought. *Psychological Bulletin, 59,* 477–488.
Isen, A., & Daubman, K. A. (1984). The influence of affect on categorization. *Journal of Personality and Social Psychology, 52,* 1122–1131.
Isen, A. M., Daubman, K. A., & Nowicki, G. P. (1987). Positive affect facilitates creative problem solving. *Journal of Personality and Social Psychology, 52,* 1122–1131.
Isen, A., Johnson, M. M., Mertz, E., & Robinson, G. F. (1985). The influence of positive effect on the unusualness of word associations. *Journal of Personality and Social Psychology, 48,* 1413–1426.
Jamison, K. R. (1993). *Touched with fire: Manic-depressive illness and the artistic temperament.* New York: Free Press.
Koestler, A. (1964). *The act of creation.* New York: Macmillan.
Kris, E. (1952). *Psychoanalytic explorations in art.* New York: Schoken Books.
Kuhn, T. (1977). *The essential tension: Selected studies in scientific tradition and change.* Chicago: University of Chicago Press.
Larson, R. W. (1990). Emotions and the creative process: Anxiety, boredom, and enjoyment as predictors of creative writing. *Imagination, Cognition, and Personality, 9,* 275–292.
Lazarus, R. S. (1991). *Emotion and adaptation.* New York: Oxford University Press.
Lipscomb, W. N. (1982). Aesthetic aspects of science. In D. W. Curtin (Ed.), *The aesthetic dimension of science* (pp. 1–24). New York: Philosophical Library.
Lombroso, C. (1891/1976). Genius and insanity. In A. Rothenberg & C. R. Hausman (Eds.), *The creativity question* (pp. 79–86). Durham, NC: Duke University Press.
Ludwig, A. M. (1992). Creative achievement and psychopathology: Comparison among professions. *American Journal of Psychotherapy, 46,* 330–354.
Ludwig, A. M. (1995). *The price of greatness.* New York: Guilford Press.
MacKinnon, D. W. (1970). Creativity: A multi-faceted phenomenon. In J. Roslansky (Ed.), *Creativity* (pp. 19–32). Amsterdam: North-Holland.
MacKinnon, D. W. (1975). IPAR's contribution to the conceptualization and study of creativity. In I. Taylor & J. Getzels (Eds.), *Perspectives on creativity* (pp. 60–89). Chicago: Adeline.
Matthews, G. (1986). The effects of anxiety on intellectual performance: When and why are they found? *Journal of Research on Personality, 20,* 385–401.
Mendelsohn, G. A. (1976). Associative and attentional processes in creative performance. *Journal of Personality, 44,* 341–369.
Mynatt, C. R., Doherty, M. E., & Tweney, R. D. (1977). Confirmation bias in simulated research environment: An experimental study of scientific inference. *Quarterly Journal of Experimental Psychology, 29,* 85–95.
Mynatt, C. R., Doherty, M. E., & Tweney, R. D. (1978). Consequences of confirmation and disconfirmation in a simulated research environment. *Quarterly Journal of Experimental Psychology, 30,* 395–406.
O'Quin, K., & Derks, P. (1996). Humor and creativity: A review of the empirical literature. In M. A. Runco (Ed.), *Creativity research handbook* (Vol. 1, pp. 223–252). Cresskill, NJ: Hampton Press.
Otto, J. H., & Schmitz, B. B. (1993). Veränderungen positiver Gefühlszustände durch analytische und kreative Informationsverarbeitung [Changes in positive mood states induced by analytical and creative information processing]. *Zeitschrift für Experimentaelle und Angewandte Psychologie, 40,* 235–266.
Pine, F., & Holt, R. R. (1960). Creativity and primary process: A study of adaptive regression. *Journal of Abnormal and Social Psychology, 61,* 370–379.

Poincaré, H. (1952). Mathematical creation. In B. Ghiselin (Ed.), *The creative process* (pp. 33–42). New York: Plume and Meridan Books.
Rank, O. (1964). *The myth of the birth of the hero.* New York: Vintage. (Original work published 1932)
Richards, R. (1994).Creativity and bipolar mood swings: Why the association? In M. P. Shaw & M. A. Runco (Eds.), *Creativity and affect* (pp. 44–72). Norwood, NJ: Ablex.
Richards, R. L., & Kinney, D. K. (1990). Mood swings and creativity. *Creativity Research Journal, 3,* 202–217.
Richards, R. L. Kinney, D. K., Lunde, I., Benet, M., & Merzel, A. (1988). Creativity in manic-depressives, cyclothymes, their normal relatives, and control subjects. *Journal of Abnormal Psychology, 97,* 281–289.
Root-Bernstein, R. S. (1989). *Discovering.* Cambridge, MA: Harvard University Press.
Rosenberg, E. L., Ekman, P., & Blumenthal, J. (1998). Facial expression and the affective component of cynical hostility. *Health Psychology, 17,* 1–15.
Runco, M. A. (1994). Creativity and its discontents. In M. P. Shaw & M. A. Runco (Eds.), *Creativity and affect* (pp. 102–123). Norwood, NJ: Ablex.
Russ, S. (1993). *Affect and creativity: The role of affect and play in the creative process.* Hillsdale, NJ: Erlbaum.
Sagan, C. (1996). *The demon-haunted world: Science as a candle in the dark.* New York: Random House.
Sashin, J. I. (1993). Duke Ellington: The creative process and the ability to experience and tolerate affect. In S. L. Ablon, D. Brown, E. J. Khantzian, & J. E. Mack (Eds.), *Human feelings: Explorations in affect, development and meaning* (pp. 317–332). Hillsdale, NJ: Analytic Press.
Shaw, M., & Runco, M. A. (Eds.). (1994). *Creativity and affect.* Norwood, NJ: Ablex.
Skinner, B. F. (1953). *Science and human behavior.* New York: Macmillan.
Suler, J. R. (1980). Primary process thinking and creativity. *Psychological Bulletin, 88,* 144–165.
Wayne, J. (1974). The male artist as stereotypical female. *Arts in Society, 11,* 107–114.
Wild, C. (1965). Creativity and adaptive regression. *Journal of Personality and Social Psychology, 2,* 161–169.
Yang, C. N. (1982). Beauty and theoretical physics. In D. W. Curtin (Ed.), *The aesthetic dimension of science* (pp. 25–40). New York: Philosophical Library.

7

Affect in Artists and Architects: Images of Self and World

Stephanie Z. Dudek
Université de Montreal

Zajonc (1980) pointed out that emotional reactions are formulated in parallel with cognitive processing and occur with greater immediacy than nonemotional ones. The split in consciousness allows feelings to precede and thus establish priority (in front of thought). Aestheticians have pointed out that reuniting thought and feeling is perhaps the most important work of the ego, and this has been described as precisely the function of the finished work of art (Vygotsky, 1962). It may account for the sense of emotional unity and cohesion in experiencing great works of art, that is, the unconscious flow of cognition into feeling and vice versa, giving a sense of coming together at least for a moment. When emotion surges, perception is enhanced and enriched. Affect may be described as the life within the thought. Its presence and perception help to sustain the visual experience.

Artistic representation, projection, and perception are all invested with the dynamics of feeling, from beginning to end. They are personal and intimate. Halfway between feeling and intellect, art creates an experience in which both merge (Rose, 1980, p. 212).

How individuals process and put to use their emotions naturally depends on their temperament, their formative background, their professional skills and their formation (or deformation), and their current psychological state. The present analysis will deal with the qualitative differences in cognitive–affective processing of emotion and its expression in two distinct professional groups: artists and architects. Both groups reflect the temper of their times in ways that make symbolic forms such as art and architecture remain, to this day, the best reflections of the spirit and philosophy of the times.

According to Tolstoy, the emotional impact of looking at great art makes something accessible that was only felt vaguely before and is now understood in an integrative way, although perhaps not adaptable to verbal communication. Great art and architecture open ways of affirming a sense of self in time and place through their immediate emotional impact, opening up unconscious memories informed by experiences of "fusion and separation, pleasure and pain" (Rose, 1980). This allows the observer to attain an emotional balance without any seeming effort on his or her part. The reasons for this are obvious. Creative forms speak to the issues of their day and inevitably reflect the spirit and philosophy that brought them into being. Good art and architecture vibrate with the often hidden passion that animated their time and creation and thus guarantees their survival. Forms that do not reflect the mind and heart of their creators have no emotional weight and appeal and are unlikely to survive their time. Symbolic forms are fashioned with feeling and are symbols of emotion, living, palpitating symbols declaring their right to be taken as they are—to startle, move, or repel their audience as their creator intended they should. In short, art and architecture are meant to express emotion, thought, judgment, exultation, and not infrequently, conquest over despair.

Emotion is, by definition, an affective state of consciousness in which feeling is experienced as distinguished from cognitive and volitional states of consciousness (*Webster's Encyclopedic Unabridged Dictionary,* 1989). Zajonc (1980) defined emotion as an agitation of the feelings. According to Schachter and Singer (1962), emotion is a combination of arousal and cognition. They insisted that there is no universally accepted definition of emotion. Berlyne's (1974) preoccupation with arousal was, in effect, a preoccupation with the reticular activity that the brain releases. The person immediately experiences arousal in response to a stimulus. The affective response is set in motion by collative variables such as complexity, novelty, and incongruity, all of which may be called cognitive. It can also be released by inner thoughts and feelings with no external stimulus in evidence.

Although the cognitive–affective bond is inseparable, it is possible to focus on affect alone in describing the emotional patterns of a particular group of persons. In the present study, I analyzed the emotional patterns of artists and architects who have been recognized by the collectivity as making important contributions to their profession. (Dudek & Hall, 1991; MacKinnon, 1962).

Why look for differences between these two groups of creative people? Because artists and architects have different goals and make different uses of themselves and their talents. Modern art deals with the tensions of the unconscious and attempts to purify them. Architecture deals with the real world and aims to create a more comfortable and attractive external environment. Artists feed on themselves; their emotions are their raw material. Architects have a trade, and their profession makes use of the sticks and stones around them to project their dreams of a resplendent world. However, whatever their goals, both artists and architects have to use their emotions to ply their trade, and it is clear that human beings have developed unique structural systems for the processing of emotions. Such systems are meant to respond to the needs of the organisms and of the professions to which they apply their energies.

The created object may be seen as a replica of the emotional structure, woven into shape through an active intellect. Architects are somewhat more removed from the turmoil of their own affect. Creating a real world is their major concern, although both professionals aim to give birth to their innermost dreams.

In keeping with the demands of each profession, it is logical to assume that persons choosing such different professions as art and architecture necessarily develop different patterns for coping with their own emotional needs. However, for both artist and architect one of the primary motivations for work is to leave a symbolic memento of themselves behind. Both artists and architects are aware of their time and place in ways that other professionals and laypersons cannot intuit. They both develop unique structural systems for processing their emotions in the service of their art. Their primary goal is to express personal needs within the framework of society's constraints. In this way, an image of the social time and place is inevitably reflected through the forms created.

Although one would expect the vision and experience of 20th-century reality to be the same for everyone, persons with different professional formations appear to experience reality in different ways and express it in forms true to their own perception. Hence the variegated images of the times. An analysis of the Rorschach protocols of artists and architects reveals that their visions of reality are indeed different, as are their personal goals in life.

In this chapter, I demonstrate differences in perception and artistic expression revealed in an analysis of the personalities of the creators, and specifically through an analysis of their affective structure. This was attempted by an analysis of the responses that artists and architects gave to the inkblots of the Rorschach test. The Rorschach test is a well-validated instrument for the study of personality and the creative process. An analysis of the responses to the Rorschach test by both artists and architects allows the psychologist to arrive at a picture of their psychological world, their attitudes toward themselves, and their desires for self-expression as creators.

My report is based on the psychological testing of two groups of renowned artists and architects at the same point in time (between 1958 and 1965). The architects were evaluated at the Institute of Personality Assessment and Research (IPAR) by MacKinnon (1962) and his associates. I interviewed and tested the artists and the professional group.

The control group consisted of persons who were selected to provide an adequate control group by nature of training, socioeconomic status, age, and experience. All the control participants were successful in professional careers that did not have, as their goal, the construction or production of so-called creative objects or artifacts.

THE 20th-CENTURY SOCIAL SCENE

In the first half of the 20th-century, the initial appearance of an art of devastation produced a shock of revulsion even within the art milieu, but before the century was half over, the eyes of the public had become dulled to the now dominant landscape of the age. While the novelists and philosophers attested to an existential despair, and the artists' interpretive energy and frenetic dynamism called attention to the presence of both pain and the possibilities of an incredible richness, complexity, and freedom of expression never before experienced in any form, the architects had a predominantly optimistic view of their place and time.

The nihilistic philosophies underlying the dematerialization of the object and the deconstruction of form in the arts that have continued from early Dada to the present have produced an art that tells a story of bitterness and disillusion. Architecture had been animated by an entirely different philosophy—a philosophy of unbridled optimism that persisted, with some dissenting voices, until the late 1960s (Heyer, 1966). Unlike literature and the plastic arts (Dadaism, conceptual art, minimalism, the theater of the absurd), which moaned about the futility of all human gestures while continuing to make them, architecture moved with confidence and its achievements in 20th-century architecture were magnificent. Buildings more than 100 stories high scratch the sky, bridges span the rivers and bays, and rockets of remarkable industrial design reach for the planets. Even with the rapid obsolescence of buildings and the continual growth and attempted redevelopment of slums, architects retained their positive attitude.

However by the late 1960s, even architecture had to face the fact that its rosy dreams of designing a better world had not resulted in beauty and order. The ugliness of modern cities, the alienation and dehumanization engendered by high-rise housing and office buildings, and the cagelike construction of factories had to be acknowledged.

In less talented hands than those of its originators, modern architecture produced dense, cagelike, and beehive constructions in which the human being felt imprisoned, anonymous, mass-produced, rigidified, and alienated from his or her individuality. Jencks (1973) expressed an opinion that is increasingly current: "If architecture concretizes the public realm and if that realm has lost its credibility because it is founded on a false idea of what allows men to govern themselves, then its whole expressive nature, and therefore its essence is thrown into doubt" (p. 380).

Toward the end of the century, both architects and artists are laboring under a burden of remorse, uncertainty, and confusion. For the artists, it is more of the same turmoil, but for the architect it is an about-face. It has become clear that the bright new world that architecture had predicted (Heyer, 1966) has unfortunately emerged with a look of impoverishment, if not actual chaos. "In its most abstract form, architecture of course, played a certain role in the impoverishment of the environment" (Frampton, 1980, p. 9). This is a modest assessment compared to Pichler's 1962 statement: "The machines have taken possession of it and human beings are now merely tolerated in its domain" (Pichler, quoted in Conrad, 1970, p. 118).

The spiritual world situation about which artists and architects had such different opinions prior to the 1960s now appears to have a more unified voice of gloom. Graf (1979) summarized it in these words: "Our increasing inability to comprehend our reality, combined with our growing suspicion of modes of comprehension that seem reductive, dogmatic, or tied to a coercive politics, has provoked a crisis of rational understanding" (p. 238).

On the symbolic level, the arts at the turn of the century had already presented eloquent testimony of the impending chaos, pointing at the same time to its genesis: humankind's mounting disillusion, anger, and unwillingness to care. The trajectory from the urge to spiritual self-destruction (Marinetti, 1941 in *Futurist Manifesto*) to the growing urge for material self-destruction is a direct one. The meaning of the aggressive new art was clear within the first two decades, but the true significance of the new architectural forms (e.g., Bauhaus and the International Style.), created with an almost messianic spirit ("The great epoch has begun. . . . There is a new spirit: it is a spirit of construction and synthesis guided by a clear conception" [Corbusier, quoted in Jencks, 1973, p. 32]), did not become clear until some time later.

Jencks (1980) pointed out that the modern movement in architecture "had its Heroic Period in the twenties and its Classic Period, its dissemination and commercialization, in the Fifties. By the late Sixties, it has lost much of its ideological power, and, with the death of Le Corbusier in 1965, it had lost much of its moral and spiritual direction" (p. 10). In fact, Jencks dramatically declared the death of modern architecture as follows:

> Modern Architecture died in St. Louis, Missouri on July 15, 1972 at 3:32 p.m. (or thereabouts) when the infamous Pruitt-Igoe scheme, or rather several of its slab blocks, were given the final coup de grace by dynamite. Previously it had been vandalized, mutilated, and defaced by its black inhabitants, and although millions of dollars were pumped back, trying to keep it alive (fixing the broken elevators, repairing smashed windows, repainting), it was finally put out of its misery. Boom boom boom . . . Pruitt-Igoe was constructed according to the most progressive ideals of CIAM (the Congress of International Modern Architects) and it won an award from the American Institute of Architects when it was designed in 1951. (1973)

The goal of the psychologist is to explain how two groups of artists and architects who began with radically different aims both arrived at an image of the world as spiritually impoverished and moving toward Apocalypse.

PERSONALITY AND CREATION

The differences between artist and architect at the level of personality and attitude are great. The modern artist, lost in a self-consciousness of enormous proportions, perpetually defying social acceptance, puts him- or herself at risk unflinchingly and unreflectingly with each serious act of creation. Aware at the time of making a professional commitment that a pragmatic society has no place for artists, he or she begins defiantly and welcomes the philosophy of existential despair. Whatever the functions of art prior to the 20th-century, modern art is dedicated to "displeasing, provoking or frustrating its audience" (Sontag, 1962, p.7) The writers and philosophers have stated the facts, as they see them. "The work brings neither certitude nor clarity. It assures us of nothing, nor does it shed any light upon itself" (Blanchot, 1982, p. 233). And yet, the artist continues the lonely travail.

The architect's awareness of place within a materially evolving social structure has been entirely different. City planner, builder of environments, designer of space in which humans can feel free and expansive, he or she plans the future with a sense of power and enthusiasm, watching dreams and designs take larger shape (and undergo faster demolition) than ever before in the history of the world. Architects are self-confident, free of the doubts that beset the artist.

> Hard as I try, I see no chaos in our time. Just because a few painters do not know whether they should paint realistically or in the abstract, or whether they should paint at all, does not mean chaos. Our needs seem clear, the possibilities limited only by us. The main thing is that we act whenever a need appears and use our strength to find an economic and coherent solution. (Breuer, quoted in Heyer, 1966, p. 265)

There are also important differences between the attitudes of the two groups toward industrialization and the socioeconomic order (without which the modern enterprise of architecture would be impossible). Whereas the artist at the turn of the century was essentially opposed to technology and industrialization (with a few notable exceptions, e.g., the Russian constructivists and the Italian futurists) and contrives today to oppose technology, the modern architect found him- or herself in tune with the spirit of the age. Architects accepted the economic order, technology, science, and the power of the masses; they were eager to work within these constraints in the service of a new, vigorous architecture (and for a self-identity to match it).

"We want a clear, organic architecture . . . adjusted to our world of machines, radios, and fast motor cars" (Gropius, quoted in Jencks, 1973, p. 109).

As Smith (1977) pointed out, "architects who were with it" insisted on constructing buildings in line with the rest of contemporary industrial life. Their goal is "to build houses as Detroit builds automobiles" (p. 39).

On the other side of this coin is architects' awareness of social responsibility. The concern for human welfare has never been absent. The architect's explicit design philosophy has always been to build a better world through intelligent design. Le Corbusier and many of his generation constantly aspired to place architecture on a cosmic scale, to work toward the utopia they felt society should and could become. These ideals were behind Le Corbusier's Villa Radieuse and Unité d'Habitation; they guided the design of La Citta Nueva de Sant'Elia, as well as Buckminster Fuller's Dymaxion World. Humane conditions were behind the model-city programs in the United States and the Welfare State Housing of Great Britain. Aldo Van Eyck's projects in Holland are examples of attempts in this direction. The plans of CIAM and Team 10 between 1953 and 1963 were directed toward humanizing architecture and establishing the bases for human identity. The emphasis was on architecture that shows its respect for the traditions of a locale and a multivalence of meaning to achieve a sense of place. However, by the mid-1960s, while many of America's most established architects were still expressing optimism (Heyer, 1966) and Fuller was organizing a world community of scientists to make the world work through design, many others were disillusioned and at a loss.

The failure of 20th-century architecture is evident in both the external surface and the internal structure of buildings, whether commercial, residential, or public. "The contradiction between technical and visual excellence on the one hand, and the undeniable banality of the building task on the other, became so obvious in the early sixties that the curtain wall and its related aesthetic fell into disrepute, to be replaced by other approaches" (Jencks, 1973, p. 42).

THE PRESENT STUDY

Method

To arrive at an understanding of affect in artists and architects, I examined Rorschach data collected on eminent modern artists and architects. All of my inferences are based on this data.

Forty architects were interviewed and tested during a 3-day weekend at IPAR. Six psychologists administered the tests. The artists and the professional comparison group were individually given the Rorschach tests by me between 1960 and 1967. In view of the fact that I did not interview the 40 IPAR architects, the focus of my Rorschach analysis was on qualitative rather than quantitative material. The psychograms of all three groups were used to identify degree of productivity, psychic complexity, Erlebnistyp or experience balance, form level, and number of popular responses (i.e., the standard criteria). An intensive psychogram analysis was not attempted.

I scored all the Rorschach protocols of the artists, and professionals. They were rescored by two other experienced psychologists. Agreement between us ranged from 85% to 95%.

As mentioned, the focus of the present study was on drive sources of creative energy, of which affect is the chief identifying component. Creative works are replete with affect. They call attention to themselves through their emotional energy, which projects itself in forms that may appear harsh or ugly to eyes unprepared for images of novelty and challenge.

Imagery is, by definition, closer to the unconscious sources or drive energy, and its forms have been labeled the raw material of art. As such, imagery reflects drive in form, symbol, image, and built form. The creative person is expected to manifest a significantly greater tendency than the average person to transform unstructured raw drive material into form wherever the opportunity arises.

Thus the unstructured inkblots of the Rorschach test offer the creative person the necessary raw material to manifest this transformative drive. The goal of the present study was to analyze the Rorschach responses of creative artists and architects elicited during a research project on creativity. The study of architects was carried out at IPAR (1958–60) at the University of California. The study of the artists was carried out by me in Montreal.

The Rorschach test encourages and thus elicits imagery, which is by definition closer to unconscious sources and thus more easily reflects the presence of drive—the raw material necessary for creative transformation.

I analyzed the Rorschach protocols in terms of the determinants that are considered key factors in interpretation: the human movement response, the color response, and the cognitive approach. The large number of responses; the high development of movement, color, and shading; the adequate number of popular responses; as well as the excellent form level indicated that the sample consisted of imaginative, sensitive, relatively uninhibited persons in good contact with reality and able to experience a high degree of self-actualization. There was certainly evidence of conflict, tension, and sensitivity, but the basically adequate balance on the psychogram suggested that problems were generally under manageable control.

Participants

The Architects The original research study of the architects at IPAR was carried out by MacKinnon and his collaborators (1962). The selection of 40 of the most creative male architects in the United States began with a nominating jury of five professors of architecture, each working independently. Sixty-four names were finally retained, and the 40 who agreed to come to IPAR were assessed during an intensive weekend of testing and group interaction.

The Artists The artists of the present study were nominated by a jury of three experienced artists selected for the task by the editor of a prominent Canadian art journal. The 60 artists named were considered to be among the best painters and sculptors in Canada. The final selection of 30 artists (5 refused to participate) were all from the East Coast (because of lack of funds for travel, the West Coast artists were not interviewed).

Table 1 Rorschach Psychograms of Four Groups: Mean Scores

Response	Architects	Artists	Superior normals	Normals (Exner, 1978)
n	40	20	30	325
R	34.2	37.5	36.0	21.7
W	14.6	13.2	10.2	7.0
Human movement	5.5	4.5	4.4	3.4
Animal movement	3.8	4.8	4.6	2.3
Inanimate movement	3.1	2.5	2.4	.73
F %	34.0	40.0	42.0	45.0
Sum C	5.2	5.6	4.6	3.7
Sum shading	5.6	6.2	4.9	2.6
Popular	7.2	6.2	7.0	6.4

Note: The typical Rorschach psychograms for artists, architects, and superior normals (university-educated professional groups) I evaluated from 1958 to 1965. The sample from Exner (1978) reflects a more "normal" group of persons within which the "superior" group would represent approximately 15%.

The Professional Group The professional group ($n = 32$) consisted of practicing doctors, lawyers, engineers, university teachers, administrators, biologists, and one translator. They were matched by virtue of professional status. They were all roughly middle-aged (40 plus years old).

Results

See Tables 1, 2, and 3 for the Rorschach psychogram data for the three groups.

The Movement Response The human movement response reflects a tendency to sublimate affect through fantasy (Beck, 1945), sometimes to defer action altogether. Piotrowski's (1965) definition of the movement response is concept of role in life, that is, the image a person has of him- or herself. It is generally an image acceptable to the ego as an accurate reflection of the self, whether it is negative or positive. It may also reflect an ego ideal. It describes behavior that the person sees as characteristic of the self. It goes without saying that it also reflects the perception a person has of other people and the built-in expectations that go with that perception. At the cognitive level, it reflects the imaginative resources.

Architects The architects projected a large variety of human movement responses, and they were mainly of a lively, energetic, friendly, good-humored, and cooperative but detached nature. Typical descriptions of people were comedians, jesters, pantomimes, conjurers, minstrels, and dancers—that is, all varieties of performers. There were also frequent projections of "humorous caricatures."

The movement response was seen with clarity. There was no hesitation or hedging. The situation and the interpersonal contacts were pleasant. The affect

Table 2 Rorschach Variables

Variable	Architects M	Architects SD	Artists M	Artists SD	F
R	35.20	15.27	37.23	23.54	1.94
W	15.60	6.58	10.85	4.12	.48
Human movement	4.27	2.82	5.69	3.38	3.17
Animal movement	4.93	3.31	7.39	6.79	6.24*
Inanimate movement	2.80	2.15	2.39	1.98	.11
SumC	4.23	2.40	2.46	1.94	2.99
Sumc	3.63	1.93	3.41	2.67	.57
Popular	8.13	2.75	5.23	1.59	6.65*
F %	35.60	13.92	37.46	11.20	.03
P %	25.40	9.56	18.31	8.74	15.40**
R (8–10%)	37.60	10.49	34.46	11.46	.16
A %	41.67	7.99	39.62	14.82	.01

Note: The psychograms of 20 artists and 20 architects (matched for age, socioeconomic status, and professional training). The only significant psychogram difference that emerged was the projection of more animal movement responses and fewer popular responses. This finding was consistent with my interview impression of greater expressive vitality in the artist population and a marked tendency to avoid popular (i.e., stereotyped) concepts and ideas.
*$p < .05$ ($n = 19$). **$p < .01$.

Table 3 Holt Content Scores for Primary Process (Percentage)

Variable	Architects M	Architects SD	Artists M	Artists SD	F
Primary process	19.87	8.52	23.77	12.73	4.20*
Density	1.45	.27	1.60	.43	.89
Contents	58.7	14.69	61.9	16.10	1.40
Level 1	6.1	6.32	13.4	14.0	3.11
Level 2	52.6	10.84	48.5	11.31	.02
Libidinal	37.2	15.66	55.2	15.12	1.84
Libidinal Level 1	12.9	13.90	26.5	19.50	.87
Libidinal Level 2	61.6	16.80	42.2	16.30	3.91
Aggressive	62.8	15.66	44.8	15.12	1.83
Aggressive Level 1	1.1	2.00	2.65	.10	3.72
Aggressive Level 2	24.3	13.10	28.7	12.70	.21
Form level	5.19	.47	5.07	.56	.13
Defense demand	2.59	.80	3.40	1.38	1.72
Defense effectiveness	.98	.52	.93	.36	.73
Controls and defenses	8.07	5.38	10.85	7.58	2.98
Poor defenses	1.20	2.57	2.62	2.14	3.81
Regression in service of ego	2.54	1.70	3.18	2.22	.02

Note: The artists projected significantly more primary process content than did the architects, but they clearly did not differ from the architects in the distribution of libidinal and aggressive contents and in the quality of the form (5.1 vs. 5.0). Overall, both artists and architects had free and easy access to both libidinal and aggressive primary process energy and used it in the service of the ego equally well. The percentages of primary process content for both artists and architects were much greater than is generally evident in the Rorschachs of "normal" controls (Dudek, 1996).
*$p < .05$ dl = 19

was joyful. The activity was primarily constructive and pleasurable. There was, however, one qualification. Sixty percent of the M responses were described in ways so as to place a psychic distance between themselves and others. (There were on the average 3.0 movement responses per person of this nature, out of a mean of 5.0 movement responses). The responses were not only mildly distant, but also highly exhibitionistic. The architects saw themselves as active, energetic, socially aware but playing a "game," enjoying it and successful at it. It was a game where an audience and its positive response were required. Often the people seen were caricatures, indicating a derogatory attitude, but there was no nasty or direct aggression. The architects were both involved and detached. In other words, they were always in control of the situation.

Artists The artists, on the other hand, projected persons in movements that carried a much greater fantasy quality. They were much more introverted and self-referential as a group. In their descriptions of the human actions, seen alone or with others, the people lacked human proportions. They tended to be seen abstractly, more like objects or forces. Sometimes, what started out to be a description of a person ended up as a painting, a design, or a lit-up sculpture. The following response to Card I is a typical response: "It's kind of anthropomorphic—a conflict between some forms which suggest people, human, or some biological forms of the natural, more accidental landscape quality. [Inquiry: "What do you see?"] It's a woman. It's hard to say . . . she looks so inhuman. Maybe it's more like a mythological construction, a projection of what she is or could represent—something symbolic. [Inquiry: "What is it?"] . . . It's a kind of flight from the self . . . getting away from the self. Such a strong dynamic quality of the design because the body is so static!!"

The artists visions were multivalent, pulled every which way. The boundaries between figure and ground fluctuated, and sometimes the quality of movement was lost in reflections about its reality. The artists were not engaged in direct relationships, even from a distance. They allowed hidden scenarios to intrude and intermingle with the existing reality. Viewer and viewed were lost from sight. Concepts were often superimposed on real situations in incompatible ways. The following response to Card III is again relatively typical: "I see a humorous heraldic crest of two figures which are hermaphrodites—female breasts and male penises; both touching the skull of a strange animal out of which is emerging a butterfly; and [in the side red] I see a scientific diagram of their stomachs."

Comparison of Perceptual Modes of Artists and Architects In the artists' responses, a form of concrete association took over in response to the precise areas of the blot. The artists moved from one area of the inkblot to another until they encompassed them all into one concept. Incompatible images were arbitrarily forced together and the result was absurd theatre. The architects seldom lost contact with the task set by the Rorschach, although they, too, could project disquiet. However, by comparison, it was low key; for example, "Some person bearing down on something. It might be a person in motion. It's a dance; flying or about to leap. Ominous!" Self-referential comments of a highly personal nature, however, were rare in the architects' fantasties. The content generally did not strain the imagination, although flights of pleasant (and unpleasant) fantasy occurred. Consider, for example, one architect's response to Card IX: "Ritual fire dance. Peer Gynt in the hall of the mountain king." The imagery revealed the scene occurring on stage. The pink at the bottom of Card IX represented the footlights; Peer Gynt became "two figures or gnomes dancing underground, little devils, not vicious devils." The scene was contained within the blot stimuli and made good sense in terms of the structure of the blot. The reference to a fairy story was appropriately justified by context. The architects were also more prone to use simple denial than were the artists (e.g., "these are not vicious devils").

When the artists showed flights of fantasy, they often took on weird proportions that did not have literary references. Consider this response to Card X:

> I'm trying to force myself to see one object in the middle. It's like a mythical king of some kind. I'd like it to have a face, but it has two faces; one body, though. The impression is awfully strong. Might have a beard, a collar, and two breasts. No face, but has ears and a mustache and here I see a little angel jigging along inside his brain. This is very beautiful. It's going up. It's going to bomb and destroy this sexual symbol. It's located in the brain of this being.

The whole justification was strained, the resulting form was poor, and the affect was inappropriate. This response is taken from the record of an accomplished and productive artist who had achieved international recognition (he taught part-time in the art department of a large urban university). It became evident that the response to stimulus-pull and the use of common sense were quite different in the content of artist and architect.

Comparison of Cognitive Approaches of Artists and Architects Nowhere was the difference between the artists and architects more evident than in their cognitive approaches to the organization of the whole blot. Both were able to organize the blot easily, but they did it quite differently.

The architects' responses generally took account of all the stimulus variables in a complete and intelligible way. In fact, the story line left nothing to the imagination. The people were well seen, the concept of firelight explained the red color of their faces, the splash of red paint justified the poor splotchy form of the red legs. The black shading in the dark areas was seen as a shaggy fur coat. The response accounted beautifully for form, color, and shading. The form level of the response, and the finesse in elaboration could not be improved upon. There was even the projection of strong and happy affect, expressing a joyous energy, but also pointing to the undercurrents and presence of a more complex, earlier emotional state. The response came immediately. There was no hesitation, no fumbling for words. The whole response demonstrated a high level of intuitive intelligence, an easy and first-rate synthetic ability, and a capacity to project appropriate affect.

The artists' responses were also immediate and complete, accounting for all areas of the blot. However, the approach resembled a patchwork quilt. The associations came quickly and easily but did not end in a synthesis; each part remained discrete, and parts were strung together arbitrarily. What relevance any of the objects had to each other was never explained. There was no sense of closure, and it did not engender in the audience the same admiration the architects' clever syntheses evoked. It remained absurd theatre.

Interpretive Inferences What do these responses tell us about the creative processes of two highly creative and socially successful individuals? The architects' treatment of the blot material was brilliant and their work was finished when they stopped talking. The reality they created could not have been better elaborated. All the details fit; nothing more needed to be done. But there was no surprise, no mystery; all questions had been answered. It was a banal story that we already knew, with emotions we recognized and accepted. The admiration was for the organizational skill and the easy interpretation. Neither the content nor the form offered room for, or required, creative redefinition. In the artists' responses, the work had barely begun. There was both surprise and dismay. Questions abounded. We were left with the mystery of percepts that had no ordinary logical explanation. It was our job to do the work of redefinition—of creation. There was no clue to the mystery, no indication of the affect that could or should accompany the tale. The contents emerged out of the artists' immediate internal state, without a tight definition. Projection was not given any specific form. It was a spontaneous outpouring. In contrast, the architects instinctively felt the need to tell a logical story, to take from the bolt what would fill it out best and what would evoke a commonsense, comfortable closure. All that in a few seconds!

Each projection may be taken to depict the actual creative reality of both persons. In his creation, the architect must respect the sticks, stones, and icons that describe a house as a sheltering place. The artist's mission is to sell a dream; question a reality; disrupt expectations; transform the ordinary into the unusual; and, in so doing, effect an extension of consciousness. Whereas the artist poses new problems, the architect feels compelled to resolve the existing ones. The artists looks for secrets buried in the recesses of the human mind; the architect organizes space so that human activity can proceed in effective, useful, and pleasurable fashion.

The architect's vision must be precise, concrete, aware of the details but focusing on the larger gestalt. Architects cannot permit themselves to live in the chaos of ferment that is artists' fertile storehouse of raw inspiration. The artist's job, on the other hand, is to not let one stay easy in one's skin. He or she tries to confront, attack, excite, redefine, transvaluate, and push beyond the limits of existing knowledge and beyond the limits of mind—not a very comfortable occupation.

The artist's affective drive forces a perceptual restructuring, in which the intrusion of the unconscious is always a welcome challenge to form. Whereas for the architect, the careless intrusion of the unconscious, in the wrong place and at the wrong time, endangers a professional career, for the artist it is labeled a "creative spell." The architect is protected against unconscious slips by working with a hard-nosed team—the engineer, the business manager, and the generally conservative client. The artist's flights of provocative fantasy are encouraged by peers, art dealers, and the audience.

The Color Response—Affect The quality and availability of feelings are more clearly revealed in responses to color in the Rorschach test. The different types of feelings that offer themselves for interpretation in response to color indicate what kinds of emotional needs press for symbolic (or direct) expression. Color responses in the Rorschach cannot be meaningfully evaluated without also considering the movement responses, that is, the concept of role that will determine how the affect will be lived out or sublimated.

Architects The architects gave strong responses to color, projecting a wide range of content, from highly socialized to violent. On the whole, however, the quality of the color responses tended to be pleasant and positive. Their color responses came early (in Card II) and were often associated with movement.

When movement was combined with color, the contact was generally described as vigorous, pleasant, enjoyable. Although aggressive contacts were also evident, they were less frequent. Here are two typical examples from Card II:

> Two dancers with red turbans. They stepped into a pail of red ink. [Inquiry: Tell me more about them.] They are playing patty cake. They're happy. They have some kind of hats and capes. [Inquiry: Why happy?] The color.
>
> They have Oriental eyes—two clownlike figures facing each other with black coats, and the feet are red. [Inquiry: why sad?] It suggests blood. They have red hats, white faces; their palms are together. They're kicking; it's blood because it's red; hurt themselves.

Both responses are multiple determinants.

The color responses were generally earthy, appropriate to the action, and set in common or natural settings. They implied emotions the participants were in touch with and accepted as normal.

Artists The color responses projected by the artists showed a basically different quality (although there was obviously some overlap). There were a larger number of sex and blood responses described with evidence of tension or conflict. (Blood, however, was mentioned by roughly 30% of participants in all three groups.) The artists differed from the architects in the intensity of affect. They often projected a wild and undisciplined energy held under tense control by the ego. The quality of the color responses was then crude and unsocialized, and their form level was often poor. The artists were much less comfortable with Cards II and III than were architects. Many gave sex responses in these cards with obvious discomfort and often without color. Hermaphrodite responses were not uncommon (and almost never found in the comparison group of professional persons). Only 14.7% of the artists, as opposed to 47.5% of the architects, were able to combine movement with color in Cards II and III. Whereas color (affect) seemed to stimulate the architects to see positive human interaction in these cards, it had no such effect on the artists. In fact, there was reason to believe the opposite. Thirty percent of the artists, as opposed to 7.5% of the architects, did not interpret color until they reached the last three cards, and then they often projected a forced, that is, arbitrary use of color (e.g., on Card X; "A face with yellow eyes and red hair"). At other times, the initial naturalness of a response disappeared in its elaboration, changing into a design, a painting, or a fabric rather than remaining a real-life object. Such signs of dissociated affect were frequently evident in the artists. For example, the following response to Card IX confuses the images of fountain and phallus.

> Bouncing out—a central stream. Seems to be a fountain. Coming up and streaming gaiety. Bouncing up with excitement. The pink at the bottom is gorgeous. Bouncing up with sunlight: Nice and free and easy. A nice big play either between two people, or two groups, or two anything. Nice, indeed. [Inquiry] Can be sexy or spermlike. Gaiety, joy, freedom. By the play of the fountain. It's a very happy situation. This response was given by an internationally famous painter.

The quality was one of narcissistic rather than shared enjoyment, a quality that distinguished artist from architect. The artist was indifferent as to whether it was the fountain or the inferred phallus that was streaming. His feeling was that the play can be "either between two people, or two groups, or two anything." The symbolic and the real merged into each other and the human element was lost. The joy he experienced was more likely to be sublimated into art than shared with people, since they have no greater pull than inanimate objects or forces.

Images of pain were as frequent in the Rorschachs of the artists as pleasure was in the records of the architects. Expression of neither pain nor pleasure were much in evidence in the Rorschachs of the professional group. The artists often showed an emergence of formal deviations of thinking, as seen, for example, in this response to Card X: "Looks like Vietnam bleeding. Suffering is going on there." The elongated pink shape in Card X suggested the image of Vietnam as a country and because it happened to be pink, this renowned artist interpreted it as Vietnam bleeding.

Not all the color responses given by the artists projected confusion, dissociation, or detachment. The artists, like other people, can experience gentle and tender emotions, for example, the following response given to Card VIII by a female artist: "This is very pleasant. Very reminiscent of an enlargement, close-up of a blossom. [Inquiry] Gives feeling of some of those delphinium or snapdragons which have an intricate form. Not the daily type. The center would be the pistil." However, even here we are dealing with a vision one step removed. The artist is seeing an enlarged version, that is, a picture of a blossom. Her need to analyze and perhaps to make the scene symbolically larger than it is, rather than to simply enjoy, places a distance between self and object and, by extrapolation, between self and others.

On the whole, the aggressive content of the artists' color responses stood out compared with the content of the architects' color responses. The artists did not appear to be interested in intimate, friendly relations, although they were not incapable of them. They preferred to take issue, to argue the negative side, to feel isolated, to savor loneliness and pain, or to brood about being at the mercy of indeterminate forces. The artist's primary stance was as one who contests, finds fault, feels the pain and fear inherent in closeness, in living in a world where ambivalence and existential despair are the mode. The concept of role in life, however, was not that of aggressor. The artists were primarily detached from social affairs but active and busy with present projects. However, the quality of the artists' human movement responses were, on the whole, more positive than negative.

The Control Group: Movement and Color Responses The realistic and commonsense movement and color responses of professional persons of high educational level (lawyers, engineers, administrators, and physicians) paled into insignificance when compared with the intellectualizing and phantasizing of the artists and architects. The productive professional person appeared to be more interested in going about the business of everyday working and living without giving way to extravagant fantasies. An intense involvement with a generally rewarding profession did not seem to cloud a vision of day-to-day reality shared with the typical man/woman (compared with whom the professional felt fortunate by virtue of having an absorbing profession).

The movement and color responses of the control group were to the point, appropriately articulated, sparingly elaborated. Even when elaboration was rich (Card VIII), the response stuck to a realistic mode of enrichment. By comparison with the other two groups, the responses were more banal and less complex. They lacked the elements of imminent change and unpredictability that the artists' Rorschachs revealed. They were closer to the Rorschachs of the architects but often lacked the personal and imaginative touch. A look at the psychograms of the professional group reassured me that this group did not lack complexity. However, qualitative analysis indicated that they had chosen not to develop the same degree of openness to and contact with their inner resources (less evidence of primary process, fewer affective terms, less indecision, and more popular responses). They did not feel the same need to structure and articulate a personal perception of reality.

In short, elaboration, fantastic free association, Level I primary process thinking, painful ambivalence, indecision, and dissociated affect were in slim evidence in the Rorschachs of the professional group. The high-level professional person, efficient and productive at a chosen occupation, did not abhor the stereotype and often bordered comfortably on the cliché. Divination and theory construction, even on an intuitive, diffusely articulate level, was not a stock-in-trade. This does not mean that such a person is uninteresting. The interest he or she holds for others is more in terms of creature comforts or professional know-how and less in flights of revelation or philosophical rumination. However, if such persons become mentally ill, there is no guarantee that the archetypes of Jung's collective unconscious will not emerge with the same overweaning complexity that is the storehouse of all humankind (although I would conjecture, even here, that they would be clothed in garments of a more tightly woven fabric).

Another Rorschach characteristic that differentiated artists and architects from their professional colleagues was the density of their imaginative perception and articulation. Multiple determinants in the Rorschach were significantly more frequent in the artists group and less common in the control group. For example, a response that is scored simultaneously for movement, bright color, dark color, shading, and inanimate movement may certainly be said to be more complex, more opaque, more highly differentiated, and more difficult to interpret than a simple determinant response (e.g., human movement). A profusion of determinants, containing elements that are often self-contradictory (e.g., human movement and inanimate movement), informs a psyche that is complex indeed, and by that token more creatively interesting.

In short, whereas the psychograms described the three groups as having equal amounts of energy (similar quantitative proportions), qualitative analysis revealed how amazingly different were the constructions of their inner and outer realities. Without the use of qualitative analysis, the psychogram in this study would not have reflected the complexity of personal and private worlds.

To the extent that all three groups had constructed lives reflecting some degree of active self-determination and considerable actualization of potential, they may all be described as successful.

The artist puts him- or herself at great risk in undertaking to restructure society's spiritual direction. There is no team that can diffuse responsibility, as is essential to put in motion the architect's vision. Both artists and architects as creators are called on to give expression to something new, something demanded by the needs emerging from the actual realities of a particular time and place. The artist's self-chosen task of transvaluation sets him or her against society, whereas the architect tends to work with it.

The architect has the job of expressing the meanings that a culture finds significant and is willing to underwrite in dollars and cents. If the architect is a visionary, he or she tries to create new areas of significance. The task is challenging, but it does not necessarily require a high degree of self-consciousness. The external reality, that concerning the immediate needs of others, is expected to take priority over the personal vision. "You cannot approach a large design project as a field for personal expression" (Smith, 1977, p. 32). The professional person (e.g., doctor, lawyer, or merchant) also assumes responsible roles in relation to society, but what is primarily demanded is effectiveness and productivity. Invention, although desirable, is not essential and often not relevant. (This does not apply to the research scientist.) The professional's job is best done without the essential tension of doing battle against structures that ask only to be maintained at optimum level.

CONCLUSION

Affective drive and attitude toward the world differed between artists and architects. While the artists were enmeshed in a profound spiritual travail, always close to the existential and apocalyptic despair identified by the philosophers at the turn of the century, the architects saw both the self and the world situation in positive terms. The challenge was seen as one of building a brighter future for humankind and a personally pleasant and rewarding one for oneself. The artists seldom emerged from the self-absorbing gloom long enough to consider consciously a present or a future. These black-and-white positions for artists and architects were true at the extremes, but, to be sure, the more accurate picture lies in the many shades of gray that are in between. The contribution of the personologist is to try and understand the inner affective forces that normally play a large part in shaping the artists', architects', and others' views of the world in word, image, and built form.

REFERENCES

Beck, S. J. (1945). *Rorschach's Test II. A variety of personality pictures.* New York: Grune & Stratton.
Berlyne, D. E. (1974). *The new experimental aesthetics.* New York: Hemisphere.
Blanchot, M. (1982). *The writing of the disaster* (A. Smock, Trans.). Lincoln: University of Nebraska Press.
Conrads, U. (Ed.). (1970). *Programmes and manifestoes on 20th century architecture.* Cambridge, England: Cambridge M.I.T. Press.
Dudek, S. Z. (1996). (need reference for table 3, p. 23
Dudek, S. Z., & Hall, W. (1984). Some test correlates of high level creativity in architects. J. Personality Assessment, *48,* 351–359.
Dudek, S. Z., & Hall, W. B. (1991). Personality Consistency: Eminent architects: 25 years later *Creativity Research Journal, 44,* 213–231.
Frampton, K. (1980). *Modern architecture: A critical history.* London: Thames & Hudson.
Graf, G. (1979). *Literature against itself.* Chicago: University of Chicago Press.
Heyer, P. (1966). *Architects on Architecture: New Directions in America.* New York: Walker.
Jencks, C. (1973). *The language of postmodern architecture.* London: Academy Editions.

Marinetti, F. T. (1941). In S. Cheney, (Ed.), *Futurism: The story of modern art.* (pp. 250–257). New York: Viking Press.
MacKinnon, D. W. (1962). The nature and nurture of creative talent. *American Psychologist, 17,* 484–495.
Piotrowski, Z. A. (1957). Perceptanalysis; a fundamentally reworked, expanded, and systematized Rorschach method. New York: Macmillan.
Rose, G. J. (1980). *The power of form.* New York: International Universities Press.
Schachter, S. Z., & Singer, J. (1962). Cognitive, social and physiological determinants of emotional style. *Psychological Review, 69,* 379–399.
Smith, C. R. (1977). *Supermannerism. New attitudes in postmodern architecture.* New York: Dutton.
Sontag, S. (1962). *Against interpretation.* New York: Delta Books.
Vygotsky, L. S. (1962). *Thought and language.* New York: Wiley.
Webster's Encyclopedic Unabridged Dictionary of the English Language. (1989). New York: Portland House.
Zajonc, R. B. (1980). Feeling and thinking: Preferences need no inferences. *American Psychologist, 35,* 151–175.

8

Feeling Creativity Through *Deep Listening*

Kimberly A. McCarthy
Columbia College, Chicago

Einstein did not speak until age four. We know he was listening. What was he hearing? (Oliveros, in press)

This chapter examines the role of affect and attention in creativity, using as illustration a form of music improvisation entitled Deep Listening (Oliveros, 1990, 1998). In addition to creativity in general (Sawyer, 1992), music improvisation provides a particularly rich medium for the study of affect and attention for two reasons. First, the power of music to influence our thoughts, feelings, and behaviors (in a largely affective, nonverbal capacity) has been reviewed from a variety of fields (Tame, 1984), the practical side of which is well represented in the music and sound-arts therapies (Beaulieu, 1987; Bejjani, 1993; Bruscia, 1987; Newham, 1993). The perception of sound relies heavily on a variety of forms of affect (for a review, see Radocy & Boyle, 1988). The definition of affect used in this chapter encompasses feeling, emotion, mood, and temperament as interpreted through psychophysiology or phenomenology (Goleman, 1995; LeDoux, 1996).

Second, music improvisation refers to the process by which verbal and nonverbal information is received, sent, or exchanged during the act of performance. Music improvisation is a multimodal, multisensory form of decision making, a highly complex, feedback-dependent medium (Schwartz & Godfrey, 1993). Much of the discussion surrounding music includes both reflective and agenic volition (Tame, 1984) in intrapersonal (within oneself) and interpersonal (among people) affective (Foucault & Boulez, 1994; Boretz, 1994) and aesthetic experiences (for a review, see Rahn, 1994). An ability to detect, differentiate, symbolize, and utilize affective perceptual relationships is advantageous in intrapersonal and interpersonal decision making (Gardner, 1983; Goleman, 1995; Sawyer, 1992). Consequently, the ability to moderate affect and attention facilitates creativity in music improvisation, not to mention the advantage of enhanced creativity for overall psychological health, a topic that remains of high interest.

The question then is twofold: In what manner are affect and attention related, and how does this relationship effect creativity in music improvisation? Research in affect (e.g., Goleman, 1995; LeDoux, 1996) and attention (e.g., Baars, 1988; LaBerge, 1995; Posner & Raichle, 1994) has identified some of the implicit and explicit mechanisms through which automatic and volitional capacities of affect and attention interact. Of particular interest are the detection, activation, and maintenance of novel affect, especially those features responsible for the enhancement or potentiation of affective and attentional states.

The work of LeDoux (1996) is particularly relevant here as one of the few investigations into auditory perception and affect that did not rely on language and vision. Attention studies tend to focus on visual perception and language (see Posner & Raichle, 1994); aural perception may be mentioned, but usually in relation to language. Affect, if mentioned at all, is usually limited to terms of neuroanatomy (e.g., hemisphericity, amygdala, and anterior cingulate gyrus) or pathology (e.g., alexithymia, amnesia, anxiety, depression, and bipolar disorder). Perhaps visual perception, verbal language, and pathology are easier to define and measure objectively in terms of lexical, behavioral, or neuroanatomic stimuli and response. Many of the existing music studies on auditory perception and affect have relied on an understanding of western European music theory, which tends to be equated with verbal language. More important, research (Aiello, 1994; Deutsch, 1975; Gardner, 1993; Reisberg, 1992) has identified distinct processing mechanisms for language and music, and suggests a promising future for nonverbal auditory perception and affect research.

As will be shown, Deep Listening provides an effective medium for the illustration, examination, and development of affective and attentional elements that operate within creativity. Oliveros's use of prose notation gives an opportunity for the reader to experience directly the creative sound process involved in Deep Listening. One advantage of Deep Listening proposed here is the enhancement of auditory imagery (Reisberg, 1992), which influences and is influenced by affect and attention.

Unfortunately, direct empirical research on Deep Listening has yet to be conducted. But as does Oliveros (1985), the current chapter draws from existing theories and research on cognition and affect as support for the proposed structures and functions of Deep Listening.

To illustrate this largely theoretical analysis, a theme and variations has been created entitled Creative [Absolute][2] [Rational][3] Ear [CARE] that will be discussed throughout this analysis. CARE provides a mechanism for the direct experience of affect and attention in the creative process involved in Deep Listening. CARE also functions as a musical score providing an opportunity for the manifestation of a creative musical product equal to other professional musical forms.

The analysis begins with a review of Deep Listening and the role of attention as outlined by Oliveros (1998) and the working example CARE. The structures, functions, and interrelationships of attention and affect are then presented, followed by a discussion of their role in creativity in Deep Listening and illustrated in CARE.

THE POWER OF SOUND: DEEP LISTENING AND CARE

Developed by composer Pauline Oliveros (1990), Deep Listening refers to "a meditative exploration of listening and sounding, designed to help people [musicians and nonmusicians alike] gain flexibility in as many forms of listening as possible."[1] It is a form of creativity using simultaneous listening, composing, and sounding in consideration of oneself, others, and the environment.

Understanding sound as a powerful change agent, Oliveros (1998) composed the Deep Listening improvisational pieces as tools for healing, personal growth, awareness, and emotional and intellectual development—in other words, self-actualization. Sound serves as both the vehicle and the outcome of self-actualization, often resulting in the enhanced creative musical product. Improvement is concomitant with an ability to cooperate with others and compete with oneself. Reception and volition are inherent in the creative process of Deep Listening.

The Deep Listening pieces consist of attentional strategies for listening and sounding in solo and ensemble situations (Oliveros, 1998). Each piece focuses on some aspect of global and focal attention as applied to sound and music (and space and time). *Global attention* refers to the unlimited, nonlinear perception of the field of sound. Attention is globally expanded by defocusing the ears as one would the eyes for a wider field of vision. In contrast, *focal attention* refers to the perception of a point in the field, a linear process within a limited capacity.

Global and focal attention operate within two types of listening: receptive and active. In *receptive listening,* attention is global, expanding in all directions without commitment to any particular sound, receiving any and all sound. *Active listening* refers to purposeful, intentional listening, meeting the stimulus with sensual, emotional, intellectual, or intuitive energy for the purpose of interpretation or participation.

Attention is attracted by or directed to two types of stimuli: *internal,* such as memory and imagination, and *external,* such as environmental (Oliveros, 1998). The bridge between memory, imagination, and environmental stimuli lies

---

[1] For more information, contact the Pauline Oliveros Foundation at http://www.deeplistening.org.

<u>The Creative [Absolute][1] [Rational?][1] Ear</u>

Following [focal attention][23] the sound passageways [outer ear (air conduction): pinna & auditory canal][2] I wobble in full resonance [empathy][3] with the mammoth vibrations [air pressure][2] of the tympanic membrane [eardrum][2]. On the sound wave I ride through the shuddering porous membrane [metaphor][3] teetering tottering balancing with the undulating phenomena [sinusoidal stimulation][2]. Adventure [affect][3] on the other side [middle ear (bone conduction): ossicles, oval window][2] I narrowly escape the pounding hammer [malleus][2] as it thumps the anvil [incus][2]. Thrilling [affect][3] I glide through the oscillating archways [metaphor][3] of the stirrups [stapes][2]. Plunged [through the oval window][2] into the spiraling fluid of the inner ear [(fluid conduction): cochlea, organ of corti][2] I float marveling [affect][3] at the fleeting echoes in the bony chambers [semicircular canals][2] of the sea shell like cochlea [metaphor][3]. I sink to the most secret [affect][3] basilar membrane protected by the hardest of bone armor [metaphor][3]. Among a myriad field of precious hair cells [approx. 28,000][2] I grow curious and strum [traveling wave][2]--fairly fainting at the harmoniousness [affect][3] of this microscopic harp of my being [metaphor][3]. Suddenly [temporal resolution][2] the journey accelerates as I am slung into space [auditory nerve][2] by a quickening neuron [generation of action potential][2]. Weightless I experience a celestial calm [affect][3] accompanied by the tiniest pings and pongs [weights of facilitation and inhibition][2] over a rippling subtle harmonic drone [self][3] making [creativity][3] the most comforting [affect][3] music [sound][2]. Traveling simultaneously fast yet slow [janusian process][3] my still yet moving alternate body [neural network][2] sings a wordless and wondrous song ["tuned" neurons][2] in the company of my multitudinous self [distributed representation][2].
(Oliveros, in press, pp. 47-48; [ ] added)

Figure 1: a CARE theme

in the self-referential nature of bodily sensory systems: The body may serve as both independent and dependent variable, sometimes simultaneously. In this way, affect may be experienced psychophysiologically and phenomenologically, as stimulus or response. Attention and affect with the body and to the body (e.g., focused breath work and body movement work) are essential to Deep Listening.

The Specifics of CARE

The various versions of CARE illustrate the continuum Figure 1 shows a CARE theme with its variations from verbal and visual modes of perception, based primarily on language, to the nonverbal and aural modes of perception, which are more likely to use affective measures. They also illuminate those features that distinguish the enhanced affective capacity, and thereby unique creativity, of Deep Listening from the more familiar, traditional, or conventional scholarly and artistic products. Peruse CARE, noting the pulls on global and focal attention, and receptive and active listening, especially any feelings or bodily sensations.

CARE is varied through the inclusion or exclusion of bracketed information to represent a continuum from the conventional scholarly essay, to the conventionally artistic sound/text piece, to the relatively unconventional Deep Listening

FEELING CREATIVITY THROUGH DEEP LISTENING   133

piece. An excerpt of Olivero's writings forms the theme of CARE, "Poetic Prose," and is experienced by excluding all bracketed information, as shown below. Poetic Prose straddles the "Absolute" interpretation as factual information about measurable phenomena and the "Rational?" interpretation as poetry.

> Following the sound passageways I wobble in full resonance with the mammoth vibrations of the tympanic membrane. On the soundwave I ride through the shuddering porous membrane teetering tottering balancing with the undulating phenomena. Adventure on the other side I narrowly escape the pounding hammer as it thumps the anvil. Thrilling I glide through the oscillating archways of the stirrups. Plunged into the spiraling fluid of the inner ear I float marveling at the fleeting echoes in the bony chambers of the sea shell like cochlea. I sink to the most secret basilar membrane protected by the hardest of bone armor. Among a myriad field of precious hair cells I grow curious and strum—fairly fainting at the harmoniousness of this microscopic harp of my being. Suddenly the journey accelerates as I am slung into space by a quickening neuron. Weightless I experience a celestial calm accompanied by the tiniest pings and pongs over a rippling subtle harmonic drone making the most comforting music. Traveling simultaneously fast yet slow my still yet moving alternate body sings a wordless and wondrous song in the company of my multitudinous self. (Oliveros, 1998, pp. 47–48).

Figure 2: Poetic Prose

CARE and Poetic Prose function as two versions of the example. The second variation or the third version of CARE, "Scholarly Essay" is experienced through the linear incorporation of scientific or technical, material information such as that suggested in the bracketed "[ ][2]" information (see below). If the subjective (e.g., "rational?") information within and preceeding bracketed "[ ][3] information as shown in CARE is to be included, it must be redefined in objective terms (e.g., "absolute").

> The process of listening encompasses the excitation of hair cells which leads to the generation of action potentials in the neurons of the auditory nerve (Gregory & Colman, 1995). This sensory information is first processed at the midbrain (which orients attention) and again

at the thalamus (which filters out irrelevant features or distractors) (Goleman, 1995; Laberge, 1995; Ledoux, 1996; Posner & Raichle, 1994). At this point the information is passed onto two distinct paths: (a) the amygdala, the source of emotion as proposed by Goleman (1995) and Ledoux (1996); and (b) the neocortex, the cite of...

Figure 3: Scholarly Essay

Sound-Text is realized by freely interpreting any printed information in CARE (e.g., letters, words, punctuations), as sonic cues emphasizing pitch, timbre, duration, and volume as equally important (or more important) than semantics. Duration is indicated graphically, each line is five seconds long. The placement of the phonics or letters indicated the approximate timing. Volume is indicated

"Sound-Text," the third variation and the fourth version of the CARE, is shown below, to be practiced freely with expression:

fa fa fafafaFAFAFAFAFAT!!   Soooop p p p p pa! pa!

PA!   SsssSsssaaaaaaaaaag g g g geeeeee   wa——

wa——   wa——   wa——ay   ssssSSSSSSSSSSSSSSSSSSAH

HAha ha ha ha   bull!   bull!   fafafafa BULL!   Iiinnn furrrrrrr rrr Rrrr

rrreeEEeeeessssssss   RRRrrreeeessssoooooonnnn   nnnnn nnnn nnn nnnzzz

ping pong ping pong ping   pong!   mmmm

mmmmmmmmmmmmmmmmmmm   sssssssssseeeeeeceellllllllllffffffmaaaahhh

Figure 4: Sound-Text Piece

by the size of the letters. Blank areas indicate silence. The text below has been extracted from the letters and words of CARE.

The score for "Deep Ear," the fourth version and third variation of CARE does not use either graphic or traditional music notation, but instead consists of a series of instructions for improvisation. "Deep Ear" provides the greatest degree of creative freedom for the composer/performer/listener, who again, under the auspices of *Deep Listening,* is one and the same.

Figure 5: Deep Ear

Peruse CARE as written above, a single composite of four versions. Listen to the space between you, the page, the letters, the ideas and feelings as you wander through the versions. Alternate between listening to the sounds filling those spaces and sounding the sounds, feeling those spaces. Continue until the overall space feels and sounds at rest.

Ambiguity and Temporality in CARE

The theme and variations encompass different levels of ambiguity, incongruency, or novelty, which in turn evoke different levels of affective and attentional response. Oliveros's original excerpt provides a high degree of familiarity in both form and content as Poetic Prose. The current context of Scholarly Essay introduces a degree of ambiguity that might be significant were this not a chapter on creativity—scholarly essays on creativity are somewhat more accepting of unconventional (e.g., "rational?") ideas. The exclusion of "rational?" terms and the linear incorporation of "absolute" terms reduce ambiguity regarding an interpretation of CARE as anything other than Scholarly Essay and fortified by the current context. An emphasis on sonic interpretation is fairly conventional for a Sound/Text piece but unconventional (e.g., too "rational?") for a Scholarly Essay, especially one aimed at scientific audiences. The Deep Ear version presents increased ambiguity (e.g., nontraditional notation and abstract imagination) relative to the Sound/Text piece, even more so as a Scholarly Essay (unless it's an essay for philosophers!). The degree of ambiguity is related to the duration of attention needed to process the information. It is through affect that the unexpected or ambiguous is characterized as something to be desired or avoided (LeDoux, 1996).

CARE also incorporates a temporal element (which I shall return to), in that both the Sound/Text and Deep Ear versions exist as musical scores (an Inpotentia version) and as such cross three time dimensions: the past and the future, through memory and imagination, and the here-and-now, as live music and by some as versions of Visual Art. With the addition of Inpotentia and Visual Art, CARE consists of six versions and the ambiguity is increased. Intermittently return to CARE, noticing any changes in your overall affective and attentional response. What evokes feelings, captures attention, or triggers memory or imagination?

In what way, if any, does your response change as a result of reexposure or learning?

AWARENESS OF EXPERIENCE THROUGH AFFECT AND ATTENTION

The Basics of Attention

Focal and global attention as described by Oliveros finds support in the attention research of Posner and Raichle (1994). The continuum between conscious and unconscious perception is mediated by attention through a series of connected networks, including (but not limited to) orienting, detecting events (e.g., executive attention network, which brings information into consciousness), and maintaining the alert state (e.g., vigilance network). The process of attention includes automatic (without awareness) and volitional (with awareness) functions.

Initially, before attention is engaged, all sensory signals excite internal memory, an "automatic activation" process not requiring conscious attention (for a brief review, see Posner & Snyder, 1975; for an in-depth, updated review, see Posner & Raichle, 1994). Consequently, pathways in the memory system that are associated during activation may receive facilitation from processing signals without widespread inhibitory consequence. Perception without action can be infinitely ambiguous.

Once action is required in terms of transferring this information to long-term memory, attention is engaged and a limited number of information units are selected through a process of facilitation and inhibition. When the activated information is attended to, signals not associated with the initial information are inhibited and subsequent facilitation processes are enhanced. It is through inhibition that selection is made; inhibition occurs only in the presence of attention.

The probability of perceiving a particular signal increases when that signal and memory are highly associated (as in the case of habit or learning), but it greatly decreases, relative to the automatic activation process, when an association is not shared (e.g., a novel experience) (Posner & Raichle, 1994). In the case of novel or competing signals, attention and its effort to activate inhibition may be evaded, resulting in an experience of altered consciousness.

Martindale (1995) referred to this state as defocused attention (Oliveros's global attention), a second level of awareness in which a larger number of associational networks are activated but to a less degree than in focal attention. Moderately activated networks have yet to commit to being on or off. They exist in a state of potentia, increasing the possibility of an unusual or unexpected response. Focused or focal attention, in having fewer nodes activated, tends to detect quickly expected or learned associations; defocused or global attention presents more opportunity to detect the unexpected or novel association.

The subtleties of focal and global attention and their relation to affect are indirectly delineated through LaBerge's (1995) distinction between attentional expectation and preparation. In preparation, a state of arousal is activated in anticipation of a significant event and the body readies itself for more effective processing, especially those neuroanatomic structures and functions related to the general anticipated context. An expectation refers to an item stored in long-term or working memory that codes an event in terms of its content and spatial and temporal characteristics. Expectation, an expression of memory, may occur in the absence of preparation. Preparation, the expression of attention, always includes the activation of arousal, regardless of the presence or absence of expectation.

For example, consider the phenomena of telling and understanding jokes (LaBerge, 1995). The joke is successful to the extent that the listener anticipates the unfolding events of the joke so that when an unexpected event occurs (e.g., the punch line), it produces an intense surprise effect. Preparatory attention is often activated when the expected event does not occur but could occur. Following the delivery of a joke without anticipation of the ending reduces the surprise effect. The joke works to the extent that the listener values novel experience enough to maintain attention in the face of expectation and ambiguity of both learned and novel stimuli.

Sustained performance, the kind necessary to process novel, emotionally significant, or ambiguous information (e.g., joke telling, and CARE) requires a balance between attentional capacity and the demands of sensory and response selection (LaBerge, 1995). Attending to multiple tasks entails stimulus sampling to create response strategies, which in turn creates changes in response tendency. The orientation or shifting of attention represents automatic and volitional mechanisms based on detected incongruities between the current environment and some sort of internal representation of the environment that is maintained in working memory (LaBerge, 1995).

Attentional capacity is to some extent within the control of the person's energetic properties, for example, arousal, motivation, and effort. Volition manifests as the conscious execution of an instruction and the recognition of a stimulus and its value at that particular moment as determined through the independent mechanisms of cognitive evaluation and affective appraisal (LeDoux, 1996).

The Basics of Affect and Emotion

The basic emotional unit consists of a set of inputs, an appraisal mechanism, and a set of outputs (LeDoux, 1996). Emotional responses are hardwired in the brain; people have little direct control over their emotional reactions. Appraisal is the first step in the initiation of an emotional response and refers to the mental evaluation of the potential benefit (felt tendency toward) or harm (felt tendency away from) of a situation. Emotional appraisal systems are directly connected with the systems that control emotional responses. The process of appraisal is unconscious and can occur before a person knows exactly what something is. It is the content or effects of appraisal that are experienced consciously as feelings. Automatic responses of appraisal are programmed by evolution to detect certain stimuli (e.g., natural triggers) relevant to the function of the network. Volitional responses are learned through association with natural triggers.

Emotional feelings involve more brain systems than thoughts, but the repertoire of responses is smaller compared with cognition (Goleman, 1995; LeDoux, 1996). Emotion organizes and synchronizes the brain's activity much quicker and with more strength than does cognition. Emotional appraisal performance and response control are moderated by the same system; once the emotional appraisal is made, an emotional response occurs automatically. The response is quicker but less accurate than that after cortical processing.

Affect can influence sustained attention as a form of motivation or reinforcement. For example, recall the temporal experience of "flow" as outlined by Csiksentmihalyi (1990), an influence particularly advantageous for creativity. Although any novel stimulus will evoke arousal, only the emotionally significant novel stimulus results in amygdala activation and the consequent prolongation of arousal (LeDoux, 1996).

Joke telling and music improvisation (e.g., CARE) are similar creative mediums in that the creative process and product unfold within the same ontological temporal space; memory and imagination are coactivated in a much shorter time frame relative to non-performance-based creativity. Creativity is the value of novelty, including attentional and affective components. Creative joke telling and music improvisation provide effective mediums from which to study, across sustained attention, the structures and functions of attentional preparation and the varying degrees and qualities of affect. Each involves an expectation regarding the temporal significance of affect and the affective significance of the temporal event. Affect illuminates the distinctions between psychological and ontological temporal experience (for a general review of temporal experience, see Slife, 1993).

LeDoux's (1996) distinction between the memory of an emotion and an emotional memory clarifies the role of temporality in attention and affect as used here. The memory of an emotion is an explicit, declarative memory, a state of perception that may be activated through conscious recollection and expressed verbally. Explicit memories about emotional situations are derived through the hippocampal system, the pooled relations among stimuli forming the emotional context. In contrast, an emotional memory is an implicit memory, a state of emotion that does not require perceptual representation and eludes verbalization. Implicit emotional memories are derived through the amygdala system. Unlike the explicit memory, which is notoriously forgetful and inaccurate, the implicit memory, a fear-conditioned response, not only is durable, but often increases in potency over time via Eysenck's "incubation of fear" (as cited in LeDoux, 1996).

The ways in which emotion systems learn and remember are essential to this discussion and include automatic and volitional mechanisms. In fact, one of the brain's most powerful and efficient learning and memory functions is the ability to rapidly form memories of stimuli associated with danger, hold onto them for long periods of time (perhaps eternally), and use them automatically when similar situations occur in the future (LeDoux, 1996).

The Separate Interactions of Affect and Attention

New technologies and theories of neuroscience have identified three possible meeting points of volitional and automatic mechanisms in affect and attention: structurally through the amygdala in terms of emotion (Goleman, 1995; LeDoux, 1996) and the anterior cingulate gyrus in terms of attention (Posner & Raichle, 1994) and functionally through working or short-term memory in terms of the enhancement of and by affective or attentional states (Baars, 1988; LaBerge, 1995; LeDoux, 1996; Posner & Raichle, 1994). Again, I return to the body as affective and attentional stimulus and response.

According to LeDoux (1996) emotion and cognition are "separate but interacting mental functions mediated by separate but interacting brain systems" (p. 69). The perceptual representation of an object and the evaluation of its significance are separate brain processes. The difference between the state of perception and the state of emotion is not the system that represents conscious content (e.g., feeling or color), but "the systems that provide the inputs to the system of awareness" (LeDoux, p. 19). The thalamus–amygdala circuit provides a pathway in which emotional responses and learning can occur without the involvement of the higher processing systems of the brain, systems believed to be involved in thinking, reasoning, and consciousness.

From Sound to Emotion to Attention to Action: Automatic and Volitional Paths

For example, the process of listening encompasses the excitation of hair cells, which leads to the generation of action potentials in the neurons of the auditory nerve (Gregory & Colman, 1995). This sensory information is processed first at the midbrain (which orients attention) and again at the thalamus (which filters out irrelevant features or distractors) (Goleman, 1995; LaBerge, 1995; LeDoux, 1996; Posner & Raichle, 1994). At this point, the information is passed onto two distinct paths: (a) the amygdala, the source of emotion as proposed by Goleman (1995) and LeDoux (1996), and (b) the neocortex, the cite of the anterior cingulate gyrus, the source of attention as proposed by LaBerge (1995) and Posner and Raichle (1994).

The connection between the thalamus and amygdala is quicker than that between thalamus and neocortex (LeDoux, 1996). Consequently, the amygdala may evoke a response (e.g., arousal systems) to stimuli before cortical processing. This evocation may be the source of emotional response the individual does not fully understand, a result of implicit memory formation and retrieval.

The thalamus–amygdala circuit provides a pathway in which emotional responses and learning can occur without the activation of brain systems believed to be involved in thinking, reasoning, and consciousness.

Meanwhile, the majority of sensory information is relayed by the thalamus to the neocortex for more thorough processing—particularly the prefrontal lobes and hippocampus, the source of explicit memory formation and retrieval (LeDoux, 1996). This more informed interpretation of the initial stimulus is then recycled back through the amygdala, the final analysis of which includes low-level, sensory-specific information from the thalamus; high-level information resulting from sensory-specific cortical analysis; and analysis of the emotional context by hippocampal formation (e.g., context in terms of the relationships among stimuli).

Emotional responses (the amygdala path) are hard-wired in the brain in terms of a bias toward response evocation (LeDoux, 1996). When the interpretations of the amygdala and cortical paths match, the response initiated by the amygdala is appropriate. When the amygdala and cortical interpretations do not match, as in the case of ambiguous or novel stimuli, the function of the cortical path is inhibitory in overriding the activation of the amygdala path in the event of an inappropriate response.

The anterior cingulate gyrus has been identified as one important area of the cortical path and the possible source of attention, the meeting point between bottom–up (automatic to volition) and top–down (volition to automatic) processing (Posner & Raichle, 1994). While waiting for a nonspecific target, the orienting system of attention is tuned so that it responds faster to information in the object recognition pathway. When attending to the possibility of target detection, information from the environment is inhibited so as not to interfere; the anterior cingulate gyrus is quiet. Alertness is maintained through the vigilance network (the right frontal and parietal lobes), which influences emotional arousal, sleep, and mental disorders.

As in affect, the situation is complicated when stimuli are ambiguous, complex, or novel. While defocused attention of vigilance is prime for the detection of novel stimuli, novel features of stimuli increase activation of the anterior cingulate gyrus and subsequent inhibition, a function that serves to block the automatic response so that other features may be detected. The creative response requires a delicate balance between vigilance and attention, some of which may be achieved through volition.

For example, four situations or tasks associated with increased activation of the anterior cingulate gyrus are (a) simultaneously evaluating multiple attributes of targets; (b) performing on Stroop test trials; (c) passively listening to (but not watching) spoken words; and (d) processing novel information prior to automatization, or when novel combinations of actions are required (Posner & Raichle, 1994). These same characteristics are often present during creativity. How, then, in the face of complexity and ambiguity, can volition function to maintain vigilance and control attention at levels conducive to creativity?

Attention serves the two goals of behavioral action and experiential enhancement (LaBerge, 1995). A behavioral goal of attention is the ability to take quick, appropriate action based on accurate decisions reflective of the environment. Toward experience, attention may include an ability to potentiate or enhance affective mental states, as seen in the relationship between decreased ability to focus and shift attention and increased feelings of depression and anxiety (Posner & Raichle, 1994; Schwarzer & Wicklund, 1991). The creative experience requires a delicate balance between experiential and behavioral attention, a balance influenced by affect.

For example, one result of rehearsal or learning is the automatization of a sequence of behaviors, thereby requiring less attention to behavior (e.g., music technique) and increased attention to experience (e.g., musical expression) (LaBerge, 1995). In turn, experiential attention may be subsumed within a current behavioral goal of attention, along the lines of LeDoux's memories of emotion and emotional memories. In this manner, affect may also be automaticized and function as intrinsic motivation.

In creativity, extrinsic motivation in part may result in a decrease of intrinsic motivation (Amabile, 1996). Behavioral attention can overide experiential attention, as in performance anxiety, when behavioral attention serves to inhibit experiential attention (LaBerge, 1995). Likewise, experiential attention can inhibit behavioral attention, as in the case of anxiety.

Creative ideas rarely hatch in completed form, and creative behavior seldom emerges in productive measures on first effort. Vigilant attention and affect are necessary in the face of ambiguous ideation or behavioral action. In fact, it may be affect that signals the ambiguous experience in terms of the presence or absence of incongruities between the current environment and its internalized representation. And because of automatization, an ability to change the behavior, environment, cognition, or affect may not be readily available (LeDoux, 1996). The individual may simply report a "feeling-of-knowing" (Metcalfe & Shimamura, 1994), "tip-of-the-tongue," or "feeling-of-warmth" experience (e.g., Baars, 1988; Neisser & Winograd, 1988; Shaw & Runco, 1994; Russ, 1993), which might stem from implicit, state-related or mood-dependent memory (e.g., Berry & Dienes, 1993; Christianson, 1992; Graf & Masson, 1993).

Volitionally, in certain situations people are able to imagine what bodily feedback would feel like if it occurred, what Damasio (cited in LeDoux, 1996) called "as if" loops. "As if" feedback may be cognitively represented in working memory and can influence implicit and explicit processes of attention and affect. Bloch (Bloch & Lemeignan, 1992; Bloch, Orthous, & Santibanez-H, 1987) noted a volitional relationship between facial expression, body posture, and affect, and the actor Richard Gere (1993) cited the need for actors to beware of "emotional hangovers" influenced by pretending or imagining emotion as part of their job. Using explicit emotion to activate behavior may lead to the activation of implicit emotion.

Again, it is creativity that helps to distinguish the life-enhancing response from the dysfunctional one. Novelty or ambiguity is valued in creativity, at the very least, as an intrinsically significant temporal experience, whereas in psychopathology, the novel is apt to be viewed either as insignificant, thereby releasing cognitive activity (e.g., reorienting), or as significant but to be avoided, thereby leading to dysfunctional behavior (for a review, see Taylor, 1989). If the primary expectation is one of temporal experiential significance (e.g., ambiguity between psychological and onotological temporal experience is tolerable), the habit response may be controlled long enough for creative activity to occur, including the positive affective experience.

AFFECT AND ATTENTION IN CREATIVITY THROUGH DEEP LISTENING

The live performance of Deep Ear is proposed to offer the more intensive creative experience in terms of exposure to novelty through both listening and sounding, especially when performed by two or more people. Recall the directions for Deep Ear. The orienting system of attention and the appraisal mechanisms of affect are activated by the directions to listen, notice, and feel the sounds, feelings, and spaces experienced while perusing CARE. No direction is given in regard to specific types of sounds (e.g., physical, emotional, cognitive, phenomenological, and environmental), only that a representation of temporal significance be kept in working memory. This requires the delicate balance of sustained affect and attention, setting the stage for auditory imagery and subsequent creative sounding.

Deep Ear calls into demand the mechanisms of visual and auditory memory and imagination, especially auditory imagery (Halpern, 1992). Auditory imagery differs from auditory perception in that the latter refers to the interpretation of a physical stimulus outside the perceiver, whereas the former refers to the subjective sustained auditory experience in the absence of direct sensory stimulation of that experience or the auditory after-effects from a just-vanished auditory stimulus, including one constructed from long-term memory fragments (e.g., popcorn popping) (Smith, Reisberg, & Wilson, 1992).

The maintainance of auditory imagery occurs via an "articulatory rehearsal loop" between subvocal rehearsal (e.g., inner voice) and phonological (e.g., inner ear) store (Smith et al., 1992). Subvocalization refers to the silent pronunciation of auditory information and the interpretation of kinesthetic cues resulting from covert lip and tongue movements. With auditory presentation, access to the phonological store is immediate. With visual presentation (e.g., Inpotentia), subvocalization is used to load information into the phonological store. In both visual and auditory presentation of information, subvocalization operates in the maintainance of information in the phonological store, a cycle that must be repeated periodically for action or the transfer into long-term memory.

The performance of Deep Ear can facilitate creativity in that it requires both listening to and making sounds. Although the inner voice (e.g., subvocalization) and inner ear (e.g., phonological store) are necessary for the generation of auditory imagery in general, the necessity of the inner ear in acting on nonverbal auditory imagery has yet to be confirmed (Smith et al., 1992). In this manner, an imagined or creative auditory event may be generated through affect. Attention serves to enhance target features of the imagined auditory event while inhibiting interference from the inner voice until the imagined event has a chance to become sufficiently identified for a motor plan to activate. Affect, in all its definitions, performs an important role in the generation of auditory imagery and its resultant organization into creative music improvisation, from both psychophysiological and phenomenological sources.

CONCLUSION

People who are unable to identify, express, and tolerate emotion and feelings may find creative participation in CARE, especially Deep Ear, difficult. For some, a single request to "sound" is enough to provoke extreme anxiety (Newham, 1993). Ambiguity or novelty is amplified through the quantity and diversity of experiential and behavioral choices perceived via the two channels of attention and affect, including unexpected choices arising through implicit mechanisms.

The degree to which affect and attention interrelate in the experience of creativity in music improvisation is to some extent self-determined. The individual who is open (e.g., sees high emotional significance) to the creative process of music improvisation (e.g., novel or ambiguous stimuli) influences the degree of affect he or she experiences through the control of attentional state (e.g., preparation, expectation, prolongation, and potentiation). The delicate balance of affect and attention can be conditioned so that an optimum level is maintained. As suggested by Berlyne (1971), imbalance may result in arousal levels that preclude optimum performance. Performance, regardless of outcome, influences one's affective experience. An opportunity exists in Deep Listening to experience a range of affect through attention manipulation and a range of attentional states through the manipulation of affect.

The development of skill in listening and sounding promises increased creativity and mental health (Newham, 1993). I hope I have shown how some of the mechanisms of learning (e.g., perception and control of affect and attention, including musical training) can enhance the creative experience and affectively manage some of the possible detractions. Deep Listening provides one method to tap into the nonverbal, affective components of creativity of which so much remains to be understood.

REFERENCES

Aiello, R. (with Sloboda, J. A.). (Eds.). (1994). *Musical perceptions.* New York: Oxford University Press.

Amabile, T. M. (1996). *Creativity in context.* Boulder, CO: Westview Press.
Baars, B. J. (1988). *A cognitive theory of consciousness.* New York: Cambridge University Press.
Beaulieu, J. (1987). *Music and sound in the healing arts.* Barrytown, NY: Station Hill Press.
Bejjani, F. J. (Ed.). (1993). *Current research in arts medicine: A compendium of the MedArt International 1992 World Congress on Arts and Medicine.* Chicago: MedArt International.
Berlyne, D. E. (1971). *Aesthetics and psychobiology.* New York: Appleton-Century-Crofts.
Berry, D. C., & Dienes, Z. (1993). *Implicit learning: Theoretical and empirical issues.* Hillsdale, NJ: Erlbaum.
Bloch, S., & Lemeignan, M. (1992). Precise respiratory-posturo-facial patterns are related to specific basic emotions. *Bewegen and Hulpverlening,* 1992 (1), 31–39.
Bloch, S., Orthous, P., & Santibanez-H, G. (1987). Effector patterns of basic emotions: A psychophysiological method for training actors. *Journal of Social and Biological Structures, 10*(1), 1–19.
Boretz, B. (1994). Interface I–V: Texts and commentaries on music and life. In J. Rahn (Ed.), *Perspectives on musical aesthetics* (pp. 116–142). New York: W. W. Norton.
Bruscia, K. E. (1987). *Improvisational models of music therapy.* Springfield, IL: Charles C. Thomas.
Christianson, S. (Ed.). (1992). *The handbook of emotion and memory: Research and theory.* Hillsdale, NJ: Erlbaum.
Csikszentmihalyi, M. (1990). *Flow: The psychology of optimal experience.* New York: Harper & Row.
Deutsch, D. (1975). The organization of short-term memory for a single acoustic attribute. In D. Deutsch (Ed.), *Short-term memory* (pp. 108–151). San Diego, CA: Academic Press.
Foucault, M., & Boulez, P. (1994). Contemporary music and the public. In J. Rahn (Ed.), *Perspectives on musical aesthetics* (pp. 83–89). New York: W. W. Norton.
Gardner, H. (1983). *Frames of mind: The theory of multiple intelligences.* New York: Basic Books.
Gere, R. (1993). Dealing with emotional hangover: cool-down and the performance cycle in acting. *Theatre Topics, 3*(2), 147–148.
Goleman, D. (1995). *Emotional intelligence.* New York: Bantam Books.
Graf, P., & Masson, M. E. J. (Eds.). (1993). *Implicit memory: New directions in cognition, development, and neuropsychology.* Hillsdale, NJ: Erlbaum.
Gregory, R. L., & Colman, A. M. (Eds.). (1995). *Sensation and perception.* White Plains, NY: Longman.
Halpern, A. R. (1992). Musical aspects of auditory imagery. In D. Reisberg (Ed.), *Auditory imagery* (pp. 1–28). Hillsdale, NJ: Erlbaum.
LaBerge, D. (1995). *Attentional processing: The brain's art of mindfulness.* Cambridge, MA: Harvard University Press.
LeDoux, J. (1996). *The emotional brain: The mysterious underpinnings of emotional life.* New York: Simon & Schuster.
Martindale, C. (1995). Creativity and connectionism. In S. M. Smith, T. B. Ward, & R. A. Finke (Eds.), *The creative cognition approach.* Cambridge, MA: MIT Press.
Metcalfe, J., & Shimamura, A. P. (Eds.). (1994). *Metacognition: Knowing about knowing.* Cambridge, MA: MIT Press.
Neisser, U., & Winograd, E. (Eds.). (1988). *Remembering reconsidered: Ecological and traditional approaches to the study of memory.* Cambridge, England: Cambridge University Press.
Newham, P. (1994). *The singing cure: An introduction to voice movement therapy.* Boston: Shambhala.
Oliveros, P. (1985). *Software for people: Collected writings 1963–80.* New York: Smith.
Oliveros, P. (1990). *Deep Listening pieces* [music scores]. New York: Deep Listening Publications.
Oliveros, P. (1998). *The roots of the moment.* New York: Drogue Press.
Posner, M. I., & Raichle, M. E. (1994). *Images of mind.* New York: Scientific American Library.
Posner, M. I., & Snyder, C. R. R. (1975). Facilitation and inhibition in the processing of signals. In P. M. A. Rabbit (Ed.), *Attention and performance V* (pp. 669–682). San Diego, CA: Academic Press.

Radocy, R. E., & Boyle, J. D. (1988). *Psychological foundations of musical behavior (2nd ed.).* Springfield, IL: Charles C. Thomas.
Rahn, J. (1994). *Perspectives on musical aesthetics.* New York: W. W. Norton.
Reisberg, D. (Ed.). (1992). *Auditory imagery.* Hillsdale, NJ: Erlbaum.
Russ, S. W. (1993). *Affect and creativity: The role of affect and play in the creative process.* Hillsdale, NJ: Erlbaum.
Sawyer, K. (1992). Improvisational creativity: An analysis of jazz performance. *Creativity Research Journal, 5,* 253–263.
Schwartz, E., & Godfrey, D. (1993). *Music since 1945: Issues, materials, and literature.* New York: Macmillan.
Schwarzer, R., & Wicklund, R. A. (Eds.). (1991). *Anxiety and self-focused attention.* New York: Harwood Academic.
Shaw, M. P., & Runco, M. A. (Eds.). (1994). *Creativity and affect.* Norwood, NJ: Ablex.
Slife, B. D. (1993). *Time and psychological explanation.* Albany, New York: State University of New York.
Smith, J. D., Reisberg, D., & Wilson, M. (1992). Subvocalization and auditory imagery: Interactions between the inner ear and inner voice. In D. Reisberg (Ed.), *Auditory imagery* (pp. 95–119). Hillsdale, NJ: Erlbaum.
Tame, D. (1984). *The secret power of music: The transformation of self and society through musical energy.* Rochester, VT: Destiny Books.
Taylor, S. (1989). *Positive illusions: Creative self-deception and the healthy mind.* New York: Basic Books.

9

On The Role of Affect in Scientific Discovery

Melvin P. Shaw
Birmingham, Michigan

It is generally accepted that creative artists, writers, and musicians often demonstrate signs of intense emotionality and troubled childhoods; the artistic professions are frequently associated with feelings and emotions and are accepting and integrating of such personalities (Ludwig, 1995). On the other hand, creative academicians, scientists, and politicians often have rather stable and emotionally sound childhoods and develop in a mature and coherent fashion into adulthood. Because of this, the role of affect in scientific creativity tends to be given short shrift. That is, because the personalities of this latter group do not often display mental disturbances or turmoil, and cold logic is believed to be a requirement of these professions, the emotional state of scientific thinkers is considered irrelevant to their creative work. I have recently shown that this is not the case (Shaw, 1989, 1994). The reason for this transcends the issue of mental turbulence and pain. Rather, it is because people's feelings will always be part of them and intimately linked to their rational components (Damasio, 1994). People should be aware that in order to make rational choices in life, it is important that they learn about their feelings, understand their nature and causes, not be overwhelmed or controlled by them, and use them as signals that can aid them in making appropriate decisions.

In this chapter, I address the problem of how to understand and use the role that feelings and emotions, or affects, play in the process of thinking creatively in a scientific fashion. Creative scientific thinking is a timely topic to discuss, because much recent work has been devoted to the general problem of creativity (see e.g., Runco & Albert, 1990; Shaw & Runco, 1994). My goal is to identify and examine the normal feelings (Damasio, 1994), conscious or otherwise, generated by the various stages of the creative scientific thinking process. How does a creator feel during its more mundane phases? Can he or she tolerate the frustration of failing and being unsuccessful most of the time? What is the real joy of achievement, success, and ultimate acceptance by one's peers in a given field?

First, however, I look into what makes people creative in general, with the goal of illuminating underlying mechanisms that couple affect to creativity. Family background and mentorship are very important, and linked to these is the concept of appropriate mirroring via the support and encouragement that in many cases are required. The converse is also significant, in that sometimes the lack of appropriate mirroring is also a motivating factor. (The combination of major pathological personality features, such as depression or manic–depressive states, with other stabilizing components within one individual is sometimes noted.) It seems that the identification of creative thinkers often shows the common human trait of *and,* rather than *or.* Individuals feel this way *and* that way, exhibit a broad spectrum of behaviors, and are commonly capable of a wide variety of different moods, feelings, and emotions. They deal with them in their own style, and at the present time, psychologists ability to *predict* based on these styles is at a primitive stage.

Many professionals involved with the tasks of research and development in science and engineering, and the production aspects of engineering and technology, might agree that a reasonable view of the creative thinking process is that it progresses as follows: Find the "mess," find the facts, find the problem, find the ideas, find the solution, find the acceptance, find the new mess. Further, recent results from a variety of disciplines (e.g., Runco & Albert, 1990) seem to be consistent with the view that there are at least three major features of the creative process from the standpoint of the individual: ideational fluency (the ability to generate many ideas), affect tolerance (the ability to tolerate negative feelings), and intrinsic motivation. Ideational fluency is important for finding the problem, generating ideas (divergent thinking), and arriving at a solution. Affect tolerance is required if one is to persist long enough to find the solution and have it accepted by one's peers, and intrinsic motivation is fundamental to the process as a whole. It is also important to stress that the process transcends the individual. The domain, field, and individual are all linked in a complex manner (Csikszentmihalyi, 1990). In my recent studies, the domain was the area of creative thinking in making mathematical models of natural phenomena, the field was represented by scientific peers and reviewers, and the individual was represented by someone who has the talent and motivation to work effectively in this specific field (Shaw, 1989, 1994).

Although the above parameters appear to be important in describing major requirements of the creative thinking process, it is likely that human behavior, both personal and collective, is best described by processes of deterministic chaos (Shaw, 1989). If this is the case, the occurrence of creative thinking in an individual or social system will always contain unpredictable elements.

THE MODEL

Over the years, a great deal has been written on the creative process. Some authors have suggested that creativity is similar in a wide variety of disciplines, such as visual art, literature, science, and music. Ghiselin (1952) edited a compendium of contributions from a broad spectrum of creative people. Their views, dating back through the eighteenth century, seem congruent with many features of extant models of the creative process. However, in the majority of the existing studies and models, the role of affect, emotions, and feelings has clearly been a secondary concern. To help fill this void, I presented a structural model (Shaw, 1989) for the integrated affective and cognitive components of the creative thinking process in science and engineering that was based on a study of 12 internationally known research scientists and engineers. On the basis of my findings, I developed a process flow diagram (Figure 1) in which the emotional texture was overlaid on the cognitive structure. In some ways, the model is a superimposing of the functions of the left and right sides of the brain, or an overlay of its cortical and precortical components. It represents an integrated view of the various important components of the creative thinking process: flow (Csikszentmihalyi, 1990), illumination, and acceptance. I developed the model by focusing on both the *thoughts* and the *feelings* reported by the scientists and engineers as they recalled their experiences during creative investigations. The process involves the phases of immersion (schooling and learning), incubation (subconscious), illumination (eureka!), explication, and creative synthesis. Validation processes (personal and collective) are also vital.

Four unipolar (positive or negative) and four bipolar (positive and negative) affective components are contained in the structure. The positive unipolar components are the illumination and acceptance phases. The components that exhibit negative polarity are the blocks to illumination and the blocks to acceptance (not being able to "get it" and not having one's ideas accepted). The emotions associated with the positive unipolar components range from neutral to positive feelings; negative unipolar components range from neutral to negative feelings. The immersion and incubation phases are strongly enmeshed with each other, as are the explication and creative synthesis phases. In fact, the incubation phase seems to be embedded in the immersion phase. (These bipolar modes seem to be synonymous with the *flow* states described by Csikszentmihalyi, 1990.) Some of the many themes identified in the study have major affective components associated with them, including getting stuck (anger, fear, sadness, and shame), emotional reactions to illumination and body sensations ("walking on air," good feelings in the stomach and chest, and euphoria), rejection, validation, external pressure, and failure (depression, anxiety, and self-deprecation).

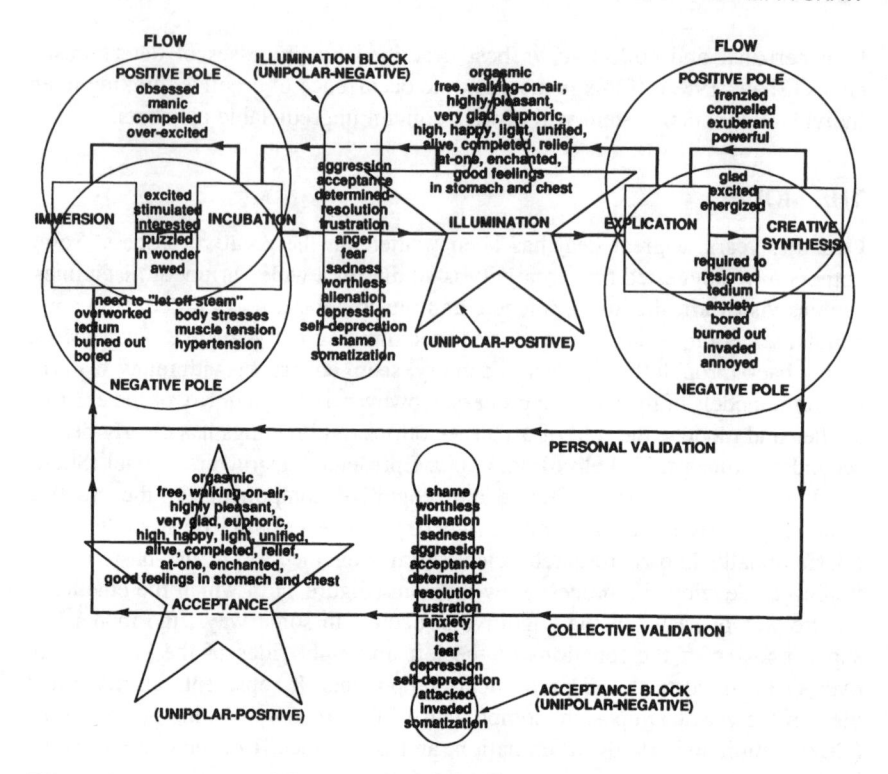

Figure 1

There is a constant interplay between conscious immersion and unconscious incubation. The incubation phase flits around inside the immersion phase like a bubble in a very viscous liquid filling an enclosed container. Illumination occurs at the instant the bubble touches the surface. Here, the blockage evaporates and everything falls into place.

The enmeshment of the explication and creative-synthesis phases is not as dramatic or dynamic. These phases occur after the first unipolar positive phase and are often anticlimactic. The next blockage or resistance appears only when collective validation is sought. Because acceptance by others is often a fundamental need, if individuals do not receive appropriate acceptance, they can use their own egos, if they are firmly established, to sustain them during those trying times, but this is not an easy thing for people to endure for a prolonged time.

Figure 1 is an integrated view of the various important components of the creative process: flow (the bipolar components), illumination, and acceptance. As mentioned, I developed it by focusing on both the thoughts and feelings reported by the scientists and engineers as they recalled their experiences during creative work. They were asked to address the question, What is the experience of making a mathematical model of a natural phenomenon? I used a formal heuristic procedure to gather and analyze the data, tape recording and transcribing their responses, and then searching for general themes and viewpoints. One of the more significant features of the study were the raw affective data; in the following sections, I present a small selection of them and reexamine the potential comprehensiveness of the model. I then discuss the implications, applications, and conclusions.

THE HANDLING OF THE DATA

Here I describe how I analyzed the transcribed tapes of the interviews (more than 200 pages of transcriptions) to determine what the experience of mathematical modeling actually is. The reader should be aware that complete objectivity was not possible. My own prejudices and experiences surely interfered as I examined significant features of the data, as well as during the interviewing process. Such interference is intrinsic to heuristics. Further, working in a heuristic fashion allows for a substantial degree of freedom of choice in methods of inquiry. Douglas and Moustakas (1985) noted that "as a conceptional framework of human science, heuristics offers an attitude with which to approach research, but it does not describe methodology" (p. 42).

As the study began, the first thing that I became aware of was how much experience I already had in the heuristic method without being aware of it. It was the way in which I had always done physics. I had attacked every physics problem heuristically and also had often been aware that I wanted to understand the *process* that I was going through. Indeed, I have been immersed in the problem and question for more than 30 years, most of the time in an unconscious manner.

The choice of the 14 male scientist and engineer researchers to whom I wrote for help was dictated primarily by the ease with which I could interact with them and by their international reputations. I focused on colleagues in the Detroit metropolitan area for obvious reasons. About a week before the interviews, I called the researchers and asked them to think about the question in their spare time. I conducted the interviews in my own home (which I was able to do with all but 2 researchers). This setting was warm, congenial, and open; I believe honest exchanges occurred in all of the interviews that I conducted. The interviews lasted no more than 90 min. They were tape recorded and then transcribed.

At first I believed that I would need 10 to 20 interviews in order to get a clear picture of the feelings that surfaced during the process. I was surprised to find that after 5 or 6 interviews, I had obtained most of the data that I needed; the last few interviews revealed little more than what I had obtained during the first few.

After the data were gathered, the specific interaction with each participant was deemphasized as I undertook a search for themes. These were relatively easy to describe and often were connected intimately to or overlapped with other themes. Once this was accomplished, a model emerged that seemed to describe the essence of the experience in a fairly compact manner.

The themes fell into the two broad categories: structural (the form of the process) and textural (the feelings and emotions associated with each component of the process). Two structures emerged. The first (cognitive) is reflected in the structure of the basic heuristic model with feedback (Shaw, 1989). Superimposed on this structure is the structure of the feelings evoked during the experience, the essence of the experience: the polarities, blockages, bipolar components, and unipolar components. Finally, the textural quality appears primarily as the components of emotions and feelings associated with the complete experience (Figure 1). The emotional structure is then a description of how the texture is organized. Because we have a cognitive structure here too, then thinking clearly plays an important role in the study. The interviewees' thoughts took a variety of forms: images, symbols such as mathematics, and words. Sometimes, some of them thought in more than one way at once. However, the study did not focus on this feature, which is a subject of considerable interest. Rather, it focused on an equally important problem, one that is often neglected at the peril of our species: emotional reactions (Goleman, 1995; Russ, 1993). The results of my interviews and the study of Russ (1993) clearly show that creative thinking involves much more than just thinking in a conscious sense. Unconscious processes and the conscious awareness of feelings are also of utmost importance.

After I had transcribed all the material, an assistant and I read it for specific themes; 19 stood out, some major and others minor. The themes are discussed briefly in the next section. A more comprehensive treatment can be found in Shaw (1994).

In general, the responses obtained during the interviews began with the theme that the creative process in science follows a vague methodology that cannot be clearly delineated or defined. From that starting point, I often directed the interview with a sketchy outline of some of the preliminary features of my personal views of what occurred—the heuristic process. All of the interviewees responded to this lead, when given, in a positive fashion. After a short while, the feelings they recalled experiencing during the different stages of their work started to emerge. I found little or no opposition to my preliminary portrait of the workings of the process, from either a cognitive or an emotional perspective. My personal views were generally either supported or embellished.

The basic contributions of each interviewee, the part of the process that predominated for each, and the highlight of the experience for each did not emerge as fundamental contributions to the work. Rather, the similarities and congruencies between the experiences were overwhelming. Indeed, the major feature was how similar the interviewees' experiences were. However, specific parts of some interviews were sufficiently different from my personal experiences that they are worth noting. In several cases, it was surprising how much the interviewee belittled himself in comparison to someone whom he considered "really" smart. One person said the highlight of a dignified career occurred when a deep understanding emerged from a standard, but complex, textbook problem. Another interviewee insisted that he was unaware of his feelings and completely unemotional; yet his interview belied that self-image. Another debated everything that was said, whether he agreed with it or not. He noticed that his wife often complained about this aspect of his personality. She would say, "Hey, how about not qualifying something, anything, just once?" He said "yes, but" constantly. "Just think," he said, "maybe we'd make better lawyers than lawyers."

Two interviewees, both of whom had previously been in therapy for difficult situational problems in their lives, were good at describing how they felt and had actually thought about the process quite a bit in the past. They needed little prodding. Most of the time, a surprising mix of feelings of arrogance, humility, humbleness, and narcissism was presented.

RESULTS

Ten major themes emerged quantitatively from the interviews: the requirements for becoming immersed, trusting one's intuition, the role of unconscious incubation, getting stuck, letting go and the use of recreation, illumination, emotional and body reactions to illumination, explication and creative synthesis, rejection, and validation and acceptance. Five minor themes emerged: recognizing the problem, pushing for a solution, external pressures, failure, and the general subject of creativity.

Competitiveness and aggression were themes that arose only sporadically during the interviews. This is surprising, because a large number of scientists and engineers are intensely competitive. Perhaps these issues did not emerge because the interviewees' felt ashamed of their aggressive drives or had been taught that the expression of these feelings is taboo or is such a natural part of people that it is implicit in their behavior.

Major Themes

The following quotes represent the major themes that I culled from my data. The linkages are obvious, and are clearly suggested by the heuristic model with feedback shown in Figure 1.

The Requirements for Becoming Immersed

Why hadn't I known of this work? When I saw it I devoured it. Damn, it had the ring of truth to it. I couldn't believe what I was reading. He was right, and I felt it. There is a warmth in the stomach that begins when you know something is correct, some data are important. I had the warmth.

We only develop tremendous skills through hard work and study. It is no different in that sense from the guy who likes sports, or painters. What happens if you're good at something is that you like to do it, because for you it feels easy to do. It's not a struggle. So, once we develop our skills in science, then we like to do science.

Trusting One's Intuition

People have tried models that seem inadequate. I feel that I know something, or have a technique or idea that no one else has had. I feel confident that I might make some progress. I have a technique, I think, which intuitively I feel may lead to something in the problem, even though I don't know exactly how to apply it yet. At this point I reject everything else ever done before. I feel that I understand what has already been done.

So there are two parallel processes. One of the artisan, and the other of the poet or "matchmaker," or whatever you're doing . . . they go together, and the pleasures you get from each other. You might formulate the problem, come up with an equation, and then you feel you don't know how to solve it . . . [you feel like] you failed on one side but put together a good model.

The Role of Unconscious Incubation

That often [just] comes to me. It's like I'll be doing this assimilation process . . . this will sort of brew for a while. Typically, the answer will come to me when I'm at home, doing something else, or if I've had a good night's sleep and came to it very fresh.

Sure, it's like a crossword puzzle. Sometimes the word will come to you when you're not involved with the puzzle. Once you've got your mind in a certain framework of thinking and looking for a word, it's hard to get yourself off a certain track.

Getting Stuck

You stop. You can't get anywhere. Everything stops. You feel that you are ready to come apart. There is a sense of agitation. Frustration starts to appear, along with some anger.

Usually I go through a period of [being] just real bitter. A lot of times I'm so intensely caught up that I start dreaming about it. I have sort of wild fragmented dreams. I think I have solutions, and I don't have solutions. There's a frantic pace to the dreams that is almost a kaleidoscopic kind of thing. It's just going round and round and nothing seems to go. I can't grab anything. I can't contour it. I can't make any sense out of it.

Letting Go and the Use of Recreation

So you're playing [a sport], but you're not playing well, because, unconsciously, you feel that you're still worrying about something else. So your unconscious mind is not focused on the game, which would allow you to play well if it was. You would be playing well if your unconscious were focused on the game, but it is focused on the problem.

I will be stuck on something, so I just go to bed. I may have worked many, many hours, and felt very, very stuck. But then in the morning somehow I know.

Illumination

But if you have that one orgasm, which is "seeing this thing" ... then creative people don't necessarily need drugs. They turn themselves on their way.

Great! That's really exciting. That's fantastic. It's like when you play music or something. You get in a whole lot of practice, and you always miss a note or do something wrong, and then, suddenly, you play it right. Then you feel that you can play this right forever. That feeling is great.

Emotional and Body Reactions to Illumination

... and then you go up again, and then you understand. Sometimes on the down slope you go through a disappointing period of really understanding and realizing that it may not be important. But then you think again that it might be important. So you have all these wavy kind of emotions that you go through, and these wavy emotions often reach a fairly high amplitude, both up and down.

You've heard Paul Simon's album "Graceland." ... He describes a feeling of doing something very, very nice. It's like climbing Mt. Everest. ... At one point he says, "turn around jump shot." I empathize with Dennis Rodman [ex-Detroit Piston] ... with his fists up in the air. I mean it's exactly that feeling. You realize that it's not the end of life. It's something you might have to do again. It's not unique, but it's something you've done, not exactly a lay-up, although it counts as much as a lay-up. But in your mind it counts much more. And that's the feeling you get after the feeling of relief has gone by.

Explication and Creative Synthesis

And commingled with that is the building of another sense of anxiety and a sense of purpose. It's the anxiety that comes with purposeful direction. You know that you got a job ahead of you now ... you got to roll up your sleeves and go to work. The fun is over with.

You could get dejected again, depending on the significance of what you're doing. The dejection stage may very well last longer than the euphoric phase. After a while you get pragmatic. You become involved with the nitty gritty of writing it up, publishing it, presenting it. The worst part of writing a paper is looking up references.

Rejection

They cut me out of the program. I wouldn't be on TV. I felt like shit, really worthless. I had very high expectations, and then suddenly, nothing. Really worthless. I was angry and sad, but it was more worthlessness. I do have the sense of enormous fear of publishing stuff and being held up as a fool . . . on many things.

I sent the papers to the wrong journals and got brutal reviews. That sent my blood pressure so high that I had to go on some blood pressure medication. I hate to admit just how much it affected me.

Validation and Acceptance

I need more feedback in order to get to the next stage. . . . The first stage is where I do something, and then there's the second stage which is feedback from other people, which is becoming to me more and more important.

Ah, wait till I tell the son of a bitch. Wait till I show him this . . . you know, that's part of the arrogance of I'm better than you are.

Minor Themes

Recognizing the Problem

There is a constant unconscious and conscious involvement with this frustration, which you put before yourself. It keeps going and going, and then you see the problem. It's like tennis. You've been practicing all the time, you make a lot of mistakes, and then hit a great shot.

If nothing excites me, I'll go start reading literature. This can go on for anywhere from a day to several months. Then I'll grab hold of something and say, "This sounds like an interesting problem."

Pushing for a Solution

[He would say to his 3-week-old daughter, perched on his desk,] "How the hell do I solve this equation? Come on, tell me; don't sit there like a dummy."

I really don't have it. I was dancing around. I was sparring: one right thing; one wrong thing. A lot of things were being sparred. I had to think about it. And what happened was I went to bed thinking about it. I had a lousy night's sleep.

External Pressures

Distraction factors. If there are too many other things happening—personal life, social life, too many different jobs being input—that seems to slow it down. But too few things seem to slow it up also. There's like an optimum number [for each person].

Negative emotional experiences come mainly from funding pressures, not the scientific pressure. There is this getting money to support the thing; people then consider it as not "real" research work because there's no money attached to it . . . that frustrates me sometimes.

Failure

[When you fail, it's] a total case of despair and disappointment and sadness, incredible sadness. We once thought we had the world by the tail, but it didn't work . . . and we got sadder and sadder and sadder and sadder . . . and it was a very bad moment for all of us. It was as if a pot of gold at the end of the rainbow suddenly turned to brass.

Failure is a more personal involvement than success.

The General Subject of Creativity

A lot of people are smart—high IQs—but they are not creative.

You know, I'll tell you one thing, that sort of education is not what the students get at all. So, maybe, if they were made aware at a younger age of what really goes into scientific creation, and that indeed it is creation, just like a painting is a creation, they would appreciate more the powers that they have to develop, and you would get more creative people trying it.

IMPLICATIONS OF THE FINDINGS

Several implications arise after some reflection on the findings. Those that come to mind immediately address the following questions:

1. Is there a unified process associated with the experience of creative behavior of all types?
2. How fundamental to people's basic needs are the concepts of illumination and acceptance?
3. What is the significance of the difference between personal and collective validation?
4. What is the role of affect tolerance (Krystal, 1988) in the creative process?

It is clear from the discussion so far that there may well be a dominant, preferred, or even unique natural process (Douglas & Moustakas, 1985) at work when a human being is acting in a creative fashion: the heuristic mode, the structure of which is outlined in Figure 1. Ghiselin (1952) stated,

The creative process is not only the concern of specialists, however; it is not limited to the arts and to thought, but is as wide as life. Or perhaps, it would be more correct to say that invention in the arts and thought is a part of the invention of life, and that this invention is essentially a *single process*. (p. 24, emphasis mine)

There are substantial and exquisite differences between individuals, families, tribes, and cultures. However, it is not difficult to imagine that since people's body parts are all similar and function essentially in the same manner, regardless of whether they're an Eskimo or Aborigine, their brains might also *process* input in an identical manner. If so, the concept of a unique creative mode is not as farfetched as one might think.

With regard to the concept of illumination, an interesting view was put forth by May, Angel, and Ellenberger (1958), who saw it as "the moment when eternity touches time." It occurs when *meaning* is given to events that have occurred in the past or are capable of occurring in the future. In this interpretation meaning ("aha!") is dominant. In other views, such features as *completion, euphoria,* or *orgasm* are used. Whatever the personal feeling, there is clearly the implication that both illumination and acceptance by the relevant community are unipolar positive modes; individuals rarely, if ever (except perhaps in pathological personalities), have negative feelings when they are illuminated or accepted. Hence, one might expect that there is a drive toward these positive unipolar modes akin to the natural biological drive toward orgasm. People can live without it, but without it they react to their blockages, which are unipolar and can led to emotional discomfort and, ultimately, pathological behavior. They get no *relief* but can get temporary *release* by letting off steam, which is often self-abusive or abusive to others. Lastly, the proposed similarity between the sex drive and the drive toward illumination is consistent with Freud's controversial view that it is a simple matter to redirect libidinal energies into nonsexual arenas. The payoff is similar. That is, when one is immersed in an exciting creative act that is not sexual, one's sex drive might well be diminished.

I would also like to propose that the collective modes of validation and consciousness offer more rewards than the personal modes. First, the collective mode contains the unipolar positive mode of acceptance, whereas the personal mode does not. Second, the collective mode allows for more rewards (positive strokes) from fellow humans; this concept is a means toward establishing a more satisfying life. Indeed, Freud (1-1950) pointed out that

> the asocial nature of neuroses has its genetic origin in their most fundamental purpose, which is to take flight from an unsatisfying reality into a more pleasurable world of phantasy. The real world, which is avoided in this way by neurotics, is under the sway of human society and of the institutions collectively created by it. To turn away from reality is at the same time to withdraw from the community of man. (p. 74)

Of course, there are other ways to attain peak experiences, such as the runner's high, which is certainly a personal validation. Appropriate drugs will provide one with similar feelings of power and euphoria and so-called mystical experiences. These experiences, too, are forms of personal validation. However, they decouple individuals from the collective consciousness. Indeed, they often alienate the individual, separate him or her from the local and nonlocal communities and provide few or no strokes from others. They ultimately fail because of this deficiency. All the drugs, running, and self-indulgence imaginable will not substitute for the basic need for bonding, which is physical closeness and emotional openness with our fellow humans. As humans, we *need* to be autonomous, to show *others* what *we* can do, and to have *them* accept *us*.

The last implication lies in the area of affect tolerance (Krystal, 1988), one of the three major personal parameters of the creative process that I identified earlier, the others being ideational fluency and intrinsic motivation. The present results identify rejection and failure as critical components of the creative process, a view consistent with the findings of various researchers. (The issues surrounding failure are perhaps best summarized in a review of Epstein's, 1990, work by Runco & Albert, 1990.)

Rejection as a form of failure and failure itself commonly produce the negative feelings outlined in Figure 1: anger, fear, worthlessness, depression, shame, and so on. To be able to work through these feelings in a way that allows them to be encapsulated or controlled by the meanings and lessons of the failure appears to be a vital component that lets the individual stay on track and continue along the creative path. In this regard, perhaps a primary educational component should be the *teaching of the affective features of the creative process*. Imagine all the talent wasted by those who are ignorant or unappreciative of the role that feelings play in the process.

APPLICATIONS OF THE FINDINGS

With regard to applications, possibilities exist in the areas of education, understanding human behavior, psychotherapy, and motivation. In terms of educational process, institutions have always focused primarily on the immersion phase, where assimilation dominates, and it is clear from the present study that to be creative, scientists must be knowledgeable. They don't have to be as knowledgeable as possible, but they must have a clear, uncluttered view of the field and be skilled in the use of its tools so that ideational fluency is optimized. In contrast, teaching about creativity has been sorely lacking in the educational system. Perhaps one of the reasons for this is that the subject appears to be intimately connected to emotional state, to the right side of the brain, and the mood of the 20th century is predominantly logical and scientific. The acceptance of the role that emotions play in the process could lead to an enhanced educational environment for young people. They might learn that it's quite acceptable to sometimes live inside the feelings of the unipolar negative pole of the blockages, to feel aggression, frustration, anger, anxiety, fear, worthlessness, alienation, shame, and depression. Everyone, even the greatest creative talents, has some or all of these feelings at one time or another. Humans are apparently *born* with the affects of anger, pleasure, sadness, and fear. It is not acceptable, appropriate, or in the individual's best interests to deny their existence and the role they play in the most creative parts of life. Young people would do well to learn to accept and appreciate their feelings and to learn affect tolerance, that is, not letting their normal negative feelings impede their development. In this way, they can learn to trust themselves, feel good about themselves, and believe in themselves. It is invaluable for them to learn that being able to express and use their feelings is as important to their creativity as the fundamental need to immerse themselves deeply in an appropriate knowledge base that fits their temperament, intellect, and desires (intrinsic motivation). Toward this end, people need to understand their behavior via a two-pronged attack—thoughts and feelings. When they learn to further their understanding of who they are, individuals can learn to trust themselves and their intrinsic powers.

Finally, one might inquire into the implications of the results in the area of psychotherapy. B. Miller-Shaw (personal communication, May 1987) suggested that her experience as a psychotherapist has led her to view therapy as a multistep process. Her steps include awareness of a problem or pain, incubation, insight, self-explanation, decision, action, and integration. In the heuristic structure, the awareness lies in the immersion phase, the decision and action phases are the creative synthesis, and the integration is the validation feedback loop. Change does not occur in the person unless the learning experience is integrated into the personality, unless the person *grows,* reaching a new level of knowledge. More significantly, the structure may provide a reason why insight-oriented therapy sometimes, if not often, works. In this therapeutic modality, the key is the insight or peak experience. The attainment of peak experiences (eureka!) has exceptional results in many cases. Maslow (1968) stated,

> The person in the peak experience feels more integrated (whole) than at other times ... more at peace with himself ... more efficiently organized ... more able to fuse with the world. (p. 104)

This can be interpreted as a feeling of oneness with the greater human condition. It is therefore suggestive that blocks to insight presented by repressed material and strong defenses in psychotherapy may be similar to blocks to creativity in general. Erasure of early negative "tapes" and repressed material and effective reprogramming (working through) might have a more useful application than previously imagined. The identification of the above structure with loops also leads one to muse about specific psychopathologies. Loops, of course, can produce knots, internally or externally. However, because the loop process can be one of growth, with the individual reentering the immersion phase at a higher level, the structure might more appropriately be modeled as a spiral. It is easier to visualize helices enmeshing than to envision closed loops. Helices might be the preferred embodiments by which psychopathology can best be modeled in patients who appear to be stuck or trapped.

With reference to the problem of motivation, it is important for managers and leaders in business enterprises to understand that creativity is far from simply a cognitive process. It involves human processes that have deep feelings, both positive and negative, associated with them. If productivity is to be optimized, workers' emotional needs will have to be met. This means learning to appreciate and work with feelings and to be aware that negative feelings are a normal part of the process. It is also important to realize that great highs come from both illumination and acceptance and that acceptance usually means not only a personal statement that the work is really appreciated, but also an appropriate financial remuneration.

One might also point to similarities, rather than differences, between individuals as well as between groups to find further justification for the above considerations. For example, sufficient similarities exist between religions, cultures, and psychotherapies to suggest the existence of a human creative process. As mentioned earlier, although individuals are unique and different, the *processing* of information might well be the same for all members of the species. Even the constant battle between political philosophies can be thought of within the creative process; rugged individualism (personal consciousness) versus socialism (the collective consciousness). One can see that a proper balance must be struck between developing freedom without exploitation and societal control without restricting personal creativity.

In this chapter, I have proceeded through three different categories. Firstly, in the Introduction I noted several parameters presently in use to describe creative behavior and developed my own descriptive model. In comparing and contrasting my model with others, I showed that there is significant overlap with specific features of several other models (e.g., Ghiselin, 1952; Runco & Albert, 1990; Russ, 1993; Weisberg, 1986), suggesting that the present one is worthy of attention. My model seems to be congruent with others in enough areas to be reasonably comprehensive in scope, especially when it focuses on the areas of intrinsic motivation and, in particular, affect tolerance. However, given that one of my guideposts is the suggestion that human beings are probably governed by the laws of deterministic chaos, the model might ultimately be considered simplistic.

I then reported on my analysis of the interview data and presented excerpts to convey some of the richness of the emotional experiences described by the interviewees. The utility of this is obvious, and it should be especially helpful to all students, particularly graduate students, in that they can feel the ultimate human qualities of these eminent scientists and engineers. It might aid students substantially to know that the process they are involved in is similar for all practitioners, no matter what stage of development they are in.

Lastly, I discussed the implications and applications of the study. I concluded that there might be a unified process associated with all types of creative behavior; that acceptance by one's peer group is a fundamental need, and hence that collective validation is generally more significant than personal validation; and that affect tolerance is a critical parameter in allowing for the development of personal creativity.

REFERENCES

Csikszentmihalyi, M. (1990). *Flow: The psychology of optimal experience.* New York: Harper & Row.
Damasio, A. R. (1994). *Descartes' error.* New York: Avon Books.
Douglas, B. G., & Moustakas, C. (1985). Heuristic inquiry: The internal search to know. *Journal of Humanistic Psychology, 25,* 39– .
Freud, S. (1950). *Totem and taboo.* (Original work published 1913 [Vienna, Hugotleller]) New York: W. W. Norton.
Ghiselin, B. (Ed.). (1952). *The creative process.* New York: Mentor Books.
Goleman, D. (1995). *Emotional intelligence.* New York: Bantam Books.
Krystal, H. (1988). *Integration and Self-Healing.* Hillsdale, NJ: Analytic Press.
Ludwig, A. M. (1995). *The Price of Greatness: Resolving the Creativity and Madness Controversy.* New York: Guilford Press.
Maslow, A. H. (1968). *Toward a psychology of being.* New York: Van Nostrand.
May, R., Angel, E., & Ellenberger, H. F. (1958). *Existence.* New York: Basic Books.
Runco, M. S. & Albert, R. S. (Eds.). (1990). *Theories of creativity.* Newbury Park, CA: Sage.
Russ, S. (1993). *Affect and creativity.* Hillside, NJ: Erlbaum.
Shaw, M. P. (1989). The eureka process: A structure for the creative experience in science and engineering. *Creativity Research Journal 2,* 286–298.
Shaw, M. P. (1994). Affective components of scientific creativity. In M. P. Shaw & M. A. Runco (Eds.), *Creativity and affect* (pp. 286–298). Norwood, NJ: Ablex.
Shaw, M. P., & Runco, M. A. (Eds.). (1994). *Creativity and affect.* Norwood, NJ: Ablex.
Weisberg, R. W. (1986). *Genius, creativity and other myths.* New York: W. H. Freeman.

Part Three

Creativity, Psychopathology, and Adjustment

10

Tension, Adaptability, and Creativity

Mark A. Runco
California State University at Fullerton

Happiness in intelligent people is the rarest thing I know.—Ernest Hemingway (1986, p. 97)
Relish the struggle, that's the way.—Dick Francis (1987)
Never regret a genuine show of feelings.—Shamus Archie Goodwin in *Bloodied Ivy* (Goldsborough, in press, p. 41)

One of the most interesting cases of creative work is that of the Wright brothers. Their case shows the relevance of Zeitgeist, for example, as well as the benefits of persistence and a willingness to take risks. It also shows how judgment can be mistaken. After all, although Orville and Wilbur's original flight was in 1903,

> the original Wright Flyer spent 25 years under dustcovers in a Dayton shed. When no institution in the United States wanted it, it was lent to the science Museum in London and displayed there from 1928 to 1942. Not until 1942 did the Smithsonian at last accept that the Wrights were indeed the creators of powered flight, and not until 45 years after the historic flight was the craft at last permanently displayed in America. (Bryson, 1994, p. 327)

The Wright brothers' case also demonstrates the usefulness of what is often called *strategy,* but should probably be viewed as *tactical creativity.*

Parts of this chapter were presented in a symposium at the 1994 annual meeting of the American Psychological Association, Los Angeles, California.

The Wright brothers used several tactics of creativity: They looked for *analogies* (e.g., the wing of a bird and the wing of a "flying machine"), and they did this through *visualization*; they *broke a large problem into smaller ones* (i.e., weight, power, and control of the aircraft); they *sought out useful information* (writing others who were working on the problem of flight); and they *collected plenty of data*. They collected data in various ways, even building their own wind tunnel to do so.

Perhaps most surprising was the strategy they used with one another: They argued. They worked in their bike shop and later in their workshop in Kitty Hawk, Wilbur taking one side of some technical problem and Orville taking the opposing side (Combs, 1979). They yelled and debated—and then switched sides and argued again. The fact that they switched sides of the argument at hand confirms that the Wrights were using this technique intentionally and tactically to solve the problems of flight. It also distinguishes their efforts from competition, which can inhibit creative work (cf. Abra, 1989; Shalley, in press).[1]

Very likely, the argument tactic used by Wilbur and Orville forces individuals to follow a line of thought to its logical conclusion. It probably also leads to a questioning of assumptions and a consideration of other perspectives. The questioning of assumptions and openness to different perspectives represent widely accepted techniques for creative problem solving (Parnes, 1985). Most generally, argumentation probably creates constructive tension. This tension may in turn motivate a change of perspective and the questioning of assumptions.

The huge success of the Wright brothers suggests that other creators might benefit from tactical argumentation. Then again, arguing and tension have potential costs, as well as potential benefits. With tension comes the potential for stress. Is it worth it? Do the benefits outweigh the costs? These questions are addressed in this chapter.

Given that so far I have cited only the Wright brothers as evidence, the first question here concerns whether or not there is in fact a reliable relationship between tension and creativity. I address this question not only by reviewing creative efforts that seem to have been influenced by tension, but also by examining evidence for an association between the adaptability that is elicited by various forms of tension and creative efforts.

Adaptability and various forms of tension have each been tied to creativity. Cohen (1989), K. Gardner and Moran (1990), Flach (1990), Rothenberg (1990b), Runco (1994), and Valliant and Valliant (1990) have, for instance, suggested

---

[1]Tension is used tactically not just in the sciences. At least one kind is used in the arts. I am referring to the practice, most common in literature and poetry, of counterpoint, which is "any artistic arrangement or device using significant contrast or interplay of distinguishable elements" (Kuiper, 1995, p. 275). Counterpoint may of course by used for an effect other than creativity, but, then again, more specific effects (e.g., contrast and thereby a new perspective) may be related to creativity. As an example of counterpoint, Kuiper (1995) described "motions in dance juxtaposed rhythmically and visually against music or against other motions by parts of the body or groups of dancers" (p. 275). Thus, just as the Wright brothers were strategic about arguing for insights, artists too, can use tension via counterpoint.

that creative efforts are often motivated by the need to cope with these various forms of tension, and the development of creative skills is often described as a response to trauma and challenge (e.g., Goertzel & Goertzel, 1962). If these views hold up, creativity might be defined as a special type of coping or adaptability. This possibility is important for many of the same reasons that the association of creativity with general intelligence is important. Psychometricians point to the need for discriminant validity, for example, the idea being that when two constructs are nearly perfectly related, they may be redundant. If creativity is always strongly related to general intelligence, there would be no need to measure it—researchers could simply assess intelligence and know about creativity. Similarly, if creativity is simply a kind of adaptability or coping, it might be a waste of time to distinguish between the two of them.

In this chapter, I review the research that suggests that there is a connection between creativity and tension. In this regard, the present chapter is an extention of my earlier effort (Runco, 1993a). There I found tension implied by discussions of marginality, asynchrony, resilience, disequilibrium, problem gaps, and the like; and each was related to creativity, at least some of the time. Since the publication of that review, I have found that I underestimated the power of the concept of tension; I have discovered many more theories and findings about creativity that implicitly or explicitly rely on tension. Those additional theories and findings are reviewed herein.

In addition to reviewing the research on tension and creativity and addressing the question about the distinctiveness of creativity from adaptability and coping, I offer tentative suggestions about what should be done if creativity is in fact related to tension and stress. If creativity is enhanced by the experience of stress, should stress be sought out? Should parents and teachers, for instance, intentionally introduce challenging situations to give their children and students practice adapting and creatively coping?

EXPERIENCE, TENSION AND CREATIVITY

Many common experiences have the potential to create tension. These experiences may occur in nearly any facet of one's life; they may be professional experiences, familial, or otherwise interpersonal (e.g., Albert, 1978; K. Gardner & Moran, 1991; Pritzker & Runco, in press). I begin this section with examples from the developmental research and then touch on experiences related to education and work within a career. Both interpersonal and intrapersonal tensions are described along the way, as are conflicts that might arise between individuals and social or cultural expectations.

Developmental Research

Albert (1991; Albert & Elliot, 1973; Albert & Runco, 1987), Osche (1990), and Winner (1996) each reported that stress experienced during childhood may contribute to the development of creative skills. Albert (1991) found that the creative person to be comes from a family that is anything but harmonious—one which has built into its relationships its orientation of roles and its level of communication a good deal of tension if not disturbance, what I call wobble, but along with these characteristics there is commitment to achieve as opposed to "having fun," a special focus of interest and aspirations upon the child and a great deal of family effort to see that these aspirations are met. (Albert, 1978, pp. 203–204)

Along the same lines, Albert and Runco (1987) described the parents of certain exceptionally gifted children to be "aloof." An aloof parent may allow the gifted child to develop the autonomy and independence that can in turn contribute to a nonconforming creative mode of thought. There is, however, an optimal level of distance; autonomy and nonconformity are not things parents should maximize. This must be emphasized, because autonomy and nonconformity do not necessarily lead to creative insights. Sometimes they lead to serious social and emotional disturbance. This idea of optimization will arise throughout this chapter.

In her work on gifted youth, Winner (1996) suggested that a child who experiences stress may escape into "an obsessive, solitary focus on an area of talent.... Hardship could teach lessons in perseverance and resilience, two ingredients needed for later creativity" (p. 300). Winner also suggested that stressful experiences might contribute to the child's "willingness to be different" and his or her need to work to control a seemingly unpredictable world. The control may compensate for some loss, and losses do occur with alarming frequency among the gifted (Albert, 1980).

Barron (1963) tied the experience of tension to the motives of creative persons:

> The creative artist and scientist appear, when one reads biographical accounts, to have experienced an unusual amount of grief and ordeal in life and to have shouldered burdens of pain that most commonly disable the individual.... The creative individual is one who has learned to prefer irregularities and apparent disorder and to trust himself to make a new order. (p. 157)

He added, "The motive is thus generated for searching out other situations which would seem to defy rational construction, with some degree of confidence that after much deprivation, tension, and pain a superior form of pleasure will be attained" (p. 157).[2] The result of tension, in this view, is not just tolerance or coping skill, but instead a kind of preference. Creators may see potential within chaotic situations and actually seek tension.

---

[2]There may be sex differences in this regard. I raise this possibility because Helson (1996) recently reported finding that creative women "were not comfortable with uncertainty." This seems to be at odds with Barron's (1969) idea that creative persons "have learned to prefer irregularities and apparent disorder and trust himself to make a new order." Helson and Barron used somewhat different methods, so it is possible that the difference is methodological.

How common is trauma in the lives of creative persons? In Goertzel and Goertzel's (1962) biographical study of 400 eminent individuals, the majority of participants had "in their childhood experienced trauma, deprivations, frustrations, and conflicts of the kind commonly thought to predispose one to mental illness or delinquency" (p. xii). The Goertzels found that only 52 of the persons in their sample had untroubled home lives, leading these investigators to conclude that "the comfortable and contented do not ordinarily become creative" (p. 131). There were significant group differences, with all actors (100%) in their sample experiencing developmental tension, followed by novelists (89%); musicians and composers (86%); explorers and athletes (67%); and philosophers, religious leaders, and psychologists (61%). Inventors experienced the least tension (20%). The Goertzels suggested that many creative persons benefit because they use work to compensate for the tension experienced.

Given changes in the American family (Elkind, 1981), it would be very interesting to replicate the research of Goertzel and Goertzel (1962). In fact, a replication is necessary, because of the possible biases in such biographical studies. They may be distorted by self-reports or interpretive tendencies of biographers, for example; this is especially likely because creators who succeed in the face of adversity make for an interesting biography. Descriptions of adversity and success are likely to be salient and thus more memorable. This is problematic because the creators who experienced adversity may in fact be less common than those who did not, and the association between adversity and creativity might be exaggerated by the subjective weight given to the unrepresentative but highly memorable cases. MacKinnon (1962) felt there was notable potential for bias because persons who experienced "distress" were "motivated to reveal themselves" (p. 367).

Earlier, I contrasted the tactical argumentation used by the Wright brothers with competition, but before leaving developmental forms of tension behind, I should mention what may be the more common tension reflected in sibling rivalry. Sulloway (1996) explained sibling competition in Darwinian terms, suggesting that siblings must compete for resources, including parental attention. What I am calling tension, then, would be seen in a struggle for resources. Sulloway felt that competition could explain the robust birth order effects found again and again in the creativity literature (e.g., Albert, 1980). In addition to the parallel between tension and the struggle for resources, it is interesting that Sulloway took a Darwinian tack and used adaptability to explain birth order effects. First-born children, in Sulloway's view, adapt to the birth of sibling by relying on strategies that cannot be used by their less-mature brothers and sisters. In fact, younger siblings would not use these strategies even if they could, because the objective is to find a unique niche within the family. Later born children often develop lifelong strategies and behavior patterns that lead them to original behavior, or even rebellion, because this provides them with a unique niche within the family.

Education

Roe (1963) described a conflict arising between the value system of the home and that characterizing school. Such conflict may have occurred with greater regularity in the past, when parents wanted their children to stay home because that is what they themselves had done or because there was work around the home that needed to be done. Today, the conflict is more likely to occur when parents prefer one kind of education but the teacher holds a different educational philosophy. Of most relevance would be a discrepancy between the appreciation of originality expressed by either a parent or a teacher and a lack of appreciation in the home or the school (Raina, 1980; Runco, Johnson, & Baer, 1992).

Another instance of potential conflict, also relevant to education, is implied by Simonton's (1987) claim that the best mentors are similar, but not too similar, to their students. Optimal dissimilarity may minimize the imitation that could inhibit originality and might follow from extreme similarity and compatibility. Working with the right mentor may put a student in a position where there is what John-Steiner (1992) referred to as "productive tension between social connectedness and individual immersion in one's task." This could describe the benefit for the mentor; who also gains from his or her work with (younger) students (Mockros, in press; Zuckerman, 1978).

Rubenson and Runco (1996) recently identified potential conflicts that can arise between the structure of the educational setting and the spontaneity of young students or between the expertise of the teacher and his or her young (and thus flexible) charges. These investigators described the conflicts using psychoeconomic theory, as they had done in explaining how groups can be optimized for creative work (Rubenson & Runco, 1992). Certain interpersonal conflicts are highly likely in groups and can be used to facilitate creative work. Groups should, for instance, contain individuals who have worked in the area for a long time, as well as individuals who are relatively new to the area. Those who have worked in the area for a long time will bring expertise and large knowledge bases to the group; they will, however, tend to be less flexible than newcomers. The psychoeconomic explanation for this emphasizes the magnitude of the investments the experts have made in their own knowledge bases, the assumption being that a change in thinking that might undermine their expertise would cause a kind of depreciation of knowledge. Thus it is only natural for them to be resistant to new ideas, and such inflexibility would covary with the level of investment (i.e., expertise). Confidence is also a factor, as are other individual-difference variables that have been noted in research on the rigidity of older and more experienced individuals (Abra, 1989; Barber, 1961; Chown, 1961; Diamond, 1980; Feist, 1994; Messerli, 1988; Oromaner, 1977; Schultz, Kaye, & Hoyer, 1980).

Seyle (1988) gave autobiographical evidence for this, relating his inexperience as an intern to his conceptualization of human stress and the general adaptation syndrome.

The many features of disease that were already manifest did not interest our teacher very much because they were "nonspecific"—not characteristic of any one disease—and, hence, of no use to the physician.... *Since these were my first patients I was capable of looking at them without being biased by current medical thought.* Had I known more, I would never had asked questions. (p. 257)

This case is doubly relevant. Not only did Seyle benefit from his inexperience; he also brought a concept (i.e., stress) from one domain (i.e., engineering) to several other fields (e.g., medicine and psychology). Later I discuss this technique as made possible by marginality.

Of most importance for education is that the lack of flexibility among more experienced individuals can lead to interpersonal tension in the form of debate, the benefits of which would be reaped by the younger individuals in the group. Their role in the optimal group is to be adaptable and flexible and to integrate the various perspectives offered by the experienced group members into a creative and original insight. Thus it is not just dyads, like the Wright brothers, who might systematically use debate—larger groups or committees might do so, as well, If nothing else, this is good news for academics who wonder about the time they invest in committee work! For educators, the lesson is to avoid the rigidity that may accompany expertise.

Numerous other theorists have found benefits resulting from early difficulties. Rutter (1985), for instance, described how "unpleasant and potentially hazardous events may toughen an individual" (p. 600). VanTassal-Baska (1989) wrote that "adversity appears to teach certain lessons about perseverance and achievement" (quoted in Subotnik, Kassan, Summers, & Wasser, 1993, p. 107). Ochse (1990) suggested that "creators typically suffered some deprivation and distress in childhood" (p. 81). K. Gardner and Moran (1990) concluded that family "cohesion is not necessary for creative" (p. 285). MacKinnon (1960/1983) described creative persons as often characterized by "life histories marked by severe frustrations, deprivations, and traumatic experiences" (p. 369). He felt that such a person learns to "tolerate the tension... and in life and work he affects some reconciliation of them" (p. 377). In very recent research, Helson (1996) concluded, "The creative personality is relatively consistent over time.... However, we find substantial variations in the creative vitality of individuals as they moved into or were forced to move out of an encouraging environment" (pp. 296–297). Helson found that the creative women in her longitudinal study "did not give up under conditions of adversity."

Adulthood

Much of the work just described, including the longitudinal findings from Helson (1996) and the theory of optimal groups (Rubenson & Runco, 1992), suggests that tension may influence development and adaptation that occur during adulthood. Mumford (1984; Mumford, Olsen & James, 1989) went so far as to propose that particular adult needs and experiences predispose young adults to exceptional creative insight. He pointed to the common responsibilities experienced in early adulthood (e.g., raising children or finding a job) and suggested that these can force the young adult to maintain a high level of flexibility, which in turn prepares him or her for creative work. Mumford cited the tendency for major breakthroughs in some fields to come from young adults. The assumption is that young individuals are readily adaptable because they have a large number of demands placed on them. The "late-life style" (Arnheim, 1990; Cohen-Shalev, 1989; Lindauer, 1993; Schwebel, 1993) suggests that adaptations are quite possible during later adulthood. As Lindauer (1992) described it, aging artists often need to "accommodate to life's new demands" (p. 219). Those accommodations are reflected in their artwork—hence the late-life style.

Csikszentmihalyi's (1988) theory of "abreactive creativity" assumes that although tension or trauma is experienced early in life, the effects make themselves known only in adulthood. He was explicit about early experience when he wrote that trauma

> is very prevalent among contemporary painters' memories of childhood. Whether the viewer realizes it or not and often also unbeknown to the artist, the images that form the core of a great number of modern works represent the rage or ecstasy of childhood which the artist tries to recapture in order to integrate it into current experience. (p. 219)

Csikszentmihalyi referred to "a magical synthesis of past and present, abolition of objective time, a healing through the reactivation of former pain which can now be tolerated by the mature person" (p. 219.) He referred to this kind of reexperience as "abreactive originality," which he defined as "the symbolic reordering of repressed traumatic experiences" (p. 219). He contrasted abreactive originality with "cathartic originality," which implies an immediate or current discomfort.[3]

Perhaps artists are drawn to artistic careers because they are motivated to express themselves (Jones & Runco, in press). Albert and Runco (1987) alluded to something like this, describing the prerequisites of a particular career and a possible match with the individual's cognitive and affective tendencies. Sheldon (1995) approached this empirically by studying "goal conflict," defined in terms of "personal strivings." Striving was not correlated with creativity, but subjective ratings about the ability to cope with and resolve conflict were positively and significantly related.

---

[3]Incidentally, Jones (1995) recently completed her dissertation on artists' reports of influences and found that many artists apparently have some difficulty recognizing how early experience manifested itself in their work. This is not to say that the influence was not there. Some of the influence may be preconscious (cf. Smith & Amner, 1997). Jones's findings do point to another problem with research in this area, to go along with those noted earlier (cf. MacKinnon, 1962; Winner, 1996). Selection biases are quite possible, as are those associated with subjective reports.

Tension would actually be more likely when there is a mismatch—when the individual finds him- or herself in a career that does not match personal needs, interests, or thinking styles. Surely conflict and tension can occur when persons with particular cognitive styles find themselves in a career that rewards a style that is different from their own. The "tension between tradition and innovation" that Sawyer (1992) found in jazz improvisation suggests that it may be style or simply (lack of) experience.

James, Chen, and Goldberg (1992) examined particular dispositional tendencies that might match task requirements. They suggested that when there is a match, there is no tension, but when conflict between disposition and task demands is perceived, there is an increase of creative effort. These investigators concluded that settings might be constructed such that there is a match or mismatch between dispositions and specific tasks within the setting. In this view, when there is a match, more creative work will be done. This of course fits with what Albert and Runco (1987) suggested about how disposition might fit with career area, but it seems to contradict what I noted above about tension from a mismatch. A resolution is suggested by the research on optimal matches, which are optimal in the sense that the individual is challenged but does need to adapt and grow. The research on optima was reviewed by Runco and Sakamoto (1996) and Runco and Gaynor (1993).

James (in press) reported that "conflict experiences" facilitated originality when an individual was working in a domain of his or her preference or that fit with his or her potentials. Originality was restricted in other domains. James focused on social and instrumental personality dispositions and on a controlled and impersonal kind of conflict, namely, that between an individual's disposition and a particular task; however, such controlled conflicts induced in research may not be all that indicative of those that occur spontaneously in the natural environment. This is the well-recognized concern about the external validity of findings from controlled studies (see Runco & Sakamoto, in press). Similarly, the conflicts studied in the research may not be indicative of the tensions that might actually occur in one's personal experience. Still James's work is a reminder about domain specificity.

H. E. Gruber (personal communication, August 1994) believed there is a need to distinguish between the tension associated with work and that which is associated with other, more personal aspects of life. He went so far as to hypothesize that an individual does not draw on his or her personal life as much in certain domains, like the sciences, as in other domains, such as the arts (cf. Ludwig, 1995). (Gruber proposed that psychology is right in the middle between science and art.) If this holds, interpersonal and intrapersonal tensions might be expected to have different functions in the different domains. Presumably, science is more often a social activity than the arts, and although this is not always the case, it implies that interpersonal tension might have a stronger influence in the sciences. It is also possible that tensions experienced as part of one's work may be more tolerable because they are generally sought out and thus relatively predictable, at least compared with some of the surprises presented for example, by one's children. Personal tensions may be more ambiguous and more emotional because of the unpredictability. Certainly, work can be emotional and personal lives can be intellectual, but the point is that there are different kinds of tensions, and some may be more common in one's professional life.

It is possible that an interpersonal tension currently motivates some of the research on creativity. Overby (in press), for example, suggested that there is a polarization between contemporary psychologist-artists and psychologist-scientists. His distinction parallels Kimble's, 1984, description of the scientific and humanistic cultures within psychology, but Overby focused on creativity. He concluded that individuals studying creativity should think more like artists. I recently suggested just the opposite (Runco, in press)! I raised this alternative because persons who study creativity value originality and as a result regularly place too much emphasis on original research and not enough on integrative research. The problem that might arise is fragmentation or, more metaphorically, the reinvention of the wheel. In contrast to what Overby suggested, my conclusion was that those studying creativity may be biased and not looking carefully enough at relevant work because they value the arts so much and in some ways imitate artists. My assumption was that whereas artists can often get away with being contrarian, science is inherently cumulative, and scientists should therefore carefully integrate their work with earlier research. With a little luck, tension between the two sides of this debate will elicit further research and thinking about the creativity research.

Marginality

Recall that the Wright brothers owned a bike shop and then moved to the problems of aeronautics. They were experts in one field but moved into another. That move may have helped them by allowing them to see the assumptions in their new domain and bring ideas from the old domain (the mechanics of bicycles) to the new (aeronautics). Obviously, the Wright brothers are not the only ones who benefited by working in two domains or moving from one to another. Piaget may have similarly benefited, in as much as he was trained as a biologist and then studied developmental psychology. Freud was trained in physiology and then turned to the psyche. H. Gardner and Wolf (1988) explored the benefits for Freud and viewed the movement I am discussing as "professional marginality." They also described the advantages of "cultural marginality," like that experienced by Picasso after he left his native Spain (when he was quite young).

Many individuals feel that travel opens one's mind and broadens one's perspective. Campbell (1960) thought that people's being exposed to different cultures seems "to have the advantage in the range of hypotheses they are apt to consider, and through this means, in the frequency of creative innovation" (p. 391). Lasswell (1959, p. 213) looked more generally to societal innovation and suggested an analogy between innovation and the biological concept of "hybrid vigor." He posited that the intermingling of cultures can stimulate innovation. Presumably, this applies to creativity as well as innovation.

I can jump back to development at this point, because tension should be expected during development, when a child's egocentric behaviors take him or her into conflict with cultural expectations (e.g., about cooperation, social harmony, or etiquette). It would be naive to think that socialization and enculturalization can occur without some direction and redirection by parents and teachers, and these will often go against egocentric ambitions of a young child.[4]

Thus developmental, educational, professional, and cultural forms of tension may be associated with creativity. Many of the examples I have given seemed to have their effect by forcing a shift of perspective. Recall in this regard Rubenson and Runco's (1992) description of young professionals and students as adaptable because of their flexibility, the assumption being that individuals with flexible outlooks are able to adapt because they can see alternatives or perspectives other than their own. Consider also the increase in the number of hypotheses Campbell (1960) thought would result from being able to compare and contrast different cultures and the open-mindedness he thought might result from travel. If I am correct that one benefit of tension is that it can facilitate a shift of perspective, researchers need to exercise caution when interpreting the findings and theories outlined above. It would be easy to focus on the objective experiences and specific stressors and assume that these are the primary determinants of subjective disequilibrium (and even creativity). This of course is not the case. Objective experience is not all-important. Tension often originates in subjective experience and is moderated by subjective processes. With this in mind (no pun intended), I wish to consider the role of top–down processing in the taking of a perspective and the interpretation of tension.

TOP–DOWN PROCESSING

There are numerous reasons to believe that objective experience is not the primary determinant of behavior. Top–down processing originates with cognition, rather than experience, the basic idea being that experience is potentially influential, but only after it is interpreted. Top–down processes are subjective and conceptually driven; they determine how experience is interpreted and how it influences creative functioning.

---

[4]Some recognized cultural assumptions are relevant. Gordon (1987) and Trelfa and Stevenson (1996), for example, explained educational differences between cultures in terms of adult assumptions. Gordon pointed to the tendency for Asians to "believe in personal malleability" (p. 5). This assumption leads Asian parents to emphasize motivation. They feel that their children can do better in school just by trying harder. In the United States, on the other hand, many parents believe that performance reflects ability, and this means that effort is not all-important. These parents may assume that academic performance cannot easily be improved. Tension may occur if parents believe in the malleability of personality and for that reason push for more and more effort, while the student (or the teacher) does not hold the same belief or is already doing his or her best.

The most convincing evidence for interpretation may be that demonstrating that measures of perceived stress have been found to be better predictors of health than the so-called objective (events) measures (e.g., Mraz & Runco, 1994). Recall also that James et al. (1992) emphasized perceived conflict. As a matter of fact, all research on perceptual processes assumes top–down processing. This is because perception is typically defined specifically in terms of the interpretation of sensory stimuli. Percepts thus reflect the interpretations individuals construct from their experience. Smith and Amner (1997) recently presented an overview of the research on perception and creativity.

Tension in the form of stress may occur when an individual perceives a gap, need, or challenge in the environment. It may also arise with little or no input from the environment. Conflicts may arise, for example, between one's conscious mind and logical inferences and emotions or between different emotional reactions. Schuldberg (1994) recognized the latter when he referred to the "personal access to simultaneous, contradictory emotions [which] can provide an important and even necessary component of creative work." Intrapsychic tension is also implied by the asychronies that can result from a person's having blends of intelligence. H. Gardner and Wolf (1988), for example, described how many eminent creators, including Freud and Picasso, may have benefited in this regard, Freud being strong in personal and verbal intelligence and Picasso strong in spatial intelligence but unexceptional in other areas. H. Gardner and Wolf relied on Gardner's own theory of seven intelligences, and his acknowledgment of an eighth intelligence further broadens the possible asynchronies and benefits (H. Gardner, in press).

The "essential tension" that Kuhn (1963) found inherent in the creative process seems to represent another intrapsychic form of tension. Kuhn wrote;

> Something like convergent thinking is just as essential to scientific advance as is divergent. Since those two modes of thought are inevitably in conflict, it will follow that the ability to support tension that can occasionally become almost unbearable is one of the prime requisites for the very best sort of scientific research. (p. 342)

This is an important claim, in part because it brings divergent and convergent thinking into the process. Divergent thinking has become one of the most commonly used models to describe the potential for creative thought (Guilford, 1950, 1968; Runco, 1990–91; Torrance, in press). The practical significance of Kuhn's (1963) theory lies in the fact that so many programs have been designed to enhance creativity, and they often assume that convergent and divergent thinking can be separated. They may, for instance, require that participants postpone convergent thinking in order to think more divergently. This is a dubious assumption if Kuhn was correct about the inevitable conflict. In actuality, both convergent and divergent thinking are probably required for most expressions of creativity (Khandwalla, 1992; Runco, 1993c, in press). They may work together in a complementary or even synergistic fashion, and any incompatibility may be fruitful when it creates the essential tension.

Creative persons may experience a high level of tension specifically because they have more original ideas than other individuals. Intrapersonally, tension may arise because divergent ideas are original precisely because they are distant from experience and evidence. It is tension between what is and what could be. Root-Bernstein (1984) referred to something like this in the sciences as a mismatch between theory and evidence.

Certainly, domain differences need to again be recognized. Kuhn (1963) and Root-Bernstein (1984) mentioned the sciences; but the arts have a reputation of allowing professionals (and nonprofessionals, for that matter) to use their emotions. (Recall H.E. Gruber's idea, mentioned earlier in this chapter, that a career in the arts requires more personal involvement than other careers.) This in turn implies that artists are more likely to encounter intrapsychic tension of the variety that has its basis in affect. Because emotions may be inexplicable through conventional and objective logic, a logical analysis will not well understand them. This is especially true if the individual attempts to understand the tension by relying on conscious tactics. Objective logic may not easily grasp emotional logic. For this reason, tension with an emotional basis may be the most difficult to understand.[5]

I am suggesting that tension may arise between conscious logic and emotion, but there are other possible relationships. In fact, there is an ongoing debate about the possible interplay of cognition and affect. Dudek (in press) suggested, for instance, that an "immediate response is prior to understanding," which implies that feelings precede cognition (also see Schuldberg, 1994). Rothenberg (1990a) referred to the "functional integration of cognition and affect" (p. 420) and suggested that "cognitive functions are used to express and clarify affect, and affective functions guide cognition in all creative activities" (p. 420). Russ (1993) described a "pleasurable anticipation" with "affect as a cue."

If we assume for a moment that emotions can occur without before (and therefore independently of) a logical analysis, it is possible that the individual may have a feeling that something is missing and this may function as a cue or guide. That individual may be motivated specifically to logically understand that feeling. Although this is an abstract argument, there is a great deal of research on the cues that are used by creative individuals and research on individual differences in cue usage (e.g., Baker-Sennett & Ceci, 1996; Martindale & Armstrong, 1974; Mendelsohn & Lindholm, 1972; Smith & Amner, 1997; Wallach, 1970). Moreover, a sensitivity to cues would help explain behaviors often labeled intuitive. Such behaviors may simply reflect actions that are elicited by ambiguous or subtle cues or by the tension between feeling and understanding. The

---

[5]This may explain the strong association between the arts and intrinsic motivation (e.g., Stohs, 1992). If artists devote themselves to attempting to express their thoughts, and those thoughts have some basis in their emotional life, they would be very personally meaningful. No doubt, many artists feel the need to express themselves and are able to understand the need (in the sense of traditional logic) only after the work is done.

subtle cues may be affective or aesthetic. They may be reactions to tension that is difficult to fully recognize or articulate.

James et al. (1992) explained tension by adapting the argument often used with anxiety, namely, that it is a sign that there is a problem at hand. They wrote, "Such perceptions and feelings may serve as a signal that standard patterns of thinking and behaving have not succeeded" (p. 548). The experience of tension is in this sense a signal that something new must be attempted, which is another way of saying that an original, more creative approach should be used. May (1977) and Rogers (1984) each said something very similar about anxiety.

Granted, just as it is unrealistic to assume that divergent and convergent processes are entirely distinct, so too is it unreasonable to dichotomize the mind into emotions versus logic. More often than not, it is unreasonable to separate logic and affect. It may make the most sense to view affect as relying on a logic of its own, rather than viewing it as alogical. In these terms, emotional logic is difficult to understand and may seem chaotic and unreliable. Yet the criteria of being easy to understand and reliable are only bugaboos from a perspective that relies on traditional logic. They make sense only from that perspective.

Consider here the claim occasionally made that young children are not logical in their problem solving. Of course, children may seem to be alogical when they make some of their decisions, but actually they can be quite logical, even early in life. They seem to be alogical because the kind of logic they use differs from that used by adults, to whom it may seem that children are not using any logic whatsoever. The irony is that children's lack of conventional logic can actually contribute to their creative thinking (Runco, 1996). Children may make fewer assumptions, for example, and consider more options, and they may be more mindful of experience than adults. This spontaneity can facilitate the finding of original ideas.

When thinking creatively, both children and adults can use metaphoric logic (Levine, 1984; Runco, 1996), another kind of thinking that may appear to be alogical, but only from the standpoint of conventional logic. It is quite possible that metaphoric logic is functionally related to the logic used by emotions, but this, too, may be difficult to fathom from the standpoint of conventional logic. Fortunately, here it is necessary only to acknowledge the possible logic of emotions, without delving into the specifics of how exactly it differs from conscious, objective, and conventional logic. The fact that it differs may explain certain intrapersonal tensions, seemingly intuitive behavior, and personal creativity.

CREATIVITY AS INTERPRETATION

I define creativity as "the intentional transformation of objective information into original and yet meaningful interpretations, coupled with the ability to decide when this kind of transformation is useful and when it is not" (Runco, 1996). In addition to emphasizing process rather than product, this definition favors personal creativity over creative achievement and everyday creativity over eminent creativity.

Very likely, each person constructs numerous interpretations every day—but perhaps not as many as some people think. How often do you put effort into actively constructing a new, original interpretation of your experience? For many experiences, it is easier for individuals to assume that they understand what they are seeing and put no effort into checking the details. Rote behavior is all too common. No construction there—and no originality.

Note the role of discretion suggested in my definition of creativity. This is where affect comes into play, because individuals often exercise their discretion to suit their comfort and pleasure—in other words, in accordance with their affective tendencies. Many decisions reflect this kind of discretion, and as I suggested in the preceding section, they may not be entirely logical in the conventional sense.

This is important because it supports the idea that tension may be in part a reaction to emotions and may act as a guide. Bronowski (1958/1977) described something like this when he wrote,

> The man who poses a theory makes a choice—an imaginative choice which outstrips the facts. The creative activity of sciences lies here, in the process of induction. ... To the man who makes a theory it may be as inevitable as the ending of Othello must have seemed to Shakespeare, but the theory is inevitable only to him; it is his choice, as a mind and as a person, among the alternatives which are open to everyone. (pp. 10–11)

Dewey (1933, p. 108) noted something similar in his theory of scientific work. He suggested that there is an emotional facet to initiate the process, or "what at first is merely an emotional quality of the whole situation" (i.e., a scientific problem).[6]

Mumford et al. (1996) examined what the cognitive basis for this process might be. They found that individuals with exceptional problem construction abilities were able to use inconsistent cues about problems and still produce high-quality solutions to presented problems. Individuals lower in problem construction ability did not produce high-quality solutions and were unable to use inconsistent cues. These findings strike me as pertinent because the inconsistent cues used in the experimental materials would be expected to elicit the kind of tension I described earlier. The research was controlled experimentation; but if

---

[6]The emotional basis of scientific work itself has costs and benefits. The benefits are implied in this section of the chapter and by the idea that hunches and the like often lead scientists to their most significant discoveries. The costs are apparent in the biases that sometimes arise (Runco, 1994). These were implied by Rubenson and Runco (1992) and explained as depreciations; but many other examples can be found for such bias. Of course, bias per se is not undesirable—it is a natural result of emotional involvement. The problem arises when bogus data are reported or experimental results fabricated.

I am correct about the inconsistent cues, the process is a common one in creative work in the natural environment.

Cues in the natural environment may be ambiguous, however. They may have an emotional basis and thus not be open to logical or conscious analysis, as I have already suggested. An alternative view is that the cues are only preconsciously processed. Albert and Elliot (1973), Dudek and Verreault (1989), Kubie (1958), Rothenberg (1990), and Russ (1988) each described how the creative process can benefit from access to preconscious material, and often that material will be difficult to grasp except as a somewhat ambiguous message. Albert and Elliot (1973) noted that

> preadolescent creative children are less likely to use repressive defense in recognizing a personal conflict, and, along with this, appear to have greater cognitive facility with and access to cognitive resources at different levels of consciousness than less creative people. (p. 177)

It may be a guide when creators have a hunch or feel they are getting close to their objective, but that feeling may be difficult to articulate. In the terms used earlier, the preconscious material may be more emotionally meaningful than logically cogent. In these terms, the idea of tension as a cue or guide helps explain the accuracy of feelings of warmth (Jausovec, 1994; Metcalfe, 1986; Runco & Sakamoto, in press) as well as intuition (Policastro, 1994). Feelings of warmth and intuition may depend on a tension that cannot be articulated.

Disequilibrium and Creativity

I have suggested that tension sometimes functions as a cue or signal. Creative persons are, however, not exceptional only in being open-minded and sensitive to ambiguous cues. After all, creative work is often proactive and not always reactive (Heinzen, 1994). Recall Barron's (1963) description of creative individuals as often seeking out challenges knowing there are potential benefits. Moreover, creative individuals often define problems; they do not just solve them when they encounter them. Most telling for the view that creators are proactive is the common description of intrinsical motivation. The developmental and educational experiences listed earlier in this chapter may explain how individuals develop the necessary tolerance and the coping skills, but it is also possible to offer hypotheses to explain how tension motivates creative work.

Several hypotheses are suggested by the descriptions of problem solving as a kind of disequilibrium (Piaget, 1976; Runco, 1994a; Stein, 1960). Stein, for instance, used the concept of disequilibrium to explain the sensitivity of creative persons, and Runco added that disequilibrium elicits intrinsic motivation. Piaget (1976) proposed that individuals adapt by assimilating new information and then accommodating by building or reorganizing cognitive structures. Importantly, he believed that individuals are intrinsically motivated to adapt and understand their experiences. In this way, the individual experience disequilibrium—the tension resulting from a discrepancy between knowledge and experience—is naturally intrinsically motivated to resolve the conflict. Often this requires that people assimilate and accommodate to develop a new understanding of their experience.

Piaget's (1981) thinking that individuals are intrinsically motivated by disequilibrium seems to be compatible with what Lazarus (1991) proposed about the need for a cognitive appraisal and logical understanding of tension or some problem before interest is piqued. (I would add that different kinds of logic may characterize this logical understanding.) As Lazarus described it, people appraise situations and react only to those that are important to them. They do not care much about things they do not recognize (appraise) as important. The implication is that cognition (i.e., the appraisal) precedes the affect, which includes interest and motivation.[7] This perspective is part of the debate I cited earlier concerning cognition and affect. Zajonc (1991), for example, held a different view—that affect can be independent of cognition. What is most important is the idea that the intrinsic motivation results from people's recognizing that there is a gap in their experience, a gap between what is and what can be or simply between their present cognitive state and their immediate experience. If that gap elicits what I have called tension, this same theory can explain how such tension can motivate, as well as act as a guide.

Wertheimer (1945), Henle (1977), and Torrance (1974) each described the role of a gap in creative problem solving. A gap is intriguing, because it does not refer to anything concrete. On the contrary, a gap indicates that something is missing or lacking! In these terms, creative persons may react to what is *not* there, rather than what is. Perhaps creativity is necessary to recognize such a hypothetical nonexistent thing as a gap.

In any case, it is possible that tension creates disequilibrium, which in turn motivates the individual. Then, if the individual has the necessary creative skills, he or she can apply them to the problem at hand. In this light, disequilibrium may be responsible for the intrinsic motivation that ensures that individuals apply themselves but is not responsible for any other part of the creative work. Original insights and divergent thinking may often result from such intrinsic motivation, but only because the individual has a personal investment and interest in the problem at hand: The person is intrinsically motivated. In this sense, tension is a necessary but not sufficient explanation for creative effort.

DEFINING "PROBLEM"

Some individuals may be capable of coping and confident about resolving conflicts because they have already experienced similar problems. Their history of conflicts may allow them to view apparent problems as operational challenges.

---

[7]A second implication is that intrinsic motivation is a result of a more fundamental process. This is why I wrote earlier that the concept of intrinsic motivation lacks explanatory power—it relies on deeper cognitive functions.

It is possible that creative persons are less dependent on personal histories for this kind of interpretation. Their experience may allow them to trust that their creative skills will help in novel situations and that problems can be interpreted as challenges rather than problems. Some persons apparently use their creative abilities to construct interpretations that reflect challenges and opportunities, rather than problems. In addition to the trust, it may be that creative skills are necessary for the constructive part of the process. That was implied by my earlier idea about gaps, namely, that a gap is not a thing, so it must be invented.

The point is that just as perceptions of a potentially stressful experience differ among individuals, so do perceptions of problems. Root-Bernstein (1993) saw this when he described how problems can be translated into "some internalized fantasy of a visual, kinesthetic, tactile or combined sensual form." He used the term *synscientia,* derived from *synesthesia* and *scientia* "to know" to describe successful thinking of this sort.

Creators themselves often discuss transformations of problems. Schuldburg (1994) quoted Wittgenstein on "the disappearance of problems," for example, and in fact Schuldberg described the disappearance nicely himself as a dissolving of previously insoluble personal, technical, or aesthetic problems. Of course, the problem is not really disappearing. Instead, it is being transformed into a challenge or opportunity. At one point there is a problem, but then the creator starts working on it and it may become a pleasant experience, or at least something tolerable, rather than an unpleasant difficulty. Runco (1996) proposed that a reinterpretation explains why individual creators report becoming so immersed in a project that the self is lost. Barron (1996) described this as a merger of self and nonself, or subject with object.

The idea that problems are interpretations is consistent with the theories of problem finding that are common in the creativity literature. It is not unusual for a creator to see a workable and profitable problem where others see nothing. (Again we have the notion of invented gaps.) Darwin is an example, because he saw evolution, and in particular adaptive reactions of species, in the variations among species of finches, while the ornithologists of his time—the experts!—saw only ambiguous variations (Boynton, 1996, p. 80). This example also ties the idea of interpretation to the psychoeconomic theory mentioned earlier, in that Darwin was a novice when it came to birds and was able to use the finches as his data. The experts were less open to new possibilities in their area of expertise.

The reinterpretation of problems is not just a feature of genius. Kirschenbaum and Reis found something similar in their recent investigation of artists who were women raising children. In the words of the investigators,

> Ironically, the obstacles that they encountered, such as the absence of support from spouses and parents, financial difficulties, and time necessary to raise their children, were perceived by these women as contributing in some ways to their creative process and the development of their identities as artists.

Problems may not be problematical, or they may be problematical but turn out to be problems that contribute to creativity. Creators faced with such "problems" may be happy to have them! Artists with children are good examples of this; after all, they have children to appreciate, *and* they find themselves in a situation where they must concentrate on their work whenever they have a free minute.

DISCUSSION

Admittedly, I have cast a wide net in this review and attempted to tie a large set of concepts to tension and creative adaptations. Interpersonal debate, marginality, disequilibrium, problem gaps, and problem finding and solving were each explored. Reactions to the various forms of tension were also varied, as would be expected, given the diversity of the concepts themselves and what I suggested earlier about individual differences in interpretations.

Several of the explanations for the association between tension and creative effort focused on motivation. Disequilibrium can lead to intrinsic motivation, and certain traumatic experiences elicit behaviors that may be motivated by the need for compensation or cathartic work. Other explanations suggested that the response to tension is a kind of learning or conditioning. Tension may allow an individual to develop patience or tolerance, or it may simply force careful scheduling, as was probably the case for the artists who were mothers (Kirschenbaum & Reis, in press). Perceptual explanations described tension as a guide, a means by which the individual found cues, or an opportunity to shift perspective. The benefits, then, when they occur, may be short-term (e.g., a shift of perspective or careful scheduling) or long-term (e.g., tolerance or catharsis).

Although it is easy to assume that tension is a result of experience and a determinant of creative effort or insight, it is also possible that creativity can cause tension. Think about the nonconformity that often characterizes a creative individual. Nonconformity can easily disrupt a classroom, where collaborative behaviors make instruction flow smoothly and nonconformity, daydreaming, autonomy, and several other traits common to creative persons are counter to expectations (Runco, 1984; Torrance, 1962). The autonomy that characterizes many creative individuals could similarly create tension in some families or a traditional organization (Runco, 1995b). In very general terms, creative behavior is deviant (Richards, 1996; Runco, 1996) and can easily disrupt activity that assumes a routine. Most activity is routine, if not outright stereotyped. Creative behavior can therefore cause tension, because it disrupts routine. The correlation and coincidence of tension and creativity may occur because the latter causes the former, at least some of the time.

This direction of effect would help explain why Kaun (1990) found writers to have remarkably short life expectancies. Kaun suggested that the creative writing process requires the individual to lead a unhealthful lifestyle (e.g., isolation and delayed gratification). This, along with the expectations of writers to act in an eccentric fashion, supposedly contributes to the low life expectancy. The direction of effect starts with the writing and ends with the eccentric, unhealthful behavior, much of which is simply stressful.

The same direction of effect was implied by Barron's (1963) claim that creators seek out disorder and by Rubenson and Runco's (1992) description of the "active intellectual investments" made by many creative persons. As Kaun's (1990) research demonstrates, many investments made by creative persons have the potential to elicit or create tension and stress. In psychoeconomic terms, these are the costs of creative work and efforts. Some are temporal and some psychic. Temporal costs derive from the fact that the individual doing creative work is not using his or her time for other things. Psychic costs include the stigma mentioned briefly above, which may result from being different (or contrarian or simply original), as well as the tension that can result when an individual is working on something original but does not yet have one concrete solution.

Another option is the correlational one, whereby a third factor is the causal agent for both creativity and tension. A likely agent is access to the preconscious. Creative persons may have easy access to the preconscious (Rothenberg, 1990), and this may help them in several ways. It may, for instance, help them to find creative insights that are highly original or radically divergent precisely because they are free of censorship and pressure. That same freedom can, however, simultaneously cause anxiety. After all, some of those ideas bouncing around in the preconscious are frightening. Others can elicit guilt when brought into consciousness, and guilt can easily lead to anxiety. In this light, creativity could be correlated with anxiety, but the anxiety and the creativity could each actually depend on a third process, such as access to the preconscious. There are other possible third variables (e.g., openness to experience or a general sensitivity), but the point is that creativity and anxiety or stress can be correlated without being interdependent.

If creativity and tension are merely correlated and not interdependent, certain individuals could have one but not the other. And this is true of course: some persons do experience stress but do not behave creatively in response to it. Others are creative without tension to motivate or guide them. Milgram and Hong (in press) found that individuals with "high levels of work accomplishment" reported growing up in families that were highly cohesive and supportive.

> Winner's (1996) distinction between gifted and creative youths is relevant because most of the studies showing that families of creators are stress-filled and not very child-centered are retrospective and recount families of an earlier era. Since today's families are in general more child-centered, it is possible that families of future creators are more like the families of typical gifted children. (pp. 375–376)

Winner intimated that creative children differ from "typical gifted children" in that there may be no tension and stress in the background of the latter.

Independence is further suggested by the creative persons who commit suicide (Jamison, 1994; Ludwig, 1995; Runco, in press). This is especially pertinent given findings that individuals suffering from depression have the most realistic worldviews (Heinzen, 1994) and depression is among the best predictors of suicide (Mraz & Runco, 1993). There are many creative persons who are not depressed and seem not to consider suicide. Rogers (1971) and May (1971) both described creative persons who were self-actualized and thus largely free of psychological disturbance (see also Runco, Ebersole, & Mraz, in press). That may reflect their interpretive tendencies, rather than their lack of experience with tension or trauma.

Creativity as Adaptability: Necessity Is Not the Mother of Creativity

The question of the direction of effect leads us back to the issue of creativity as adaptability. Creativity is often defined as a kind of adaptation, yet the diverse reactions to tension reviewed herein suggest that creativity does not always result in an adaptation. Some persons seem to experience tension early in their lives and then deal with that experience for the rest of their lives. One could not really say that these persons have adapted; at least, one could not say they have completed the adaptation. Granted, the process may be what is important, and creative work may give these persons a process they can use to deal with a problem.

Other evidence supports the independence of adaptability from creativity. Adaptations are typically reactive, for example, but creative work is sometimes proactive (Gruber, 1993; Heinzen, 1990). Necessity may be the mother of invention, but it is only a cousin of creative work, and not always even that. Certainly, the distinction between proactive and reactive behavior can at times be ambiguous. Richards (in press), for example, recently described "the draw of the aesthetic," which implies that what may appear to be proactive by observers may feel reactive to the creators themselves, an implication also of the various indications that tension is a cue or guide. Still, the reactive basis of creativity might also be questioned because it suggests that creativity always involves a problem. However, creativity often encompasses more than problem solving. Creativity might be a form of self-expression, for example, and the individual may not really have a problem, but may be simply doing preferred work. This kind of creativity may be the most likely in self-actualized persons (Runco et al., in press), but keep in mind the earlier discussion about the "disappearance of the problem" (Schuldberg, 1994) and the merger of self and nonself (Barron, 1995).

Perhaps the most striking differences between creativity and adaptability can be posed with a question: What would adaptable persons do in an uncreative environment? What would they do if the pressures placed on them are for conformity? If they are truly and indiscriminately adaptable, they will conform (cf. Cashdan & Welsh, 1966; Schubert, 1988). Although I am against generalizations, I am comfortable saying that comformity is never creative. Conformity goes against the most basic feature of creativity, which is originality. The birth order research supports this argument in the sense that first-born individuals are often relatively uncreative (or at least unrebellious) precisely because they adapt to a situation (i.e., birth of a sibling or siblings) with elevated levels of need for achievement. Following personality theory, it is a specific kind of need for achievement: achievement through conformity (Runco & Albert, 1996).

For that matter, what about creative efforts that are not adaptive? Creativity is often manifested as a kind of deviance (Richards, 1996), and deviance is not always adaptable, at least for the individual. The same creative work may contribute to the adaptability of a group or species in the sense that it creates variability (Gould, 1997), but the deviant individual in society is often punished, rather than reinforced, for his or her deviance. This is much the same logic used by evolutionary biologists evaluating the adaptive value of altruism, which is often not beneficial for the individual but can be advantageous to the survival of his or her genes.

The definition I gave earlier for personal creativity implies that creativity and adaptability are related but distinct. Personal creativity is manifested whenever the individual intentionally constructs a meaningful and original interpretation of his or her experience. Such interpretations are assimilatory, and as Piaget (1981) noted, assimilation is only one part of an adaptation. Complete adaptation requires accommodation and a change in structure, in addition to the assimilation of new information. This leads to the conclusion that interpretations are necessary but not sufficient for adaptations, which implies a distinctiveness.

Empirical evidence to support the conclusion that creativity is distinct from adaptability was provided by Helson (in press). She found that

> the Ego Resilence scale . . . is significantly correlated only with OCS [occupational creativity], not with any of the measures of creative potential. Furthermore, ratings of psychopathology, based on questionnaire data at age 43, were significantly correlated with two of the measures of creative potential. . . . It appears that *creative potential is not associated with recovery after setback and resourceful adaptation to the changing circumstances of life* (p.).

Helson also reported an association between "negative emotionality" and creativity and concluded that "negative feelings are an important source of originality and insight." She put it this way: "Some say that creativity is a demon to which the creative person's relationships and personal growth are sacrificed." Again, the idea is that costs are often associated with creative efforts.

Empirical findings from Russ (1988) seem to support a clear relationship between creativity and adaptability, but the correlation coefficients she found, though statistically significant, indicate that the overlap was only moderate. In particular, she found a correlation between an adaptive regression score on a Rorschach test and divergent thinking ($r = .34$, $p < .05$) and a correlation between teachers' ratings of students' coping and the divergent thinking of those students ($r = .58, p < .05$). These significant correlations were found when the scores from boys in the sample were analyzed independently from those of the girls. Coefficients for the girls were not significant. Even the largest of the significant coefficents for the boys indicated that only 34% of the variance was shared. This is a far cry from redundancy.

Conclusion

What are the implications of the evidence for some sort of relationship between various forms of tension and various expressions of creativity? There are several. One is the need for more research and new methodologies. Too much of the research reviewed herein was based on biographical or autobiographical material. Selection biases are quite possible, as are those associated with subjective reports (cf. MacKinnon, 1962; Winner, 1996). Given the similarities that seem to exist between tension and stress, it may be that the methods used to study the latter (e.g., comparisons of objective indices of stress with assessments of perceived stress) might be used in studies of creativity. A large number of relevant studies are available, so a meta-analysis would also be worthwhile.

As for applied recommendations, there are several options. At one extreme is the conservative recommendation to avoid tension, or at least to avoid intentional tension. This conclusion is based in part on the uncertainty about the association between tension and creativity. Which causes which? Or is there a third variable determining each? This recommendation is also based on a concern about sampling. Debate seems to have worked for the Wright brothers, but it would be unreasonable to assume that it would benefit everyone. The Wright brothers could be an isolated case, an exception—in fact, they obviously were exceptional—and it may be that people for whom the costs of tension outweigh the benefits far outnumber those who have experienced tension or trauma and been creative specifically because of it. A third basis for what I am calling the conservative recommendation is the observation that there may already be enough tension in the natural environment! Moreover, the amount of unintentional stress may be on the rise (Elkind, 1981). Unintentional tension may be more meaningful and appropriate than any that can be construed. The conservative recommendation, then, is simply that tension should be viewed as an opportunity when it presents itself, but it should not be courted.

There are relevant traits that can be targeted by researchers interested in enhancing creativity, but without intentional tension. Several traits common to creative individuals were mentioned above, such as sensitivity and openness to experience, but it is possible that there are other traits within the creativity complex that might be required specifically for resilience and adaptability. Ego strength comes to mind. Surely it could be targeted.

The rebuttal to this is the less conservative perspective. It suggests, first, that ego strength and resilience develop only when some tension is experienced. If children never experience stress, they may never learn to deal with it. As Valliant (1977) put it, "the human ego grows in adversity as well as in prosperity" (p.

336). Perhaps the important parts of the creativity complex, ego strength included, require tension and adversity.

These views represent the extremes, but Valliant's (1977) words hint at what may be the realistic compromise. In particular, he pointed to adversity *and* prosperity. Ego strength may grow best with a little of each. The compromise relies on the concept of optimization. I mentioned examples of optima throughout this chapter, including the match between one's disposition and the task at hand, optimal dissimilarity of mentors and students, and optimal group composition. Optima are also clearly suggested by the experimental research on stress and creativity (e.g., Toplyn & Maguire, 1991). Runco and Sakamoto (1996) found optima implied by the scaffolding of parents when they present tasks to their children that are just above current functioning levels. Scaffolding can be defined as a kind of intentional, optimized tension.

Consider next the example of aloof parents mentioned earlier (and in Albert & Runco, 1987). Surely too much distance could easily communicate to children that they are not important, undermining their sense of security or even their sense of self. This will more likely inhibit rather than stimulate children's creativity. Helson's (1996) conclusion that "the creative personality ... is tough but not unmalleable or invincible" (p. 305) is very compatible with my conclusion about optimal tension.

Interestingly, children may play an active role in such optimization. This is implied by theories of transitional objects (Albert, 1996; Miller, 1993; Ostwald, in press; Singer, in press; Winnicott, 1950). Transitional objects are most often found in a child's attachments to his or her caretakers. The child may have an object—a toy or blanket—that provides comfort and security and thereby allows exploration. The notion of a transitional object, which is often chosen by the child, not the parent, implies a gradual maturation. Even more relevant is that the quality of early attachments may determine the capacity for adaptation. If this is true, and if adaptation is at all functionally related to creativity, those same attachments may also have some bearing on the development of creative skills. Cohen (1989) presented a continuum of creativity from childhood to adulthood that relies increasingly on mature modes of adaptability.

The optimization that characterizes scaffolding and transitional objects suggests that timing is a factor. Optima are optimal only at certain times. Careful timing is also necessary so the effects do not accumulate. It might be best if tension is distributed such that the individual is not overwhelmed by any one experience or by the accumulation of disturbance and depletion of resources. Very likely the benefits of distributed practice that are so clear for learning and conditioning (Dempster, 1988) are also applicable to the timing and optimization of tension.

Generalizations about optimal levels of tension are difficult to make, because of the interpretive nature of tension. With this fact in mind, I suggest that Nietzsche's well-known dictum be changed from "that which does not kill me makes me stronger" to "that which does not kill me *can* make me stronger." It can make an individual more creative, but there is no guarantee.

REFERENCES

Abra, J. (1989). Changes in creativity. *International Journal of Aging and Human Development 28*, 106–126.
Albert, R. S. (1971). Cognitive development and parental loss among the gifted, the exceptionally gifted and the creative. *Psychological Reports, 29*, 19–26.
Albert, R. S. (1978). Observations and suggestions regarding giftedness, familial influence and the achievement of eminence. *Gifted Child Quarterly, 22*, 201–211.
Albert, R. S. (1980). Family position and the attainment of eminence: A study of special family positions and special family experiences. *Gifted Child Quarterly, 24*, 87–95.
Albert, R. S. (1991). People, processes, and developmental paths to eminence: A developmental-interactional model. In R. M. Milgram (Ed.), *Counseling gifted and talented children* (pp. 75–93). Norwood, NJ: Ablex.
Albert, R. S., & Elliot, R.C. (1973). Creative ability and the handling of personal and social conflict among bright sixth graders. *Journal of Social Behavior and Personality, 1*, 169–181.
Albert, R. S., & Runco, M. A. (1987). The possible different personality dispositions of scientists and nonscientists. In D. N. Jackson & J. P. Rushton (Eds.), *Scientific excellence: Origins and assessment* (pp. 67–97). Newbury Park, CA: Sage.
Albert, R. S., & Runco, M. A. (1989). Independence and cognitive ability in gifted and exceptionally gifted boys. *Journal of Youth and Adolescence, 18*, 221–230.
Amabile, T. M. (1990). Within you, without you. In M. A. Runco & R. S. Albert (Eds.), *Theories of creativity* (pp. 61–91). Newbury Park, CA: Sage.
Arnheim, R. (1990). On the late style. In M. Perlmutter (Ed.), *Late life potential* (pp. 113–120). Washington, DC: Gerontological Society of America.
Baker-Sennett, J., & Ceci, S. (1996). Clue-efficiency and insight: Unveiling the mystery of inductive leaps. *Journal of Creative Behavior, 30*, 153–172.
Barber, B. (1961). Resistance by scientists. *Science, 134*, 596–602.
Barron, F. (1963). The need for order and for disorder as motives in creative activity. In C. W. Taylor & F. Barron (Ed.), *Scientific creativity: Its recognition and development* (pp. 153–160). New York: Wiley.
Barron, F. (1964). The relation of ego diffiusion to creative perception. In C. W. Taylor (Ed.), *Widening horizons in creativity* (pp. 80–86). New York: Wiley.
Barron, F. (1996). No Restless Flowers; An ecology of creativity. Cresskill: Hampton Press,
Boynton, R. S. (1996, October 7). The birth of an idea. *New Yorker*, pp. 72–81.
Bronowski, J. (1977). *A sense of the future.* Cambridge, MA: MIT Press. (Original work published 1958)
Brown, H. G. (October 25, 1991). At work, sexual electricity sparks creativity. *Wall Street Journal*, p. A22.
Bruner, J. S. (1973). The conditions of creativity. In J. S. Bruner (Ed.), *Beyond the information given: Studies in the psychology of knowing* (pp. 208–217). New York: Norton.
Bryson, B. (1994). *Made in America.* New York: William Morrow.
Burke, B. F., Chrisler, J. C., & Devlin, A. S. (1989). The creative thinking, environment frustration, and self-concept of left- and right-handers. *Creativity Research Journal, 2*, 279–285.
Campbell, D. N. (1960). Blind variation and selective retention in creative thought as in other knowledge processes. *Psychological Bulletin, 67*, 380–400.
Cashdan, S., & Welsh, G. (1966). Personality correlates of creative potential in talented high school students. *Journal of Personality, 34*, 445–455.
Cassidy, D. C. (1992). Heisenberg, uncertainty, and the quantum revolution. *Scientific American, 266* (5), 106–112.

Chown, S. M. (1961). Age and the rigidities. *Journal of Gerontology, 16,* 353–362.
Cohen, L. M. (1989). A continuum of adaptive creative behaviors. *Creativity Research Journal, 2,* 169–183.
Cohen-Shalev, A. (1989). Old age style: Developmental changes in creative production from a lifespan perspective. *Journal of Aging Studies, 3,* 21–37.
Combs, H. (1979). *Kill Devil Hill.* Boston: Houghton Mifflin.
Csikszentmihalyi, M. (1988). The dangers of originality: Creativity and the artistic process. In M. M. Gedo (Ed.), *Psychoanalytic perspectives on art* (pp. 213–224). Hillsdale, NJ: Analytic Press.
Dervin, D. (1983). A dialectical view of creativity. *Psychoanalytic Review, 70,* 463–491.
Dewey, J. (1933). *How we think.* Boston: Heath.
Diamond, A. M., Jr. (1980). Age and the acceptance of cliometrics. *Journal of Economic History, 40,* 838–841.
Dudek, S. Z. (in press). Aesthetics and creativity. In M. A. Runco (Ed.), *Creativity research handbook* (Vol. 2). Cresskill, NJ: Hampton Press.
Dudek, S. Z., & Verreault, R. (1989). The creative thinking and ego functioning of children. *Creativity Research Journal, 2,* 64–86.
Elkind, D. (1981). *The hurried child.* Reading, MA: Addison-Wesley.
Feist, G. (1994). A structural model of scientific eminence. *Psychological Science, 4,* 366–371.
Feldman, D. (1986). *Nature's gambit.* New York: Basic Books.
Festinger, L. (1962). Cognitive dissonance. *Scientific American, 207,* 93–102.
Flach, F. (1990). Disorders of the pathways involved in the creative process. *Creativity Research Journal, 3,* 158–165.
Francis, D. (1987). *Bolt.* New York: Putnam.
Gardner, H. (in press). Is there a moral intelligence? An essay in honor of Howard Gruber. In M. A. Runco, R. Keegan, & S. Davis (Ed.), *Festschrift for Howard Gruber.* Cresskill, NJ: Hampton Press.
Gardner, H., & Wolf, C. (1988). The fruits of asynchrony: A psychological examination of creativity. *Adolescent Psychiatry, 15,* 96–120.
Gardner, K., & Moran, J. D. (1990). Family adaptability, cohesion, and creativity. *Creativity Research Journal, 3,* 281–286.
Gaynor, J. L., & Runco, M. A. (1992). Family size, birth order, age-interval, and the creativity of children. *Journal of Creative Behavior, 26,* 108–118.
Goertzel, V., & Goertzel, M. G. (1962). *Cradles of eminence.* Boston, MA: Little, Brown.
Goldborough, R. (1999). *Bloodied ivy.* Toronto: Bantam Books.
Gordon, B. (1987). Cultural comparisons of schooling. *Educational Researcher, 16*(4), 4–7.
Gruber, H. E. (1978). Emotion and cognition: Aesthetics and science. In S. S. Madeja (Ed.), *The arts, cognition, and basic skills* (pp. 134–145). St. Louis, MO: CEMREL.
Gruber, H. E. (1981). *Darwin on man: A psychological study of scientific creativity.* Chicago, IL: Chicago University Press.
Gruber, H. E. (1988). The evolving systems approach to creative work. *Creativity Research Journal, 1,* 27–51.
Gruber, H. E. (1993). Ought implies can implies create. *Creativity Research Journal,* Vol 6, no. 1, pg. 3.
Gruber, H. E. (1996). The life space of a scientist: The visionary function and other aspects of Jean Piaget's thinking. *Creativity Research Journal,* 251–265.
Guilford, J. P. (1950). Creativity. *American Psychologist, 5,* 444–454.
Guilford, J. P. (1968). *Creativity, intelligence, and their educational implications.* San Diego, CA: EDITS.
Helson, R. (1996). In search of the creative personality. *Creativity Research Journal, 9,* 295–306.
Hennessey, B. A. (1993). Immunizing children against negative affects. *Creativity Research Journal,* Vol. 6, no. 3, pg 297.
Hunt, J. McV., & Paraskevopoulos, J. (1980). Children's psychological development as a function of the inaccuracy of their mothers' knowledge of their abilities. *Journal of Genetic Psychology, 136,* 285–298.

James, K. (in press). Goal conflict and originality of thinking. *Creativity Research Journal.*
James, K., Chen, J., & Goldburg, C. (1992). Organizational conflict in individual creativity. *Journal of Applied Social Psychology, 22,* 545–566.
John-Steiner, V. (1992). Creative lives, creative tensions. *Creativity Research Journal, 2,* 99–108.
Khandwalla, P. N. (1993). An exploratory study of divergent thinking through protocol analysis. *Creativity Research Journal,* Vol. 6, no. 3, pg. 241.
Kirschenbaum, R., & Reis, S. (in press). Conflicts in creativity: Talented female artists. *Creativity Research Journal.*
Kris, E. (1952). *Psychoanalytic explorations in art.* New York: International Universities Press.
Kubie, L. (1958). *Neurotic distortion of the creative process.* Lawrence: University of Kansas Press.
Kuhn, T. (1963). The essential tension: Tradition and innovation in scientific research. In C.W. Taylor & F. Barron (Ed.), *Scientific creativity: Its recognition and development* (pp. 341–354). New York: Wiley.
Kuiper, (1995). *Encyclopedia of literature.* Springfield, MA: Merriam-Webster.
Lasswell, H. D. (1959). The social setting for creativity. In H. H. Anderson (Ed.), *Creativity and its cultivation* (pp. 203–221). New York: Harper.
Lazarus, R. S. (1991a). Cognition and motivation in emotion. *American Psychologist, 46,* 352–367.
Lazarus, R. S. (1991b). Progress on a cognitive-motivational-relational theory of emotion. *American Psychologist, 46,* 819–834.
Levine, S. H. A critique of the Piagetian presuppositions of the role of play in human development and a suggested alternative: Metaphoric logic which organizes the play experience is the foundation for rational creativity. *Journal of Creative Behavior,* 1984, *18,* 90–108.
Lindauer, M. S. (1992). Creativity in aging artists: Contributions from the humanities to the psychology of aging. *Creativity Research Journal, 5,* 211–232.
Lindauer, M. S. (1993). The span of creativity among long-lived historical artists. *Creativity Research Journal, 6,* 221–239.
Ludwig, A. (1995). *The price of greatness.* New York: Guilford Press.
MacKinnon, D. W. (1983). The highly effective individual. In R. S. Albert (Ed.), *Genius and eminence: The social psychology of creativity and exceptional achievement* (pp. 114–127). Oxford, England: Pergamon. (Original work published 1960)
MacKinnon, D. W. (1962). The nature and nurture of creative talent. *American Psychologist, 17,* 484–495.
Martindale, C., & Armstrong, J. (1974). The relationship of creativity to cortical activation and its operant control. *Journal of Genetic Psychology, 124,* 311–320.
May, R. (1977). *The meaning of anxiety.* New York: Simon & Schuster.
Mendelsohn, G., & Lindholm, E. (1972). Individual differences and the role of attention in the use of cues in verbal problem solving. *Journal of Personality, 40,* 226 241.
Messerli, P. (1988). Age differences in the reception of new scientific theories: The case of plate tetonics theory. *Social Studies of Science, 18,* 91–112.
Metcalfe, J. (1986). Feeling of knowing in memory and problem solving. *Journal of Experimental psychology: Learning, Memory, and Cognition, 12,* 288–294.
Mraz, W., & Runco, M. A. (1994). Suicide ideation and creative problem solving. *Suicide and Life-Threatening Behavior, 24,* 38–47.
Mumford, M. D. (1984). Age and outstanding occupational achievement: Lehman revisited. *Journal of Vocational Behavior, 25,* 225–244.
Mumford, M.D., Olsen, K. A., & James, L. R. (1989). Age-related changes in the likelihood of major contributions. *International Aging and Human Development, 29,* 9–32.
Ochse, R. (1990). *Before the gates of excellence.* New York: Cambridge University Press.
Okuda, S. M., Runco, M. A., & Berger, D. E. (1991). Creativity and the finding and solving of real-world problems. *Journal of Psychoeducational Assessment, 9,* 45–53.
Oromaner, M. (1977). Professional age and the reception of sociological publications: A test of the Zuckerman-Merton hypothesis. *Social Studies of Science, 7,* 381–388.

Overby, L. A. (in press). Enthusiasm versus self-possession: The art of psychological science. *Creativity Research Journal.*
Piaget, J. (1976). *To understand is to invent.* New York: Penguin.
Piaget, J. (1981). Foreword. In H. E. Gruber (Ed.), *Darwin on man: A psychological study of scientific creativity.* Chicago: Chicago University Press.
Pritzker, S., & Runco, M. A. (in press). In R. K. Sawyer (Ed.), *Performance creativity.* Norwood, NJ: Ablex.
Rathunde, K., & Csikszentmihalyi, M. (1991). Adolescent happiness and family interaction. In K. Pilluer & K. McCartney (Eds.), *Parent child relations through life* (pp. 143–161). Hillsdale, NJ: Erlbaum.
Richards, R. (1990). Everyday creativity, eminent creativity, and health: Afterview of CRJ special issues on creativity and health. *Creativity Research Journal, 3,* 300–326.
Richards, R. (1996, summer). Beyond Piaget. *New Directions for Child Development, 72,* pg. 67.
Rogers, C. (1980). *A way of being.* Boston: Houghton Mifflin.
Roe, A. (1963). Personal problems and science. In C. W. Taylor & F. Barron (Eds.), *Scientific creativity: Its recognition and development* (pp. 132–138). New York: Wiley.
Root-Bernstein, R. (1993, October). *Polymaths, transformational thinking, and the creative process.* Paper presented at the Chicago Academy of Sciences, Chicago.
Rothenberg, A. (1990a). Creativity in adolescents. *Psychiatric Clinics of North America, 13,* 415–434.
Rothenberg, A. (1990b). Creativity, mental health, and alcoholism. *Creativity Research Journal, 3,* 179–201.
Rubenson, D. L. (1991). On creativity, economics, and baseball. *Creativity Research Journal, 4,* 205–209.
Rubenson, D. L., & Runco, M. A. (1992). The psychoeconomic approach to creativity. *New Ideas in Psychology, 10,* 131–147.
Run, S. (1993). *Affect and creativity: The role of affect and play in the creative process.* Hillsdale: Lawrence Erlbaum Ass.
Russ, S. (1988). Primary process on the Rorschach, divergent thinking, and coping in children. *Journal of Personality Assessment, 52,* 539–548.
Russ, S. (1993). *Creativity and affect.* Hillsdale, NJ: Erlbaum.
Runco, M. A. (1990–91). Mindfulness and personal control [Review of Langer's *Mindfulness*]. *Imagination, Cognition and Personality, 10,* 107–114.
Runco, M. A. (1993a). Moral creativity: Intentional and unconventional. *Creativity Research Journal, 6,* 17–28.
Runco, M. A. (1993b). On reputational paths and case studies. *Creativity Research Journal, 6,* 487–488.
Runco, M. A. (1993c). Operant theories of insight, originality, and creativity. *American Behavioral Scientist, 37,* 59–74.
Runco, M. A. (1995). Insight for creativity, expression for impact. *Creativity Research Journal, 8,* 377–390.
Runco, M. A. (1996, summer). Personal creativity: Definition and developmental issues. *New Directions for Child Development, 72,* 3–30.
Runco, M. A., & Albert, R. S. (1996). Creativity and the personality of exceptionally gifted boys and their parents.
Runco, M. A., & Chand, I. (1994). Problem finding, evaluative thinking, and creativity. In M. A. Runco (Ed.), *Problem finding, problem solving, and creativity.* Norwood, NJ: Ablex.
Runco, M. A., & Charles, R. (1997). Developmental trends in creative potential and creative performance. In M. A. Runco (Ed.), *Creativity research handbook* (vol. 1). Cresskill, NJ: Hampton Press.
Runco, M. A., & Gaynor, J. L. (1993). Creativity as optimal development. In J. Brzezinski, S. DiNuovo, T. Marek, & T. Maruszewski (Eds.), *Creativity and consciousness: Philosophical and psychological dimensions* (pp. 395–412). Amsterdam: Rodopi.

Runco, M. A., & Richards, R. (in press). *Eminent creativity, everyday creativity, and health.* Norwood, NJ: Ablex.
Runco, M. A., & Sakamoto, S. O. (1996). Optimization as a guiding principle in research on creative problem solving. In T. Helstrup, G. Kaufmann, & K. H. Teigen (Eds.), *Problem solving and cognitive processes: Essays in honor of Kjell Raaheim* (pp. 119–144). Bergen, Norway: Fagbokforlaget Vigmostad & Bjorke.
Runco, M. A., & Sakamoto, S. (in press). Experimental studies of creativity. In R. S. Sternberg (Ed.), *Handbook of human creativity.* New York: Cambridge University Press.
Runco, M. A., & Smith, W. R. (1992). Interpersonal and intrapersonal evaluations of creative ideas. *Personality and Individual Differences, 13,* 295–302.
Runco, M.A., & Vega, L. (1990). Evaluating the creativity of children's ideas. *Journal of Social Behavior and Personality, 5,* 439–452.
Rutter, M. (1981). *Maternal deprivation reassessed.* Harmondsworth, England: Penguin.
Rutter, M. (1985). Resilence in the face of adversity: Protective factors and resistence to psychiatric disorders. *British Journal of Psychiatry, 147–598–611.*
Sawyer, K. (1992). Improvisational creativity: An analysis of jazz performance. *Creativity Research Journal, 5,* 253–264.
Schuldberg, D. (1994). Giddiness and horror in the creative process. In M. P. Shaw & M. A. Runco (Eds.), *Creativity and affect* (pp. 87–101). Norwood, NJ: Ablex.
Schubert, D. (1988). Creativity and the ability to cope. In F. Flach (Ed.), *The creative mind* (pp. 97–114). Buffalo, NJ: Bearly.
Schwebel, M. (1993). Moral creativity as artistic transformation. *Creativity Research Journal, 6,* 65–82.
Schultz, N. R., Jr., Kaye, D. B., & Hoyer, W. J. (1980). Intelligence and spontaneous flexibility in adulthood and old age. *Intelligence, 4,* 219–231.
Seyle, H. (1988). Creativity in basic research. In F. Flach (Ed.), *The creative mind* (pp. 243–268). Buffalo, NY: Bearly.
Shaw, M. P. (1994). Affective components of scientific creativity. In M. P. Shaw & M. A. Runco (Eds.), *Creativity and affect.* Norwood, NJ: Ablex.
Sheldon, K. M. (1995). Creativity and goal conflict. *Creativity Research Journal, 8.*
Simonton, D. K. (1987). Developmental antecedents of achieved eminence. *Annals of Child Development, 4,* 131–169.
Simonton, D. K. (1988). *Scientific genius.* New York: Cambridge University Press.
Smith, G. J. W. (1994, October). *The internal breeding ground of creativity.* Paper presented as part of the Symposium on Creativity and Cognition, Venice.
Smith, G. J. W., & Carlsson, I. (1983). Creativity and anxiety: An experimental study. *Scandinavian Journal of Psychology, 24,* 107–115.
Smith, G. J. W., & Van der Meer, G. (1990). Creativity in old age. *Creativity Research Journal, 3,* 249 264.
Smith, G. J. W., & Amner, G. (1997). Perception and creativity. In M. A. Runco (Ed.), *Creativity research handbook* (Vol. 1, pp. 67–82). Cresskill, NJ: Hampton Press.
Stein, M. I. (1988). Creativity: The process and its stimulation. In F. Flach (Ed.), *The creative mind* (pp. 51–75). Buffalo, NY: Bearly.
Subotnik, R., Kassan, L., Summers, E., & Wasser, A. (1993). *Genius revisited: High IQ children grown up.* Norwood, NJ: Ablex.
Sulloway, F. (1996). *Born to rebel: Birth Order, Family Dynamics, and Creative Lives.* New York: Pantheon Books.
Soth, L. (1986). Van Gogh's agony. *Art Bulletin, 68,* 301–313.
Toplyn, G., & Maguire, W. (1991). The differential effect of noise on creative task performance. *Creativity Research Journal, 4,* 337–347.
Torrance, E. P. (1974). *Torrance Tests of Creative Thinking.* Bensenville, IL: Scholastic Testing Services.

Trelfa, D., & Stevenson, H. (1996, May). *Young achievers in East Asia.* Paper presented at the International Symposium on Child Development, Hong Kong.

Valliant, G. E. (1977). *Adaptation to life.* Boston: Little, Brown.

Valliant, G. E., & Valliant, C. O. (1990). Determinants and consequence of creativity in a cohort of gifted women. *Psychology of Women, 14,* 607–616.

Van Tassel-Baska, J. L. (1989). Characteristics of the developmental path of eminent and gifted adults. In J. L. VanTallel Baska & P. Olszewki Kubliius (Eds.), *Patterns of influence on gifted learners: The home, the self, the school* (pp. 146–162). New York: Teachers College Press.

Wallace, D. B. (1991). The genesis and microgenesis of sudden insight in the creation of literature. *Creativity Research Journal, 4,* 41–50.

Wallach, M. A. (1970). Creativity. In P. A. Mussen (Ed.), *Manual of child psychology* (Vol. 1, pp. 1211–1271). New York: Wiley.

Wertheimer, M. (1945). *Productive thinking.* New York: Harper & Row.

Winner, E. (1996). *Gifted children: Myths and realities.* New York: Basic Books.

Zajonc, R. B. (1980). Feeling and thinking: Preferences need no inferences. *American Psychologist, 35,* 151–175.

11

The Subtle Attraction: Beauty as a Force in Awareness, Creativity, and Survival

Ruth Richards
Saybrook Graduate School, San Francisco University of California, San Francisco McLean Hospital and Harvard Medical School

Why do people notice qualities such as beauty, elegance, or fitness? In the widely accepted view of Kant, there is no further function; beauty is disinterested, and people notice beauty (or elegance or fitness) because it, in itself, gives satisfaction. In Santayana's (1896/1955) view, aesthetic appreciation is linked to drives in biological survival and evolution. In this chapter, I draw on an aesthetic of everyday life (Dewey, 1934) and the notion of everyday creativity (Richards, 1990) to modify Santayana's perspective. I propose an active role for aesthetics in memetic evolution, or the evolution of information. Interestingly, this "active" role is consistent with Kant's "disinterested' position. Aesthetic appreciation also has characteristics of a mindfully aware state. Parallels can be drawn, to flow states found in active creating, when attention and all capacities are mobilized in the moment and coordinated. However, in active creating, the absorptive element may be even more prominent. Flow may be optimal when challenges to the organism are being successfully met, and, in this context, the

---

This chaper is based on a paper presented at the 1996 annual meeting of the American Psychological Association, Toronto, Canada. I am most grateful for the helpful comments of Tom Greening, Thanh Nguyen, Mark Runco, Sandra Russ, Tony Stigliano, and Tobi Zausner. This piece, however, does not necessarily reflect their views, and any flaws are surely my own.

195

paper examines the role of aesthetic appreciation in the lives of persons who have coped with adversity through creative means. Finally, the paper looks at what has been called the "sublime," and its particular promise for mindful awareness and personal change. If aesthetic capacity holds such promise, it should be greatly more cultivated in education and training, and in all other areas of life.

Disinterested Nature of Beauty

This paper is about the beauty everyone sees and knows so well—and possibly takes for granted. It is about how such beauty may, at times, help individuals to adapt, create, and even survive.

What? a person might say. Beauty is supposed to be "disinterested." This widely accepted view of Kant's, which dates from the 18th century (Beardsley, 1966; Kant, 1790/1964; Sheppard, 1987), asserts that people notice certain things simply because they appeal aesthetically. There is nothing more they want from them.

But perhaps—and perhaps even consistent with this well-known view of Kant's—there *is* more. If so, we would do well to understand it.
Consider this statement by Ralph Waldo Emerson (1836/1992): "Go out of the house to see the moon, and It is mere tinsel; it will not please as when its light shines upon your necessary journey" (pp. 10–11). Or this one: "Ever does natural beauty steal in like air, and envelop great actions" (p. 11). To Emerson, physical qualities gave only one aspect of beauty and were not as important as the element of "virtue" which could be reflected. Indeed, according to Emerson, "Beauty is the mark God sets upon virtue." (p. 11).

Diverse thinkers, spanning time, geography, discipline, and school, and including Kant himself (Beardsley, 1966; Kant, 1790/1964), found higher and transcendent values in the beauty of art and of nature, beyond those of particular appearance or sensory experience. They found in nature "another mind within our own external mind" (Bateson, 1972, p. 465), and found purpose in art: "to make social the brief hope offered by nature.... The transcendental face of art is always a form of prayer" (Berger, 1985, p. 9). Some believed that "beauty is not an attribute... a necessity; it is the way in which the gods touch our senses, reach the heart and attract us into life" (Hillman, 1989, p. 302).

Indeed, think of Plato (1938a, 1938b; Hofstadter & Kuhns, 1964; Sheppard, 1987), who believed that art imitated the ideal Forms of creation, of which human sense experiences are but mere copies. In speaking of poets, Plato (1938b) proposed that at times "it is the God himself who speaks, and through them becomes articulate to us (p. 84). Compare Kant's (Beardsley, 1966; Kant, 1790/1964, 1790/1929; Sheppard, 1987) conception, going beyond beauty, of the *sublime,* which I discuss later in this chapter; the sublime may be evoked by the majestic irregularities of nature—the jagged mountain peaks, the roars of thunder. These remind us that we have "a faculty of the mind surpassing every standard of Sense" (Kant, quoted in Beardsley, 1966, p. 219).

The awareness above may certainly coexist with a "disinterested" view of beauty (e.g., Sheppard, 1987), in which aesthetic judgment is rendered apart from any personal stake. People see and appreciate and respond in the moment, however exalted or transcendental the experience. The judgment comes after the event, with its particular glory representing yet another consequence of an act already completed.

Yet what if there is also a specific function? What if people in addition mark, record, and cherish important moments, realizations, accomplishments, and obstacles overcome, to bask in their aesthetic glow in the short run (where the aesthetic even expands to include the entire encounter), so that in the future if they ever want them again, they will know exactly where, within the richness of their recollections, to look.

The discussion falls into five parts: (a) characteristics of aesthetic appreciation; (b) aesthetics as a path to awareness; (c) aesthetic roads to the evolution of information; (d) aesthetics, adversity, and creative possibility; and (e) infinity, chaos theory, and the sublime.

CHARACTERISTICS OF AESTHETIC APPRECIATION

The Disinterested Interest

Aesthetic appreciation is often said to be "disinterested" (Sheppard, 1987); yet this doesn't mean people don't care about it. Individuals are struck by a beauty, an elegance, a rightness, or a fitness that draws them in and for its own sake makes them want to look at something again. It is its own reason and its own reward. (In the arts, consider the notion of "art for art's sake." One may speak further of the morality of art, with its overriding need to be true to and complete within itself [e.g., Dudek, 1993; in press].

Consider an example from nature; let's say you see a beautiful ripe fruit, an orange. It attracts you. You're not (inevitably or only) looking because you're hungry and want to eat it. Rather, oftentimes, it's the orangeness, the roundness, the puckered surface, the organic or savory qualities, which in themselves are appealing and draw you in.

You are looking past hunger and appetite and also past a central conditioned aspect, indeed, beyond the whole range of habitual and learned responses related to culture, expectation, and conventional practice that affect how people perceive and respond. As members of a culture, people learn to respond to situations in certain ways. Yet this view suggests there is something more, something more intrinsic, culture free, and universal, more related to being human and to the direct and immediate experience of the object. This may pertain to the difference between what is called "knowing" and "having knowledge" (Puhakka, 1997):

> "Knowing" is a moment of awareness in which contact occurs between the knower and the known. This contact is nonconceptual, nonimaginal, nondiscursive, and

extremely brief. "Having knowledge," on the other hand, consists of descriptive or interpretive claims to the effect that "such-and-such is the case".... [with knowing] what is contacted are, to borrow Husserl's terms, "things themselves." The act of contact breaks out of our solipsistic representational world of images and meanings, and also out of the collective solipsism of socially determined meanings, into genuine, empathic interconnectedness. (p. 9)

Consider another example, a vista of Niagara Falls. I was recently in a plane flying over these falls; people were staring out their windows, amazed at the rush of water even at that altitude, the crashing fall of tons of water and the whitest of mists rising above. We on the plane weren't gazing at the falls because we wanted to navigate around them or to avoid their sweep of water. We just wanted to see them. As we heard from the pilot over the public address system, "It is worth a look."

The response to beauty can be contrasted to the response to a food during hunger. I'm eager to eat lunch, let's say, and I don't see any nourishment, so I go out and seek it. I find food and it looks "good." My need, or hunger, directed the search and then the consequences: the meal consumed. With beauty, I was not (necessarily) yearning for it, missing it, seeking it in any way. Yet when I see it, it stops me. And I look with appreciation. This appreciation involves an intrinsic response to the object and to the very act of looking. It is complete in itself.

Aesthetic Properties: Intrinsic and Universal

Why might something in the first place, be "worth a look"? What is the nature of the attraction of that which people call beautiful? People often think they know, but English has no general term of aesthetic commendation (Sheppard, 1987). Certain flowers may be "beautiful," wines "fine," men "handsome," mathematical proofs "elegant," movements "dainty." All, nonetheless, have an intrinsic appeal. All—be their origin in nature, in the formal arts, or in the activities of our everyday life—ask in some way for our aesthetic appreciation. They all attract in an instant, they appeal, they ask the individual to come forward and look, and to look again.

Beauty, said Santayana (1896/1955), "is value, positive, intrinsic, and objectified.... Beauty is pleasure regarded as the quality of a thing" (p. 31). It is not a perception of a fact; it is an emotion, an appreciation. An object cannot be beautiful if it doesn't give pleasure to somebody. Beauty is also potentially universal, as per Kant (1790/1964), who distinguished between the pleasant and the beautiful, maintaining that the former involves private feelings and preferences. To one person, for instance, the color violet may be pleasing; to another, it may seem faded. "Violet," one might say, "is pleasing to me." This judgment may involve contextual factors relevant to "having knowledge," as defined earlier, rather than to direct "knowing" (Puhakka, 1997).

In contrast, if one uses "taste," or "the faculty of judging . . . by an entirely disinterested satisfaction or dissatisfaction," then "the object of such satisfaction is called beautiful" (Kant, 1790/1929, p. 382). One does not say, "That color is beautiful to me." Assumed is a universality of appeal, or a "ground of satisfaction for every one" (p. 382), in a direct subjective and immediate encounter with the object, without the mediation of concepts, intellect, or any special agendas (see also Runco, 1994). Indeed, Kant's judgment can be linked with aspects of a mindful encounter, in Western Psychological writings (E. Langer, 1989), and Eastern metaphysical writings (Hanh, 1976).

Imitation, Expression, and Form

Upon what qualities might appreciation depend? I focus here on the arts, because of a later focus on creativity and expressive coping. Varied viewpoints can be included under three categories: imitation, expression of emotion, and form (Sheppard, 1987). Consider again Plato, who regarded the value of art in the imitation or representation of particulars that relate to ideal Forms such as "justice." The fullest value of such imitation lies in these ideals, toward which our concrete copies can only aspire. Or consider emotional expression, for instance the 19th century Romantics, to whom "All good poetry is the spontaneous overflow of powerful feelings" (Wordsworth, quoted in Sheppard, 1987, p. 19). Or consider Kantian-type characteristics involving balance, symmetry, contrast, proportion, and relationship. As one concrete instance, there is evidence of a human preference for bodily symmetry (Pennisi, 1995). Kant's (1790/1929) free and disinterested (vs. dependent) beauty is fundamentally attributable to the broad quality of form and its intrinsic satisfactions.

An integral view for the present purposes is provided by the philosopher and logician Susanne Langer, who united form and expression through the proposal that form can "somehow correspond to formal features of human emotions in general" (Sheppard, 1987, p. 48). Indeed, to Langer (1988), such form provided alternative and nondiscursive languages, or nondiscursive symbol systems, and through the arts in particular. She believed these provided a direct and intuitive knowledge of life patterns, through the emotions and feelings that ordinary discursive language cannot convey:

> Feeling is a dynamic pattern of tremendous complexity. Its whole relation to life, the fact that all sorts of processes may culminate in feeling with or without direct regard to each other, and that vital activity goes on at all levels continuously make mental phenomena the most protean subject matter in the world. *Our best identification of such phenomena is through images that hold and present them for our contemplation; and their images are works of art.* (Langer, p. 29, emphasis mine)

Critical here is the integration of affective experience back into the substance of human thought and experience, where it belongs. No more false dichotomies!

How complex is people's recording of their experience, integrating cognitive and affective elements, conscious and unconscious, rational and "irrational," "sophisticated" and "primitive," in a holistic blend, psychologists are only beginning to understand (e.g., Damasio, 1994; Krystal, 1981; Richards, 1992, 1994, 1996b, in press-b; Russ, 1993). First, however, people must be aware of them. Consider again Langer's statement: "images that hold and present them for our contemplation." With art and beauty, people can wake up and become aware—and of a very great deal. I shall return to this point shortly.

Where Is Beauty Found? An Everyday Aesthetic

Where isn't beauty? Objects, nature, moments, movements, and puffs of air on a sweltering day. In this discussion, I maintain that beauty is everywhere. It is not constrained to formal artistic activity, such as painting or music, or locked up in a museum pending weekend visitations (see Dewey, 1934; Richards, in press; Sarason, 1990). My conception is a broad one, consistent with the notion of "everyday creativity" (Richards, 1998), and, as elaborated by John Dewey (1934) in particular, it underlies the rest of this discussion.

Peaks, Balance, and Change

Dewey (1934) saw aesthetic experience—the experiencing of vital new balances and peak moments in the flow of life—as intrinsic to being alive. Herein one finds a reflection of the growth, change, and progress of the world and one's experience in it. It is a celebration, one could say, of reaching new balances and equilibria along the path one is taking.

Art is only one part of this picture, yet it is a critical one. To Dewey, art was an indication that people are "capable of restoring *consciously*, and thus on the plane of meaning, the union of sense, need, and impulse and action characteristic of the live creature" (Eisner, 1972, p. 5), (emphasis mine). Again, one is returned to conscious awareness; again, one is provided with an integration, a complex gestalt of meaning.

Consider Dewey's aesthetic in raw, touching everyday events, yet spotlighting moments and objects that can catch and hold one's most intense interest and enjoyment. Consider, for instance, "the men perched high in air on girders, throwing and catching red-hot bolts . . . how the tense grace of the ball-player infects the onlooking crowd . . . the zest of the spectator in poking the wood burning on the hearth and in watching the darting flames and crumbling coals" (Dewey, 1934, p. 5).

Change and Biology

To Dewey, change, transition, development, and balance were key qualities in the aesthetic of life. But what about stability, solidity, and the lack, relatively speaking, of change? One might ask. What of the massive outcrop of rock that towers permanently above one's head along the hiking trail or the veins of white rock enmeshed for millions of years in a column of marble? These have aesthetic appeal. One sees it isn't just the glint of sunlight on a marble column, but the column itself, solid and unchanging, that affects one.

Yet if we think about how the mind works, it is change to which humans best respond—for example, visual changes be it dark and light, edges, borders, or flickers of brightness, and changes in emotions, too, which register in the gut as well as the mind. If one stays happy a long time, the feeling will fade. In contrast, think of the sensation when a good experience follows a series of bad ones. With action, too, people are at their best with "fight or flight"; they respond quickly to emergencies. So disposed are people to the sudden and urgent that they can miss slowly building environmental or personal dangers—even lethal ones—if they are insidious enough (Richards, 1993, 1997).

Even with the solid marble column, a contrast may be important to the viewer's processing; aesthetic appreciation is not just for the object per se, but for the impression it makes on the beholder, including the differences and contrasts, the vast spaces between. Consider the towering rock, which diminishes one's human scale, or the smoothly polished marble, unyielding in contrast with the human flesh that explores it. Part of the appeal on occasion may involve a dynamic in time, as well as in space, in a myriad of transitions and their pull on one's sensibilities. In many ways, one has first a soaring and then a coming to rest.

How might this relate to aesthetic appreciation and creative transformation?

Human Agents of Change—Aesthetics and Creative Transformation

Dewey's aesthetic fits readily with the concept of everyday creativity. It marks key points in life's creative evolution and includes those creative points that we, as human beings, can help influence. Everyday creativity (see Richards et al., 1988; Richards, 1990, 1997, 1998) has been defined in terms of the practice and results, of human originality in diverse aspects of everyday life, at work and at leisure. In general, in creating, people first notice discrepancy, need, and room for modification. The old is transformed; the new is brought into being. People are active at the borders of change, transmuting from one state to another, they are makers of new possibilities. How important it is that people can imagine, and appreciate, these possibilities.

At times of creativity, people can at times identify and work with Dewey's (1934) vital new balances, these peaks in the flow of life. The results, at best, carry their own aesthetic fitness, rightness, elegance, and often beauty. Consider everyday events, such as making innovative home repairs on a tiny budget, conducting a successful publicity campaign, helping a child learn from bitter experience, cooking a gourmet dinner from a melange of leftovers, singing joyously with friends, rearranging furniture and decorations in a country cabin. Here, too, is Dewey's change and transformation, both intentional and productive and, in its peak everyday performance, remarkable.

Aesthetic moments in one's activity can be postulated to include glimmers of pleasure, progress, and achievement along the way, as well as a sense of fitness, elegance, or beauty. Does an aesthetic sense help guide one? Think of determining the right amount of nutmeg in a recipe. Fantastic—a memorable event. Everyday creativity is rife with aesthetic moments, for indeed may not an aesthetic judgment help shape an intuition or a decision? The same goes for exceptional creative endeavor. Consider the eminent mathematician Henri Poincaré (Ghiselin, 1952; Richards, 1992, in press), who reported how "emotional sensibility" can be essential to mathematical proofs, as reflected in "the harmony of numbers and forms, of geometric elegance.... Among the great numbers of combinations blindly formed by the subliminal self ... only certain ones are harmonious, and consequently, at once useful and beautiful. They will be capable of touching this special sensibility of the geometer" (Ghiselin, 1952, p. 40).

Here perhaps is an involved and useful aesthetic, once one is no longer a spectator but is actively participating in the creation of beauty. To what extent does this connect with a more passive aesthetic appreciation? I examine the phenomenon further below in the context of flow (Csikszentmihalyi, 1990), or optimal experience in creating, once I have addressed issues of aesthetic appreciation and conscious awareness.

Aesthetic Appreciation and Awareness

One may note the pull to conscious awareness in aesthetic appreciation and in active creativity, a phenomenon noted in the writings of the thinkers I mentioned earlier, including Dewey (1934), S. K. Langer (1988), and indeed Kant (1790/1929). In fact, as a human, one can't do anything that is conscious, purposeful, and creative until one escapes the mindless, habitual stupor that often envelops one who is going about one's mechanical routines mechanical routines (see Nhat Hanh, 1976; E. Langer, 1989). It is true that a degree of selectivity and habit is necessary; otherwise, a jumble of details would confuse one's day. But there's much information one will consequently miss. And should one assume one's taking in the "right" things? (Or imagine one even know what they are? See Richards, 1993.) Consider how much of life is overlooked. Have you noticed the furniture you are using right now? Its color? Texture? The decorations on the wall? The scene, and the weather today, outside of your window? Very possibly not.

What sorts of events, or internal signals, tend to bring people to conscious awareness and potentially to action? Certainly, those that involve self-preservation must be included. Likewise, those involving the preservation of the species must be included. How quickly one may wake up, for instance, at the advent of fear, hunger, anxiety, or anger. And let's not forget the powerful effects of a sexual longing. The ultimate effect is to get one to do something. And the ultimate goal, for the most part, is biological survival.

Aesthetic response, so very different, also wakes one up. Take an example. I am driving along. I see a beautiful landscape, with the sunlight filtering through the palm trees and the hills rolling dark in the background against a setting sun. How nice, I think, and my attention flickers briefly from the road. I become awake, conscious, aware. Is there adaptive value to this?

This encounter has qualities of a Kantian "free" (vs. "dependent") beauty (Kant, 1790/1929; Sheppard, 1992). The scene is appreciated in itself and is not impeded by a conceptual overlay of categories or of various imaginings; nor is it weighed down by thoughts of those functions it might somehow ultimately provide. It is appreciated in a direct and immediate way—it is what it is. I am making much more conscious contact with the world; and my state becomes an increasingly "mindful" one (see Nhat Hanh, 1976).

One may encourage this change of state in others, as well as attempt to prolong it in oneself. "Just look at that sunset," one might suggest to a bystander, and the two stand back to look. Here, again, one may note the break, accomplished for its own sake, from the ongoing and routine. This stands in contrast to, let's say, the alerting function of sharp pain upon touching a hot stove with one's finger. When the finger is withdrawn, the problem is solved; the discomfort is gone, and the event leaves awareness. In contrast, with aesthetic appreciation, the whole point is one's awareness—along with appreciation, the ultimate valuing of the experience.

Aesthetic experience may claim as well a universality, or universal validity, because it is not the bystander and I who will find this sunset, or this landscape, beautiful, but essentially anyone, anywhere, and anytime.

There is another result as well, a critical one. This experience, which might otherwise have been lost, once it faded from consciousness, is transformed into *a mental record* within my system of memories. There it will remain for a very long time, for my later recollection and use.

Aesthetic Appreciation and Flow

A disinterested aesthetic may be fine at the theater or art gallery, but it doesn't fit fully with an active creative process. Aspects of aesthetic appreciation still fit, including a focused attention; presence in the moment; and, in its peak instances, a transcending of self and other aspects of one's existence in the focused contemplation of the creation. Here, aspects of Maslow's "peak experiences" come readily to mind (Maslow, 1959; Wertz, 1994).

What Csikszentmihalyi (1990) called "flow," goes a step further in an explicit melding of one's total being and focused attention toward a creative goal. A challenge is sensed, one in harmony with one's capacities. One may accept this and enter a satisfying, at times joyful, state of total absorption in this task for which one is truly fit. Here are concentration, sharpened attention, and psychic energy flowing effortlessly. Concerns of self and adequacy float away; time distorts, the world recedes, and one is lost in the moment and in the task, doing what is needed, with an intense sense of enjoyment pervading the whole.

Aesthetic appreciation, I propose, is in this. Yet people may not be aware of the experience in the same way. They may slow down at times and wonder consciously at what they have seen or done. At other times—perhaps most of the time—they may be entirely too busy to notice. (With absorptive qualities, it may be profitable to think about parallels to states of *samadhi* in Eastern thought [e.g., Sekida, 1977].) Indeed, the meditative aspects of art are of interest in many ways (Franck, 1973, 1979; Ross, 1960).

AN EVOLUTION OF INFORMATION

Now let's look at some purposes that all this aesthetic activity might serve, if at times unwittingly. This regards humans' evolution as a species.

Aesthetics, Evolution, and Genes

Aesthetic appreciation and evolution? Sound surprising? Here, first, is a viewpoint based on the survival of humans' biological material of heredity: genes.

Santayana (1896/1955) colorfully derived aesthetic sensibility from an "ill-adjusted" sexual instinct. This instinct becomes conscious because people (with rare exception, he stated) fail to be drawn automatically to the "best" mate with whom to procreate biologically. Out of this "groping and waste," comes a happy generalization of affect and a "tenderness" that may, he said, carry the source of aesthetic appeal. "For," said Santayana, "it is precisely from the waste, from the radiation of the sexual passion, that beauty borrows warmth . . . and the whole sentimental side of our aesthetic sensibility—without which it would be perceptive and mathematical rather than aesthetic—is due to our sexual organization remotely stirred" (p. 38).

Hence, to Santayana, certain fumblings of the mating dance may give color to the landscapes of one's courtships, to flowers, poetry, softly sung songs, and a great deal more. This view fits, in a broad way, with a Freudian view of libidinal energy (see Richards, 1981). When this energy is diverted and disguised, it is said to power a vast spectrum of human activity, all in the service of discharge and a Freudian homeostasis.

Not Genes, But "Memes"

Let's contrast with biological evolution a different realm of growth, transformation, and, hopefully, evolution—that of the world of information (Csikszentmihalyi, 1988; Richards, 1990, 1996a, 1996b, 1997). In rough analogy to "genes,"

I speak of "memes," or units of information or of "cultural imitation" (Dawkins, 1976). Examples are an equation, a song, a poem. Like genes, the materials of biological heredity, memes can be copied, transmitted, and combined. Just think of the printing of a book or the editing of a volume of poetry. Viewed as the material of cultural heredity, memes are both replicating and evolving.

This informational and cultural process is different from biological evolution but can interact dramatically with it (e.g., consider the groups of humans who didn't freeze because they discovered fire; they also passed this news along to us). Like genetic recombination in mating, memetic recombination can occur, but in more plentiful and complex ways. It can draw without limit across time and space, and across worlds real and imagined, bringing together whatever information may be useful for a purpose.

Thus, for instance, we have Picasso's painting of Guernica, which Miller (1990) suggested contains images of brutal destruction not only from the Spanish Civil War, but from Picasso's memory at 3 years of age of an earthquake that caused his family to flee and precipitated the birth of his sister. Here, in art, and in psychic life in general, the mind flits faster than light across time and space, merging information in gestalts that have their own rules and necessity. At its most original (and meaningful), this bringing together of new ideas is what many of us mean by creativity (see Richards, 1990, 1997).

Aesthetics and Memes

I propose here, in contrast with Santayana's (1896/1955) view and consistent with more humanistic views of ongoing growth and personal development (Krippner, 1994; Maslow, 1959; Richards, 1981, 1996a; Wertz, 1994), a view incorporating intrinsic human motives to question, search, grow, actualize, and create. Here "beauty," broadly defined, may fuel a much broader and more abstract, but no less critical, type of coming together. "Fumbling" needn't be postulated in this mating dance, though surely some informational unions will be more productive than others.

The guiding hypothesis may be stated as follows: The pull of beauty, broadly defined, may be to the creation of new information (or "memes") what the pull of sexual attraction is to the creation of new organisms (or "genes").

This beauty is a more subtle attraction—an attraction that may wake one from a mindless stupor and then cause one's *mind* to change, and perhaps even develop and evolve! Even if one doesn't produce a tangible product or share the experience in any way, an aesthetic encounter can still produce a change in one. The new information will mate, as it were, with the contents of one's mind; it will alter forever the memory traces to be found there. An aesthetic moment effectively says "notice me," and thereby invites one to be changed by it, and—here is the flow—to allow it to become part of the greater open system (see Richards, 1996a) of which one's mind and it are a part. Truly, one will never again be the same.

Not So Disinterested After All

Thus a result is achieved, and a worthy one. This experiential transformation also leaves its traces in the neurons and biochemicals of the affected mind. Interestingly, this situation is not in conflict with Kant's "disinterested" view of aesthetic appreciation. It even allows a new perspective on the phenomenon of "disinterest."

Let's return to the vista of Niagara Falls. My fellow airplane passengers and I are impressed by the sight. We are moved. According to Kant, this is a "judgment of taste," occurring in the moment and for no ulterior purpose. Yet, in fact, the *judgment of taste may be the purpose.* The processing, recording, integrating, and valuing are the purpose. Now we may have developed, both consciously and unconsciously, a new relationship to falling water and perhaps, more broadly, to nature and its effects—and also, on later reflection, to the power of nature to give something special to us. We may have developed a new relationship to a great many other things as well, of which we may be only marginally aware. Our minds have been indelibly changed.

Does this occur in part because humans need to know this information? Whatever the case may be, we on the plane do now know it.

It is useful to compare and contrast this situation with physical hunger. (After all, humans are ingesting as well as gestating new information!) First, people are not necessarily searching for aesthetic nourishment—they happen upon a beauteous wonder. But, similar to hunger, once they see it, they partake of it. They process it mentally (and having done so, a part goes here, a part goes there), so that it becomes from that moment on, a part of them. When transmuted into the corpus of people's minds, it assumes a new form.

Consider, for example, a picture of a mysterious red planet, Mars, on the front page of many newspapers during the summer of 1996, linked to the at least plausible story of life on other planets. A reader thinks, what might this discovery, if it holds up, mean for humans? We are not alone. We may not be the most advanced. And on it goes, with whatever chain of associations is stimulated in each person whom the information reaches. The idea replicates, and it also evolves.

In this way, the world of information evolves just a little bit further, perhaps very locally or perhaps by a process that reaches through the media, through newspapers, radio, television, and the Internet, and speeds around the globe. The participants take part in this process because it feels right or good to do so. Perhaps there is beauty in this encounter, or perhaps fitness for a circumstance or a moment. An aesthetic aspect is present, I suggest.

If all of this is true, what are the rules? When greater beauty is present, is there also necessarily a greater need, opportunity, or perhaps merit to the encounter? Are the consequences to people more important? What are people marking? A result and particular product, or perhaps also a process? A reality beyond realities, as some have suggested? If aesthetic experience can lift humans higher, might it not also function at times to show them which way is up?

This chapter does not address these many complex questions here, although I have proposed, as one aspect at least, an importance to discrepancy, change, and challenge, as well as certain aspects of natural phenomena. I suggest later, again as one possible factor, that the fractal patterns of nature have particular "attraction" and aesthetic resonance and, indeed, perhaps a compelling necessity for humans, (Richards, 1997; see also Briggs, 1992; Gleick, 1988; Kauffman, 1995; Zausner, 1996a). Here I look at just one example of potential aesthetic influence, involving a creative response to early adversity—certainly a critical adaptive phenomenon.

AN EXAMPLE—AESTHETIC APPRECIATION, ADVERSITY, AND CREATIVE POSSIBILITY

It is remarkable how many eminent creative persons have come from troubled beginnings (e.g., Goertzel & Goertzel, 1962; Jamison, 1993; Ludwig, 1995; Miller, 1990; D. C. Morrison, 1996; S. L. Morrison, 1996; Richards, 1981, 1990, 1997; Zausner, 1996b). Clearly, not all troubled persons are able to overcome their difficulties resiliently or creatively (see Richards, 1994, 1997). All the more reason, then, to learn from those who do find ways to cope.

Adversity Transformed Creatively

How might this work? Consider a child whose parents are divorcing. She is distraught. She feels responsible. She feels neglected, is convinced she must be bad, and worries about who will be there to care for her the next day. She is angry about all of this, and underneath, she feels frightened, tiny, and alone.

This little girl is certainly conscious of her circumstance; she knows something is wrong. Luckily, there's another side to her awareness, and another possibility. This little girl has had some art exposure, and art instruction, some painting and drawing. Perhaps she has a few other advantages as well—a grandparent who encourages her, an aunt who is a role model, a home that is rich in resources (Albert, in press; Albert & Runco, 1986; Richards, 1981, 1990).

For whatever reason, this distraught little girl decides to paint a picture. It evolves into a dynamic and colorful catharsis, a child showing in deep reds and blues how awful a little girl can feel at night in a silent room with a daddy gone. Suddenly she feels a little better. Some hidden anxieties have come to conscious clarity. She looks at the portrayal of her pain exposed, the piercing lines, the clarity, this witness to her deepest wound, and she feels some warmth and respect for this picture. She runs her hand over it, this validation of her pain. Now she has a little more perspective and control. She will be much more apt, the next time, to pick up her brushes and paint again.

Now here is another little girl. She just sits and feels bad. And then she feels worse. As time goes on, and the divorce unfolds, she feels more and more responsible.

Creative Coping and "Acquired Immunity"

In the first case, a small force has bent the proverbial twig so that the branch can grow in a more expansive and creative direction. Miller (1990) gave further examples of artistic means of coping. For instance, the artwork of Kathe Kollwitz is at once a general social commentary, vividly showing ailing or needy mothers clutching distressed children, and the expression of a one-time mistreated daughter whose own mother had once lost children to death and never recovered from this. Among many other instances that have been explored are the lives of Isak Dinesen (S. L. Morrison, 1996) and Jack Kerouac (D. C. Morrison, 1996), remarkable personalities who found in writing a creative outlet, if not a resolution, for their conflicts. They transmuted their pain, gave it an aesthetic glow, and went further yet to share their discoveries with all of us.

There is increasing evidence (Pennebaker, 1995) that creative expression of conflict, with catharsis of emotions, can be both psychologically and physically healing. Indeed, there is evidence for improved immune function (Pennebaker, Kiecolt-Glaseer, & Glaser, 1988, cited in Richards, 1997) even from writing about one's troubles for as little as 20 min a day. I have proposed a model of *acquired immunity,* whereby the risks of confronting conflict creatively appear less severe in repeated solutions (Richards, 1997). At the same time, the rewards, both aesthetic and empowering, can become amplified.

Personal Growth and Public Benefit

Certain creators may eventually turn from a place of personal conflict to more universal themes and aesthetic concerns and ultimately develop a wish to help others. There is increased identification with other people who suffer and, indeed, with the human condition. Motives can evolve over time from those involving personal conflict to personal growth and more general concern. In this connection, Rhodes (in Richards, 1990) applied Maslow's (see Wertz, 1994) needs hierarchy and states of "deficiency" and "being" to a discussion of deficiency creativity. As lower needs are met, creativity increasingly occurs in the more actualized mode of being (see also Richards, 1997).

Consider for a moment whether there could be a more conscious (and self-conscious) awareness of aesthetic moments in the earlier, more deficient stages of creating, with a consequent pulling away from personal pain into the sensed immediacy of aesthetic reward, now aligned with creative transformation. In the latter being stages, there could be greater absorption in the flow state of a creative realization, where creator and creation merge more fully in the doing.

In any event, with ongoing creative and personal transformation and sharing of creative discoveries, the world of information can evolve even further, and most particularly when the expressions spread out in waves of transmission to an ever greater audience. Consider, for instance, Sylvia Plath and Vincent Van Gogh, and the ever-expanding influence of their expressions over time (Richards, 1994).

If the raison d'etre of an aesthetic isn't to keep an artist painting or a mathematician working, or to serve as a creative tour guide along the way, it has certainly ended up at times assisting in these roles. In each case, child or adult, an aesthetic door has been opened, and a psychological door as well. Difficult material has been treated consciously and transformed in a way that yields aesthetic appeal and broadens the individual's psychological range and personal potency. This time, the person produces as well as appreciates the aesthetic moment, in an alchemy that may make pain more bearable, or at least puts it at a distance. Drawing, writing, experimenting, acting, or just plain fantasizing—these may seem more powerful tools the next time around. And more attractive tools as well, because both their usage and their results carry an intrinsic satisfaction. This creator is no longer so fully victimized, but is able to escape from a difficult moment to a coexistent world of possibility.

If one can learn to notice and at the same time to transform, even if in fantasy, negative material may become positively tinged with the affective glow of hardship overcome (See Krystal, 1981; Richards, 1994, 1997, 1998), as Emerson long ago expressed. Over the years, new material, along with its potential for creative modification, may be sensed more readily. The child may become more empowered and less helpless. Over time, the tendency to segregate positive and negative affects and banish the negative response with a firm "I'm not going to think about that" may abate. This could lead to greater affective integration of diverse feeling states in memory storage (and a greater openness in general) and a richer emotional palette to work with (Richards, 1994).

If this process begins in childhood, it can grow in strength over a great many years. It can become a primary mode for coping, and some of the effects of its use and usefulness may be reflected in the individual's ongoing creative style and potential (Richards, 1993, 1994). Results could include both an enriched creative associative thought process and a greater willingness to approach, rather than avoid, difficulties and to seek creative solutions (see Richards, 1994; also May, 1975). Thus, there are potential effects on both creative *ability* and *motivation*.

In the best case, with an ongoing evolution through conflict to growth and a public expression of the journey, there may be a generalizing effect that spreads outward from influential creative individuals to appreciative others like ripples on a pond. Effects become healing for many more people than the primary individual and stimulate in turn further waves of creative change. As the process continues, the world of information—and the culture to which it contributes—continues to evolve.

Now think of American culture, which often looks at the arts as an "extra" in an educational curriculum of "serious" subjects. Soft, not hard; emotional, not intellectual. And laden with misbeliefs, myths, and false dichotomies, these languages of the deepest human self are consigned the rare elective slot at school or even in certain progressive communities, are thrown out of schools altogether. As a culture we remain, with our hard science *sans* affect, our social science *sans* soul, in an era of escalating global crisis, poverty, devastation, overpopulation, and destructive responses ranging from massive substance abuse to domestic and international violence (see Dewey, 1934; Richards, 1992, 1993, 1997; Sarason, 1990).

The situation has improved, however. Recall the frightened little girl who did find an aesthetic and creative path. In fantasy, at least, the missing parent has made contact with the child. The problem parent has become more aware and knows how the little girl felt. The situation has been worked through and transformed in a way that has led to growth. Now, as Emerson suggested (1836/1992), the moon shines more brightly upon the necessary journey.

THE SUBLIME

Could anything go beyond or transcend the *beautiful?* Kant created another, distinct aesthetic category: the *sublime*. The sublime provides a pleasure, dependent neither on a sense nor on a particular concept or understanding: "It is an object (of nature) the representation of which determines the mind to think of the unattainability of nature regarded as a presentation of Ideas" (Kant, quoted in Beardsley, 1966, p. 221). One may ask, What is this? Why is it different? Is it different? What is the meaning of the *sublime* for one's aesthetic appreciation, awareness of nature, of the borders of change, and of one's own creative evolution?

As with beauty, response to the sublime is said to have a universal validity—everyone can feel it, anytime, anywhere. Yet where beauty involves the bounded, the sublime involves the *boundless*. The response can be unsettling.

Forms of Infinity

One can distinguish two aspects of sublimity in Kant (Kant, 1790/1964; Sheppard, 1966): the *mathematical* and the *dynamical*. The first involves the maximally huge or absolutely great, which renders all else small by contrast. Contrast the massive profile of a mountain range with the human standing at its base, looking up and being struck by the immensity. The judgment made by the person is nonconceptual and noncognitive, a conclusion not of the senses, but of something within. In an intuitive process of "aesthetic estimation," the imagination reaches an upper bound in its capacity to take in the whole, which therefore appears infinite. Yet in this apparent failure of imagination is celebrated a triumph of reason, which identifies this mightiness for the individual's reflection, indeed with moral overtones. According to Kant, the individual is reminded that he or she has "a faculty of the mind surpassing every standard of Sense" (Sheppard, p. 219).

The *dynamical* sublime involves forces that seem to have absolute power over the individual. Even when one is actually secure, nature can appear fearful because of its overwhelming might, examples being lightning and thunder, hurricanes, typhoons, and volcanoes. Interestingly, Kant again viewed the individual's aesthetic response as a human triumph, looking beyond humanity's physical impotence to its moral superiority in face of these perils. "Thus, humanity in our person remains unhumiliated" (Kant, quoted in Sheppard, 1966, p. 220).

In the sublime, people are confronted with awesome hints of infinity, one aspect involving sheer number beyond the usual human scale (size, power, destructiveness). Another aspect, as is suggested below, involves as one feature the ever-changing, yet unchanging, *"fingerprints of chaos,"* the bounded infinity of forms contained in the *fractal* forms of nature. (Consider the thunderclaps that are similar from one burst to the next, yet never the same throughout all time.) In the human world of habituation and compartmentalization, the sublime may bring aspects of the ungraspable that shake us from a stupor and bring individuals to awareness and appreciation.

Sublimity and Awe

If beauty involves a universality of satisfaction, the *sublime* may involve a universality of awe. Here is the terrible, the majestic, the powerful, and the incomprehensible. Here is mystery and "obscurity" (Beardsley, 1966, p. 195), because the sublime is beyond comprehension. "Nature," said Kant, is "sublime in those of its phenomena whose intuition brings with it the Idea of their infinity" (Beardsley, 1966, p. 219). Kant's sublime in nature—the pounding of thunder, the majestic outlines of mountains rising above—is appreciated for its very lack of regularity and order (Sheppard, 1992). In a state of appreciation, with mouth wide open and neck craned backward, one can feel one's awe. According to Kant, the joy one feels comes from the reminder of "a faculty of the mind surpassing every standard of Sense" (Beardsley, 1966, p. 219).

This is a time to be consciously aware. One is positive, if sometimes tremulous, response may resemble transcendent religious states of awe that are sought and valued across cultures; indeed, it may carry a potential for personal transformation (Zausner, 1998). One response is ecstasy; yet fear may be nearby. Zausner (1998) suggested parallels between awe and panic, positing that though each is an experience of expansion, awe brings "an intimation of eternity, while panic contains the fear of obliteration." The awestruck person has an "encounter with the infinite, structured by the familiar" (Zausner, p. 4). Helpfully, in some cases, there is support of a culture, a tradition, a practice.

Perhaps, I wish to add, this response to the sublime may also be one's shame at going mindlessly about ignoring the beauty and vast incomprehensibility of smaller or more commonplace objects and appearances in one's life. Why should it take such a large dose of infinity to wake one up? Infinity is all around! If one were less conceptual and habituated, one might find greater beauty *everywhere* and respond at every turn with a gasp, a recognition, and absorption in the moment.

In any event, when individuals actually confront the sublime, it is without the usual safeguards or sense of self. They don't stand apart from this scene;

they are not looking across the road at a billboard of the Sierra Nevada Mountain Range. They are dwarfed by an actual mountain looming high above them. They gaze with mouth open, humbly present, enfolded in the immensity of the panorama. They are *involved* in *it.* They *are it,* and yet at once so tiny; such is the magnitude of their awe.

Intuitive Knowing

So vast and mysterious—yet does this scene not also somehow look familiar? Consider a mountain panorama in an Eastern work of art. Within the infinite enfoldings of receding mountains and magical mist, one may sense not only a mystery, with descriptions including "the fusion of spirit, that which pertains to Heaven, and of matter, that which pertains to Earth" (Ross, 1960, p. 98), but also a resonance, of something fundamental that is already known to one. It is not specific knowledge, because the scene is a new one. It is not intellectual knowledge either, but rather something intuited from one's own involvement and reaction. What could this be?

Let us flip around from the viewer, and think about the experience of the *creator*. Let us return to the microsublime, the mysteries writ small. Here are instructions from a book on Chinese brush painting: "Paint with joy, with the sheer pleasure of singing life's song. Paint with love and kindness for the materials and the subject portrayed, becoming one with both" (Cassettari, 1987, p. 7). Here is an instance of what Sekida (1977) called *"positive samadhi,"* a "total involvement with some object or activity" (p. 42). Here is the working of flow, in its essence. Here is a directed absorption, a meditation-in-action (see also Franck, 1973, 1993). The work captures this essence, or at least its flavor, for intimate sharing with a viewer.

In creating it, we *become it*. Consider nature again on this smaller scale—in spontaneous studies of bamboo. From catalog notes (Pope, 1961) to a bamboo series by Wu Chen (1350 A.D.): "This album might be called 'Twenty portraits of the artist as a bamboo' " (p. 152). A paraphrase follows of a statement by 11th-century painter Su Shih, "the smallest burgeoning bamboo sprout ... already contains all the knots and leaves... Some painters add knot to knot... they never succeed.... The artist should have the finished bamboo in his mind ... pursuing it as the hawk swoops down" (p. 152). The artist's painting is true, because the true artist *knows*.

Fingerprints of Chaos

How does one intuit what it's like? Try closing your eyes and picturing a mountain lake. Can't you almost see the mountain outlines, patterns of clouds, and waves on the water—at least in a general sort of way, something like a characteristic signature? Think of sunlight glinting off the water. There's an overall impression, yet it's specific as well, with points of light here and there, randomly scattered and flickering—how does this picture come about?

Is there perhaps a built-in function one uses, even if not fully conscious nor fully understood? In books such as *Computers, Patterns, Chaos and Beauty* (Pickover, 1990), one finds spectacular computer-generated pictures, including simulated landscapes with jagged mountaintops and branching trees that cover the sky above. The patterns are highly complex, yet there is underlying order, and elegant economy in the underlying rule. A rule is applied over and over again, iteratively, as the system interacts with itself and with the results generated so far. Whole panoramas can be created. As Roger Lewin said, "Mathematicians are inexorably drawn to nature, not just describing what is to be found there, but in creating echoes of natural laws" (quoted in Pickover, 1990, p. 202).

Among recursive principles are found the workings of nonlinear dynamics, or chaos theory. Results are seen in everything from the forming clouds down the jagged mountain slopes to the tossing sea. Similarly the intricate branching of a tree. Time, as well as space, can reveal such patterns, for instance, the dripping of tapwater from a faucet (e.g., Hall, 1991; Mandelbrot, 1977, Marks-Tanlow, Robertson & Combs, 1995; Murphy, 1993; Schuldberg, in press). In deed, within the bounds of a chaotic "strange attractor," a simple iterative function can generate an unending variety of patterns, as a system grows, evolves, and interacts with itself. (The trajectory in mathematical "phase space" passes endlessly through the same bounded region without repetition—literally an infinity of orbits within a finite domain, the phenomenon resulting in the "fractal," described below.) A chaotic system can also adapt dramatically to a small change in initial conditions, as in the famed "butterfly effect" (Gleick, 1988), in which (when conditions are right) a butterfly flapping its wings in Beijing could cause a storm system to erupt over New York City. Consider this rapidity and sensitivity. Now we know why the weather can be so hard to predict!

Amid this turbulence and complexity, and the sometimes overwhelming responsiveness and unpredictability of chaotic systems, one finds another, highly stable hallmark of chaotic processes: the *fractal* patterns of self-similarity. These patterns are the *fingerprints* of chaos; they persist in form despite changes in scale. Whether one looks broadly or narrowly, they will still be there, in the same holistic configuration, among ripples of water, billows of clouds, the drips from a tap, the branches of plants or bushes, or indeed the branches of one's own blood vessels and nerves. Each oak tree is unique, but in another sense oak trees are all the same. They are grounded in patterns to which such infinitely variable processes always return—the *fractal* patterns of nature.

Imagine viewing a coastline from a plane. You observe its unpredictable outline, with bays, beaches, and headlands. The coastline may be entirely new to you, yet it is somehow comforting and familiar. And it *is* appealing. Although you have never seen this coastline before, you *have* seen it, again and again. When the plane flies down closer, the coastline is still irregular. A different magnification, yet it still looks generally the same. Fly closer yet, and it still shows the same familiar sorts of contours. Even an ant, crawling along the minute margins of this shore, would find some self-similar vestiges of this pattern of bays and headlands.

Chaos and Human Lives

Patterns of chaos are not strangers to human bodies; they are found everywhere, from the beating of one's heart (Gabelli, Carlson-Sabel, Patel, Levy, Diez-mantin Robertson & Combs, 1995) to the working of the brain (Skarda & Freeman, 1987). Might chaotic input resonate through homologous structures in the human nervous system (after S. K. Langer, 1988); might there be morphic resonance (Sheldrake, 1984)? Do fluid processes at the "edge of chaos" help explain the "ah ha" of creative insight (Richards, 1996a)? When one is struck by awe, might there be chaotically destabilizing and restabilizing mental processes that leave one open to significant new forms of brain organization and personal evolution (Zausner, 1996b, 1998)? Might such chaotic phenomena—contrasting the beautiful, discussed previously, with this more breathtaking sublime—yield important neurobiological changes, another neural aftermath of Kant's (1790/1964) aesthetic *judgment of taste?*

Furthermore, might there be a biologically built-in universality of appreciation? How much difference exists, really, between the Paleolithic nature gazer by the ocean and the person looking once more at similar coastlines during a weekend at the beach today?

Imagine you are that person on the beach and you have turned around and are looking up. Rising above you are the jagged peaks of Kant's magnificent mountains, indications to Kant of the sublime. These mountains have been generated through countless millennia of calm days, mild winds, rainstorms, creatures above and below, typhoons, turbulence, sudden landslides, even volcanos. Now the mountains stand massive, complex, mighty, and seemingly eternal. They are also, once again, somehow familiar.

In the distance, you hear the booming sound of thunder. Here is Kant's incomprehensible symphony, this one never before heard by Kant or you or anyone, yet it is also like every series of thunderclaps you have ever heard—so universally familiar. This display of nature is awe inspiring, singing, *sotto voce,* the praises of the universal laws of the cosmos in their infinite manifestations. To Kant, and to me, and most likely to you, it is sublime.

Self-Similarity and Patterns of Life

With a half-smile, I have used the term "chaos clouds" with my young daughter to distinguish certain dynamic, self-similar suggestive forms in Eastern art from more predictable cloudlike "fakes." How compelling is the mystery obscured by, or emerging out of, certain cloudforms of swirling mist in landscapes of dramatic scale (e.g., Pope, 1961). Here a temple is revealed, and here a mountain, the manifestations out of formlessness in everyday reality.

THE SUBTLE ATTRACTION

Out of the fractal fringes of these artistic forms, those winding, growing, evolving clouds, come many emergent possibilities. Of interest, S. Langer (1988) noted the evident paradox of distinctiveness in even quite *similar* expressive artistic forms. These forms seem unique in their beauty, with a "semblance of organism that creates the apparent uniqueness of a piece" (S. Langer, p. 84). If it's expressive, she wrote, it seems "alive."

I again suggest that one may be seeing the fingerprints of chaos, either directly in the portrayal of natural form, as it changes and evolves, or indirectly, in the workings of that mind that fashioned the organic *unity of the creation.* Is this infinity perhaps recognizing itself? This unity, S. Langer (1988) reminded us, is "the *sine qua non* of all good art work" (pp. 83–84). In its presence, perhaps, one intuits *life.* After S. Langer, I suggest that the observer is intuiting not just a product, a portrayal of an object or organism, but a hint of the life force itself—a *process* which continues through all time.

I return to a Zen-inspired artist and the bamboo. In Sekida's (1977) *"positive samadhi,"* they become one and the same. The bamboo expresses itself in strokes of pure certainty; the artist resonates with the structure of the growing tree. The moment is ripe, the brush moves on paper. The magic is captured. Yet what is it that is captured? A wandering novice asked Master Ching Hao about rendering beauty, "the important point is to obtain their true likeness, is it not?"

Ching Hao answered, "It is not. Painting is to paint.... Likeness can be obtained by shapes without spirit; but when truth is reached, spirit and substance are both fully expressed." He further cautioned that the artist who "tries to express spirit through ornamental beauty will make dead things" (Ross, 1960, p. 91).

One does not actually expect to reveal these wonders through chaos theory! Yet might not chaos theory point the way toward a hint of this mystery, as it manifests in the world? One may turn finally to Tibetan sacred art (e.g., Lauf, 1995). Here, for instance, one sees a Great Being and a series of smaller and similar figures, seated amid sinuous organic forms, be these leaves and petals, wisps of clouds, ties of fabric, or the swirling fires of transformation. All are in motion, all seem alive; all seem embodied in the dance. One may wonder at a greater structure of unity and infinity, according to laws one may begin to sense, if not to know.

CONCLUSION

The arguments in this chapter can be summarized in five points:

1. *Aesthetic appreciation may have utility.* I suggest that, paradoxically, aesthetic experience may have an ongoing usefulness. This is perhaps one reason people find themselves drawn to aesthetic experience. Through an aesthetic pull or appeal, they become conscious and attentive, awakened in the moment, and take in some manifestation of nature

or humanity for its own sake. This experience, if it is its own reason and reward, qualifies as a *distinterested* experience, in the Kantian sense. Disinterest has persisted as a criterion of aesthetic experience since the 18th century.

Yet there need be no contradiction. The Kantian *judgment of taste*, the process that establishes aesthetic merit, may itself be *part of the purpose*. Its effects can be permanent, leaving traces in one's brain and lasting effects on consciousness. People mentally record and integrate the events that astonish, delight, and challenge them. They will never be the same again. As per Dewey, such moments of aesthetic appreciation may be found on the borders of change in everyday life, representing peaks, transitions, change points in the flow of life itself. They perhaps even include the fractal boundaries of the changing world, written in the language of chaos theory. A dancer jumps higher than ever before, pushing the envelope of human possibility. As witnesses, we gasp and admire, and we are informed about new heights to which we may aspire and where we might look for these.

2   *Aesthetics may contribute to the evolution of information.* Santayana linked aesthetic appreciation to drives in *biological* survival and evolution, a sort of libidinal theory based on the perpetuation of genes and organic life. I postulate a different type of mating, a mating of ideas, of information. The drive is not libidinal; it is aesthetic. The result is not new genes; it is new "memes" (as per Dawkins). One finds creativity in action, in nature, and by human effort, driven by the irresistable attraction of new possibility. It is a fecund process that contributes fundamentally to the unfolding universe via the evolution of *information*, representing progress of thought, ideas, and culture.

3   *Here lies a chance for everyday creativity.* Included, therefore, is the opportunity for individuals—later, if not at the moment of aesthetic appreciation—to contribute to the changing world. They can produce *original and meaningful* innovations via the multitudinous manifestations of everyday creativity in their mundane worlds of work and leisure. When their efforts are successful, they will shine with an aesthetic glow; they can attract others to contribute their own uniqueness to the elaboration of our collective creativity.

Aesthetic appreciation involves a path to awareness that may include both the mindful awareness of more passively recognized beauty or fitness and absorptive involvement in active creative production. The latter may be related to Cszikszentmihalyi's concept of *flow* and perhaps also to aspects of *positive samadhi* in Eastern metaphysical thought. Indeed, it is through artistic union with one's creation that the most authentic and revealing renderings may emerge, as in, for instance, Haiku poetry.

4   Creativity can lead to *resilient coping and increased psychological well-being*. Human creativity is often not only a meaningful and productive path, but a healthy one. Many creators have used artistic means to overcome difficulty, for instance, using the arts to cope with personal

trauma. Such coping has even been shown to strengthen immune response! Here may be objectification, confrontation, and transformation. At the highest levels of creativity, one can find the refined presentation of universal insights; these shine broadly from the creator's particular circumstance to illumine others' lives as well. Here, indeed, may be aesthetic markings of a difficult job well done. As Emerson said, "Ever does natural beauty steal in like air, and envelop great actions."

5. One can be further engaged by *The sublime, the experience of awe, and the fractal forms of nature.* If individuals are brought to aesthetic appreciation by beauty, they may be more greatly alerted and *awed* by the *sublime.* Here is aesthetic crescendo, with intimations of infinity and the unknowable, even the transcendent. Kant placed the sublime in a category quite apart from beauty. I propose there may be some mechanisms in people's encounters with the sublime that could change them fundamentally in ways they could work with, enhancing their potential to live, and to be, in this world. Chaos theory, in encompassing and *bounding* one aspect of the infinite in the plentiful and pleasing fractal forms of nature, may help individuals at least to approach this mystery. At best, it could point them toward areas for greater understanding, both in the surrounding world and in a resonant potential for change in their own minds.

REFERENCES

Albert, R. S. (in press). The achievement of eminence as an evolutionary strategy. In M. A. Runco (Ed.), *Creativity research handbook* (Vol. 2). Creskill, NJ: Hampton Press.

Albert, R. B., & Runco, M. A. (1986). The achievement of eminence. In R. J. Sternberg & J. E. Davidson (Eds.), *Conceptions of giftedness* (pp.232–257). New York: Cambridge University Press.

Bateson, G. (1972). *Form, substance, and difference: Steps to an ecology of mind* (pp. 448–466). New York: Chandler.

Beardsley, M. C. (1966). *Aesthetics: From Classical Greece to the present.* New York: Macmillan.

Berger, J. (1985). *The sense of sight.* New York: Pantheon.

Briggs, J. (1992). *Fractals: The patterns of chaos—A new aesthetic of art, science, and nature.* New York: Touchstone.

Cassettari, S. (1987). *Chinese brush painting techniques.* London: Angus & Robertson.

Csikszentmihalyi, M. (1988). Society, culture, and person: A systems view of creativity. In R. J. Sternberg (Ed.), *The nature of creativity* (pp. 325–339). Cambridge, England: Cambridge University Press.

Csikszentmihalyi, M. (1990). *Flow: The psychology of optimal experience.* New York: HarperPerennial.

Damasio, A. R. (1994). *Descartes' error: Emotion, reason, and the human brain.* New York: Grosset/Putnam.

Dawkins, R. (1976). *The selfish gene.* New York: Oxford University Press.

Dewey, J. (1934). *Art as experience.* New York: Perigree Books/Putnam.

Dudek, S. (1993). The morality of 20th-century transgressive art. *Creativity Research Journal, 6,* 145–152.

Dudek, S. (1998). Art and aesthetics. In M. Runco (Ed.), *Creativity research handbook.* Creskill, NJ: Hampton Press.

Eisner, E. (1972). *Educating artistic vision.* New York: Macmillan.

Emerson, R. W. (1992). Nature. In D. Atkinson (Ed.), *Selected writings of Ralph Waldo Emerson* (pp. 5–39). New York: Modern Library. (Original work published 1836)
Franck, F. (1973). *The Zen of seeing: Seeing/drawing as meditation.* New York: Vintage.
Franck, F. (1979). *The awakened eye.* New York: Vintage.
Franck, F. (1993). *Zen seeing, Zen drawing: Meditation in action.* New York: Bantam.
Ghiselin, B. (Ed.). (1952). *The creative process.* New York: Mentor.
Gleick, J. (1988). *Chaos: Making a new science.* New York: Penguin.
Goertzel, V., & Goertzel, M. G. (1962). *Cradles of eminence.* Boston: Little, Brown.
Hall, N. (Ed.). (1991). *Exploring chaos: A guide to the new science of disorder.* New York: W. W. Norton.
Hillman, J. (1989). *A blue fire: Selected writings by James Hillman.* New York: HarperPerennial.
Jamison, K. R. (1993). *Touched with fire.* New York: Free Press.
Kant, I. (1929). Critique of judgment. In T. M. Greene (Ed.), *Kant: Selections* (pp. 375–445). New York: Scribner's. (Original work published 1790)
Kant, I. (1790/1964). The Critique of Judgement J. C. Merideth (Trans.) Oxford: Clarendon.
Kauffman, S. (1995). *At home in the universe: The search for the laws of self-organization and complexity.* New York: Oxford University Press.
Krippner, S. (1994). Humanistic psychology and chaos theory: The Third Revolution and the Third Force. *Journal of Humanistic Psychology, 34,* 48–61.
Krystal, H. (1981). The hedonic element in affectivity. *Annals of Psychoanalysis, 9,* 93–113.
Langer, S. K. (1988). *Mind: An essay on human feeling.* Baltimore, MD: Johns Hopkins University Press.
Langer, E. (1989). *Mindfulness.* Reading, MA: Addison-Wesley.
Lauf, D. I. (1995). *Tibetan sacred art.* Bangkok, Thailand: White Orchid Books.
Ludwig, A. (1995). *The price of greatness.* New York: Guilford Press.
Mandelbrot, B. B. (1977). *The fractal geometry of nature.* New York: W. H. Freeman.
Maslow, A. (1959). Creativity in self-actualizing people. In H. M. Anderson (Ed.), *Creativity and its cultivation.* New York: Harper & Row.
May, R. (1975). *The courage to create.* New York: Bantam.
Kant, E. (1952). *Critique of judgment* (J. C. Meredity, Trans.). Oxford, England: Clarendon Press. (Original work published)
Miller, A. (1990). *The untouched key: Tracing childhood trauma in creativity and destructiveness.* New York: Anchor.
Morrison, D. C. (1996, August). *Saints and fallen angels: The creative process of Jack Kerouac.* Paper presented at the 104th Annual Convention of the American Psychological Association, Toronto, Canada.
Morrison, S. L. (1996, August). *Isak Dinesen and Romantic ideation: The quest for self.* Paper presented at the 104th Annual Convention of the American Psychological Association, Toronto, Canada.
Murphy, P. (1993). *By nature's design.* San Francisco: Chronicle Books.
Nhat Hanh, T. (1976). *The miracle of mindfulness.* Boston: Beacon Press.
Pennebaker, J. W. (Ed.). (1995). *Emotion, disclosure, and health.* Washington, DC: American Psychological Association.
Pennisi, E. (1995). Imperfect match: Do ideal mates come in symmetrical packages? *Science News, 147,* 60–61.
Pickover, C. A. (1990). *Computers, patterns, chaos and beauty: Graphics from an unseen world.* New York: St. Martin's Press.
Plato (1938a). Book X, The Republic. In L. Cooper (Ed. and Trans.), *Plato (selections)* (pp.279–360). Ithaca, NY: Cornell University Press.
Plato (1938b). Ion. In L. Cooper (Ed. and Trans.), *Plato (selections)* (pp. 75–93), Ithaca, NY: Cornell University Press.
Pope, J. (1961). *Chinese art treasures. Catalog for selected group of objects exhibited in the US by the Government of the Republic of China.* Lausanne, Switzerland: Skira.

Puhakka, K. (1997). An invitation to authentic knowing. In T. Hart, P. L. Nelson, & K. Puhakka (Eds.), *Spiritual knowing: Alternative epistemic perspectives* (pp. 5–24). Carrollton, GA: State University of West Georgia.

Richards, R. (1981). Relationships between creativity and psychopathology. *Genetic Psychology Monographs, 103,* 261–324.

Richards, R. (1990). Everyday creativity, eminent creativity, and health. "Afterview" for CRJ special issues on "Creativity and Health." *Creativity Research Journal, 3,* 300–326.

Richards, R. (1992, December). Everyday—A work of art? *Psychologie Heute* (Germany), 58–64.

Richards, R. (1993). Seeing beyond: Issues of creative awareness and social responsibility. *Creativity Research Journal, 6,* 165–183.

Richards, R. (1994). Creativity and bipolar mood swings: Why the association? In M. Shaw & M. A. Runco (Eds.), *Creativity and affect* (pp. 44–72). Norwood, NJ: Ablex.

Richards, R. (1996a). Does the lone genius ride again? Chaos, creativity, and community. *Journal of Humanistic Psychology, 36*(2), 44–60.

Richards, R. (1996b). Beyond Piaget: Accepting divergent, chaotic, and creative thought. In M. Runco (Ed.), *New Directions in Child Development, 72,* 67–86. San Francisco, CA: Jossey-Bass.

Richards, R. (1997). When illness yields creativity. In M. Runco & R. Richards (Eds.), *Eminent creativity, everyday creativity, and health.* Norwood, NJ: Ablex.

Richards, R. (1998). Everyday creativity. In HS Friedman (Ed.), *Encyclopedia of Mental Health* (pp. 619–633.). San Diego: Academic Press.

Richards, R. (in press). Everyday creativity and the arts. In A. Montuori & R. Purser (Eds.), *Social creativity: Prospects and possibilities* (Vol. 3). Cresskill, NJ: Hampton Press.

Robertson, R., and Combs, A. (1995). *Chaos Theory in Psychology and the Life Science,* Mahwah, NJ: Erlbaum.

Ross, N. W. (Ed.). (1960). *The world of Zen.* New York: Vintage.

Runco, M. (1994). Creativity and its discontents. In M. Shaw & M. A. Runco (Eds.), *Creativity and affect* (pp. 102–125). Norwood, NJ: Ablex.

Runco, M. (1996). Personal creativity: Definition and developmental issues. In M. Runco (Ed.), *New Directions in Child Development, 72,* 3–30.

Russ, S. W. (1993). *Affect and creativity.* Hillsdale, NJ: Erlbaum.

Santayana, G. S. (1955). *The sense of beauty: Being the outline of aesthetic theory.* New York: Dover. (Original work published 1896)

Sarason, S. (1990). *The challenge of art to psychology.* New Haven, CT: Yale University Press.

Sekida, K. (Ed. and Trans.). (1977). *Two Zen classics: Mumonkan and Hekiganroku.* New York: Weatherhill.

Sheldrake, R. (1984). Morphic resonance. In S. Grof (Ed.), *Ancient wisdom and modern science* (pp. 149–166).

Sheppard, A. (1987). *Aesthetics.* New York: Oxford University Press.

Skarda, C. and Freeman, W. J. (1987). How brains make chaos in order to make sense of the world. *Behavioral and Brain Science, 10,* 161–173.

Wertz, F. (Ed.). (1994). *The humanistic movement: Recovering the person in psychology.* Lake Worth, FL: Gardner Press.

Zausner, T. (1996a). The iconography of chaos in a Renaissance painting. In W. Sulis & A. Combs (Eds.), *Nonlinear dynamics in human behaviour* (Vol. 5, pp.). London: World Scientific Publishing.

Zausner, T. (1996b). The creative chaos: Speculations on the connection between nonlinear dynamics and the creative process. In W. Sulis & A. Combs (Eds.), *Nonlinear dynamics in human behaviour* (Vol. 5, pp.). London: World Scientific Publishing.

Zausner, T. (1998, August). Creativity, panic attacks, and states of awe: A model from nonlinear Dynamics paper presented at the 8th International Conference, Society for Chaos Theory in Psychology and the Life Science. Boston, MA.

12

Creativity, Bipolarity, and the Dynamics of Style

David Schuldberg
University of Montana, Missoula

In this chapter, I explore empirical and theoretical connections between clinical and subclinical features of the affective disorders, other forms of psychopathology, and creativity. My focus is on normal-range, "noneminent" creativity and subclinical affective symptoms, particularly those related to bipolar affective disorder. I refer to the literature and present data on associations between scores on paper-and-pencil creativity tests and subclinical measures of symptoms. In addition, I describe several unresolved empirical and conceptual issues. Finally, I develop a tentative dynamic model for the interaction of cognitive and affective processes in the formation of a creative product within a particular genre or style. An integrative model that includes both affect and cognition can be applied to a variety of problems in the study of creativity, including accounting for the dynamics that underlie different artistic genres and switches among styles within a single work.

Areas of particular interest and controversy include evaluating the relative roles of affect and cognition (and their associated clinical syndromes) in creativity; determining whether flat affect is detrimental or facilitative in the creative

I would like to thank Ruth Richards, Louis A. Sass, Shan Guisinger, Mark Schaller, and Melvin G. Kettner for their assistance. I am grateful to the many current and former undergraduate and graduate students at the University of Montana who assisted in gathering the data reported here, notably, Kaye Norris and Peg Plimpton. I am also indebted to Don Quinlan, John Strauss, Sidney J. Blatt, Frank Barron, and Glenn A. Hughes. Portions of this work were conducted with the support of National Institute of Mental Health Grant RO3 MH46628, which is gratefully acknowledged.

process; investigating the role of mixed affect and admixtures of thought and feeling in creativity; using dynamic, process models to replace static trait conceptualizations of creativity, health, and psychopathology; and, finally, applying concepts from dynamical systems and chaos theory to explain creativity and style. I also note the necessity of addressing the specificity question, that is, discovering the relationships, if any, between particular psychopathological symptoms and personality traits and creativity in specific areas (R. L. Richards, 1981).

EMPIRICAL WORK ON CREATIVITY AND PSYCHOPATHOLOGY

Empirical interest in the relationship between creativity and psychopathology has shifted from emphasizing the cognitive and perceptual characteristics shared by creative, schizophrenic, and schizotypal persons to examining the affective characteristics of manic individuals. Depressed affect has also been linked to creative functioning (Andreasen, 1987; Haynal, 1985; Schildkraut, Hirschfeld, & Murphy, 1994). The norm-breaking behavioral symptoms associated with antisocial individuals have been studied as well, including work on alcohol and substance abuse (e.g., Ludwig, 1990). Less attention has been paid to the relationships (possibly negative) between creativity and the affective and interpersonal deficits of schizotypy (including flat affect) and other negative symptoms. Especially intriguing is the question of whether any positive, helpful role might be played by negative symptoms in certain types of creative endeavors.

I focus here on research that treats psychopathological characteristics as well as creative potential and activity as continuously measurable traits, ones that can be studied meaningfully in the subclinical or normal range (Schuldberg, 1993). Such work investigates nondiagnosed psychopathological-like personality or behavioral characteristics as well as nondiagnosed or noneminent creativity, uses various pencil-and-paper measures of clinical and subclinical symptoms, and studies their relationships with scores on a variety of creativity measures. It has generally emerged, across a variety of samples, that there are positive relationships between psychopathological-like cognitive and affective characteristics and indices of creativity (Table 1). This work contrasts with a more traditional categorical approach of assessing psychopathology via discrete diagnostic categories and studying creativity in select eminent groups. After reviewing the findings presented in Table 1 and touching on the literature on several types of psychiatric symptoms, I discuss the implications of a continuum view for the construction of meaningful dynamic models for understanding the creative person, healthy functioning, and creative products.

DATA ON NORMAL-RANGE CREATIVITY AND PSYCHOPATHOLOGY-LIKE TRAITS

In this chapter, I present new data and review older findings; the primary new data are from the Young Adult Attitude and Experience Study (Plimpton &

Table 1—Correlations Between Affect Measures and Creativity scores in Three Separate Samples

Measure (symptom)	Revised Art Scale	How Do You Think	Gough Adjective Check List (CPS)	Domino Adjective Check List	Independent Activities Questionnaire	Peak Avocational Creativity	Alternative Uses Test
Mania							
Minnesota Multiphasic Personality Inventory-2 (MMPI–2) Hypomania[a]	.09	.43***	.13*	.34***	.26***	.09	—
Wisconsin Hypomanic Traits[b]	.11	.61***	.25***	.29***	—	—	.17***
Depression							
MMPI–2 Depression[a]	−.04	−.21***	−.30***	−.22***	−.12	−.10	—
Flat Affect							
Wisconsin Physical Anhedonia[a]	−.12	−.35***	−.16*	−.19***	−.20***	−.30***	—
Wisconcin Physical Anhedonia[c]	−.06	−.38***	−.21***	−.17***	—	—	−.17***
Wisconsin Physical Anhedonia[b]	−.07	—	−.13*	−.16***	—	—	−.16***
Anhedonia[b]							
Schizoid Taxon[a]	.04	−.07	−.20***	−.10	−.01	−.01	—
Schizoid Taxon[b]	.01	−.06	−.22***	−.03	—	—	.03
Schizoid Taxon[c]	−.08	—	−.23***	.00	—	—	−.07

Note: A dash indicates that the test was not administered. CPS: Creative Personality Scale [a] N = 198–256 (Schuldberg, 1995). [b] N = 345–491. (Schuldberg, 1990).
[c] N = 265–337 (Schuldberg, 1988).
* $p < .05$ (two tailed tests).
** $p < .01$.
*** $p < .005$.

Schuldberg, 1996; Schuldberg, 1995; Schuldberg & Norris, 1996), a study of risk factors and personal resourcefulness in a cohort of young adults. Additional data sets include samples described in Schuldberg (1988, 1990) and Schuldberg, French, Stone, and Heberle (1988; with additional unpublished data on anhedonia). The emphasis is on converging evidence, accumulating across several samples, of relationships between trait measures of affect and a large suite of measures of creativity.

Affective characteristics are measured by the Hypomania (scale 9) and Depression (scale 2) scales of the Minnesota Multiphasic Personality Inventory (MMPI = 2), Golden and Meehl's (1979) Schizoid Taxon scale, and the Wisconsin Hypomanic Traits (Eckblad & Chapman, 1986) and Physical Anhedonia (Chapman, Chapman, & Raulin, 1976) scales. Creativity tests include the Barron-Welsh Revised Art Scale (Welsh & Barron, 1963), sometimes given in computer-administered form (Schuldberg & Nichols, 1990); the How Do You Think test (Davis & Subkoviak, 1975); the Gough (1979) and Domino (1970) creativity scales from the Adjective Check List (ACL; Gough & Heilbrun, 1980); a modified version of the Alternate Uses test (Guilford, Christensen, Merrifield, & Wilson, 1978); the Independent Activities Questionnaire (IAQ; J. M. Richards, Holland, & Lutz, 1967); and the scales of Everyday Vocational and Avocational Creativity (R. Richards, Kinney, Lunde, Benet, & Merzel, 1988). (Only representative data on Peak Avocational Everyday Creativity are reported from these latter ratings.)

SPECIFIC AFFECTS AND CREATIVITY

Positive Affect: Mania and Hypomania

Currently, the most popular research area shows a higher incidence of affective disorder, particularly bipolar affective disorder and hypomania, in writers, composers, and other creative or eminent individuals (Andreasen, 1987; Andreasen & Glick, 1988; Jamison, 1990, 1993). This research is generally conducted within a categorical approach to both diagnosis and assessment of creative attainment. In contrast, R. Richards et al. (1988) studied everyday creativity, establishing a link between bipolar characteristics or subclinical mania in cyclothymes and creativity in normal activity, taking this association out of the realm of eminent creativity. Other data gathered within a continuum model indicate fairly strong positive correlations between measures of hypomanic and manic traits, the Wisconsin Hypomanic Traits scale and the MMPI-2 Hypomania scale (Scale 9), and primarily pencil-and-paper creativity tests (see Table 1). The magnitudes of these associations are generally higher than those observed for measures of the more cognitive and perceptual characteristics associated with schizotypy (see also Nadasi, 1997). This is consistent with other data indicating that nonclinical ranges of positive affect enhance creative functioning (Isen, Daubman, & Nowicki, 1987; Russ, 1993, Chapter 4 in this book; see also Isen, Chapter 1 in this book).

The study of mania and hypomania raises questions regarding the possible double-edged nature of traits in relation to positive adjustment and health. At low levels affective symptoms may facilitate creativity, and at higher levels they may be destructive; this is the inverted-U relationship proposed by R. Richards et al. (1988). Others have also argued for the importance of moderate elevated affect or suggested curvilinear relationships linking affect and creativity (e.g., Akiskal & Akiskal, 1988; Russ, 1993; Schildkraut et al. 1994). Weisberg (1994) found that in one eminent creator manic periods were associated with increased productivity but not heightened quality. This question of whether the relationship between mood, on the one hand, and creativity and adjustment, on the other, is linear or nonlinear is crucial. If the relationship is indeed nonlinear, and there are many reasons to believe that it is, dynamic models of the interaction of creativity and symptoms will be very interesting and fall within the purview of nonlinear dynamical systems theory.

Negative Affect: Depression

Depressed affect may also be associated with creativity (Andreasen, 1987; Haynal, 1985; Kaufmann & Vosburg, 1997; Schildkraut et al. 1994), although the findings are mixed. These observations now tend to be assimilated to the proposed link between creativity and bipolar disorder noted earlier (e.g., Akiskal & Akiskal, 1988). There is recent work on levels of negative mood and creative problem solving (Kaufmann & Vosburg, 1997). However, others (see Isen et al., 1987; Russ, 1993) have noted that negative affect either has no effect on creative performance or detracts from it. Russ (1993) distinguished between induced negative moods and negative affect in primary process, fantasy, and play, as well as openness to negative affect in general, all of which may be positively associated with creativity.

The analyses reported here (see Table 1) reveal negative relationships between creativity test scores and the MMPI-2 Depression scale. The magnitudes of the correlations are highest for the Gough and Domino ACL scales and the How Do You Think test. These findings provide no support for the notion that creativity increases with level of psychometrically assessed depressive symptoms. The precise role of depressive symptoms and phenomenology in the creative process remains puzzling and ambiguous.

Flat Affect: Anhedonia

Flat affect is the absence of either positive or negative emotion and is thus distinct from depression; it is generally considered to be a negative symptom related to schizophrenia. Speculations about the relationship between genius and madness have tended to focus on the flamboyant positive psychotic symptoms of schizophrenia and the elevated mood of mania, not on the withdrawal and apathy of negative symptoms. However, there is interest in the possible contributions of the "schizoid" characteristics and lifestyle to creativity in some realms;

the social alienation and disjunction from the world tapped by these symptoms may be particularly relevant to some kinds of creative endeavors (see Sass, 1994). The study of negative symptoms is potentially an interesting area and can also be connected with current interest in gifted or high-functioning autistic individuals or those with Aspberger's syndrome; whose symptoms overlap with schizophrenic negative symptoms (Frith & Frith, 1991).

In the data reported here, flat affect was measured via the construct of anhedonia or lack of experienced pleasure, as assessed with the Revised Physical Anhedonia scale (Chapman et al., 1976), one of the Wisconsin scales of hypothetical psychosis proneness (Chapman-Chapman, 1985). A sample item is "The beauty of sunsets is greatly overrated" (keyed *true*). There is also interesting recent work on social anhedonia and creativity (Cox & Leon, 1996). It also appears possible that Golden and Meehl's (1979) Schizoid Taxon scale taps a negative-symptom, rather than positive-symptom, form of schizotypy, and results for this index derived from seven MMPI items are reported here as well. Physical Anhedonia is negatively correlated with a variety of creativity tests, including the How Do You Think, the Peak Avocational Everyday Creativity rating, the IAQ, and Domino's and Gough's ACL scales (see Table 1). The Schizoid Taxon scale is negatively correlated with Gough's ACL scale.

Unpublished work also investigated normal personality characteristics and creativity test scores in a group of high scorers on the Physical Anhedonia scale. Analyses of a sample that included participants described in Schuldberg et al. (1988) compared controls and an additional group who scored 2 or more standard deviations above the Wisconsin investigators' means on the Physical Anhedonia scale. As a group, the anhedonic participants scored lower on all creativity[1] measures. This effect was accounted for by the How Do You Think test, with a trend for lower scores on Domino's ACL scale, on which male anhedoni participants received low scores. In contrast, anhedonic men scored high on the Barron-Welsh Revised Art Scale; male and female anhedonics also received ACL scores indicative of high "origence," a construct that refers to creative, nonintellective thought. This partially positive picture of anhedonic individuals is enriched by results from other personality instruments that contribute to a view of these persons as socially alienated and marching to the beat of different drummers, perhaps having positive "outsider" characteristics.

Relative Roles of Cognition and Affect in Creativity

Until about the 1970s, empirical and theoretical work linking psychopathology, genius, and creativity tended to emphasize the connection between disorders in the schizophrenia spectrum and creative work and eminence. Although some attention was paid to depression, cognitive rather than affective characteristics

---

[1]For a full description of the selection procedures for controls, as well as the instrumentation in the study, see Schuldberg et al. (1988).

were predominantly cited as accounting for the relationship between genius and madness; after all, creativity involves having new ideas, and schizophrenic persons have unusual ideas. More recently, claims have been made that the co-occurrences of creativity and psychopathology—including similarities in cognitive styles—are best accounted for as a function of the symptoms of affective disorder (Jamison, 1993). Thus, it is important to elaborate the possible distinctions between manic and schizophrenic cognitive processes and consider the specificity and match of particular cognitive and affective styles with specific fields of leadership and creative endeavor, as well as with different styles or genres of creative product.

In the remainder of this Chapter, I presume that affective and cognitive symptoms are separable and can vary independently; I develop a model of creative process and product that includes both cognitive and affective dimensions. Admittedly, this discussion does not address the question of whether or not the best diagnostic formulations for both the cognitive and affective characteristics of creative individuals will ultimately be ones emphasizing bipolar affective disorder, rather than schizophrenia-like cognitive abnormalities.

Problems To Be Addressed by a Model

A number of general phenomena must be dealt with in modeling the role of affect in creative activity. Positive and negative affects tend to occur at the same time and even mix together, a co-occurrence of different affects or different cognitive styles. For example, happiness and sadness can appear at the same time, intermingle, or interpenetrate, making it difficult to tell them apart in some situations. A theory of affect and creativity must deal with this intermixing (R. Richards, 1994; Schuldberg, 1994), which can represent simultaneously experienced affects and "mixed states" or signify incipient transitions in sequences of bi- and polyphasic affective states.

Other questions concern the optimal matches between an affective state or trait and a particular creative task, and between affect, creative work, and the more general context, epoch, and environment in which the work takes place. It seems likely that there will be a correspondence between different types of affect and cognition, on the one hand, and different types of creativity and achievement in different mediums or domains, on the other. This all occurs in the context of a particular cultural milieu. For example, an artist responds to and works on fluctuating and changing problems; genres, styles, and movements change historically, as well as being pushed along by generations of creators. Creativity is an open-systems phenomenon, embedded in history. These issues point toward a conceptualization of creativity and affect that includes temporal dynamics at many scales, ranging from a creative moment to the framework of a complete work, career, or aesthetic movement.

Dynamical Systems, Affect, and Creativity

In the next section, I develop a preliminary model for the interplay of cognitive and affective factors in the temporal unfolding of the creative process during the formation of an artistic product. In this example, it is assumed that the artistic product is one that also includes time, such as a (possibly narrative) work of literature or a piece of music. The tentative model provides a new way of thinking about the link between artistic process and artistic product. It is meant to demonstrate how cognitive and affective variables can be considered within one model, as well as how they can be viewed dynamically.

I describe general steps by which a dynamic model can be constructed when familiar cross-sectional descriptions of phenomena are available. There are a number of steps involved in this. First, the model considers at least two dimensions: in this example, one aspect of cognition and one aspect of affect. Second, the two dimensions are presumed to involve dynamic processes. This approach is in line with the increasing interest in nonlinear dynamical systems in the behavioral sciences and medicine. Some relevant examples are the work of Sabelli, Carlson-Sabelli, and Javaid (1990); the theoretical work of R. Richards (1996); the approach of Callahan and Sashin (1987); and empirical studies of the dynamics of bipolar disorder and other syndromes (e.g., Gottschalk, Bauer, & Whybrow, 1995). Particularly important is work that posits that the processes of mood elevation and mood depression operate as separate simultaneous processes (see Sabelli et al., 1990). This has deep implications, because such a conceptualization encompasses the phenomena of mixed affective states, interpenetration of affect, and simultaneous and apparently contradictory emotional processes. Process models also introduce complication—in a positive sense—into models of affect, something that will facilitate the development of interesting and complex—in a more technical sense—dynamic models.

The continuum view that I emphasized earlier in this chapter and measurement models that attend to the blurred boundary between health and pathology are also important; they facilitate a transition to thinking in terms of processes. This leads smoothly to contemporary, more formal concepts of nonlinear dynamical systems, with their properties of order, self-organization, possibly chaotic behavior, oscillation, fluctuating periods of apparent stability and instability, cusp phenomena, sensitivity to initial conditions, deterministic unpredictability, as well as fractal properties of scaling and self-similarity. This sample model also illustrates the role of possible nonlinearities in a system.

A MODEL OF THE DYNAMICS OF AFFECT AND COGNITIVE MEANING IN CREATIVITY

In addition to shedding light on the distinctions between different artistic genres and the processes of shifting among styles, this hypothetical model illustrates how a simple model can be capable of complexity and chaos in its behavior.

CREATIVITY, BIPOLARITY, AND DYNAMICS OF STYLE

At this point, however, this dynamic model is a thought experiment awaiting simulation. Starting from an existing picture of static psychological dimensions or categories, it is possible to move toward an interesting process model. Once this dynamic model is constructed, reexamining the earlier static or categorical way of thinking can illuminate how dynamics can be manifested in the static classification system that is perhaps more familiar. Categories become much more interesting when seen as manifestations of dynamic processes.

The model building starts with the choice of two relevant dimensions. These define a state space for the movement of the artistic work[2], and, viewed categorically, define a two-way table. This is followed by translating from the two dimensions to a set of dynamic processes. In the present model, the initial categories are dimensions or "types" of cognitive and affective style that can be mapped onto four artistic genres. The dimensions in this example were selected because they are clinically interesting, sample from both cognitive and affective domains, and fit nicely with one account of different aesthetic modes. This model provides a bridge between the dynamics of affect and cognition in creativity and notions of style in personality and behavior, artistic work, and aesthetic products.

Two Dimensions

The current thought–feeling split in research on creativity may not accurately reflect the human processes involved. The specific dimensions of this preliminary model include both affect and cognition: positive and negative affect and assignment of meaning. This selection is arbitrary for the purposes of a demonstration. The first of the two dimensions is a single bipolar dimension of negative and positive affect, running from depressed to manic. It taps levels of hope and optimism regarding the outcome of an endeavor, or the emotional tinge given to life and the human condition[3]. The second dimension is one of a number of dimensions that are likely to underlie schizophrenic-like thought disorder, a cognitive characteristic with theoretical and empirical connections to creativity (Keefe & Magaro, 1980). This cognitive dimension refers to a continuum of styles of assigning meaning to external objects and stimuli (Schuldberg & Boster, 1985; see also Aronow, Reznikoff, & Moreland, 1994, Chapter 8; this is Schuldberg & Boster's Dimension 1). This dimension ranges from assigning meaning on the basis of concrete aspects of the external world (concreteness) to assigning meaning based on personal and abstract cosmic concerns (grandiosity, self-reference, or bizarreness). This dimension also involves the existential meaning

---

[2] As noted below, it may be more correct and more useful to view this as a phase space.

[3] It may well be argued that positive and negative affect should not be considered a single dimension, and earlier I mentioned the importance of viewing happiness and sadness as separate dimensions (see Sabelli et al., 1990). In this simplified model, each dimension has two associated processes (signified by the springs); this is consistent with the idea of separate processes for mania and for depression, although here they are treated as subtractive and unidimensional. It is also possible to model "up" affect and "down" affect with two distinct processes each, with mania and depression as orthogonal.

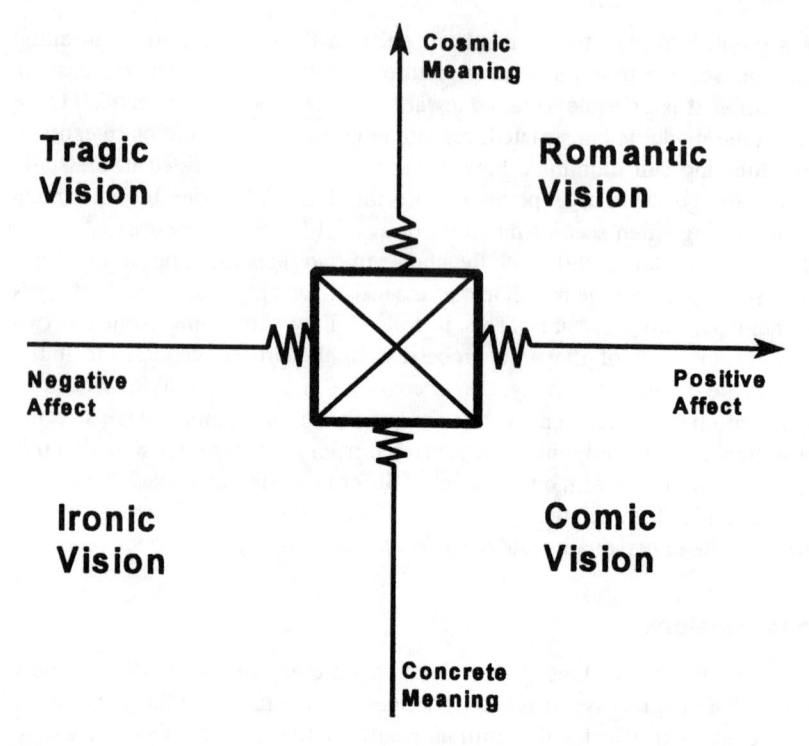

Figure 1

given to human endeavors and the world, ranging from the more mundane, overly grounded, and pedestrian to the grandiose and transcendent.

To envision the dynamic interplay in these two dimensions, consider the two-dimensional pendulum depicted in Figure 1, where the central block oscillates and traverses the state space defined by the two dimensions. Mechanical springs are depicted as attached to the block and pulling in each of four directions along the two dimensions. For clarity, issues of coupling of the different forces on the block—which are important to the qualitative dynamics of the block's motion—are omitted from this simplified description[4].

Style and Genre as Attractors

The model demonstrates how it is possible to account for existing conceptions of style using dynamic terminology. The notion of style is an important one,

[4]An important component of the model is omitted in this discussion; this is the coupling of the processes represented by the four springs. To carry on with the visual presentation, the central block could be viewed as composed of four separate blocks, coupled together by four additional (possibly nonlinear) springs. The quivering of the central block system in such a model represents an important part of the system's behavior.

and this model supports the argument that style itself is a dynamic phenomenon, the result of coupled temporal processes. It is also useful to think of any particular artistic product not simply as an example of one particular style, but as composed of different stylistic moments, or different constituent subgenres. These genres are the result of coupled cognitive and affective creative processes.

A two-way table formed by splitting the two dimensions in Figure 1 defines quadrants in a state or phase space, and four genres emerge as regions of the space. Thus, one can view the model in Figure 1 as constructed in computer software (half-facetiously called "Genre-Maker"), defining and simulating a dynamical system that could have several (possibly chaotic) attractors corresponding to four types of artistic product[5]. Although the present example emphasizes literature or the formation of a story, this model could also be applied to creativity in other endeavors, including painting, music, and the phases of scientific discovery.

Roughly speaking, an "attractor" defines a region of the space in Figure 1 where the block will tend to go and will tend to linger. The four quadrants in Figure 1 include the romantic, tragic, comic, and ironic visions discussed by Schafer (1976) and Frye (1957), a framework that is also useful for describing different visions of reality relevant to psychotherapy (Messer & Warren, 1995; Schafer, 1976). Such a model can link definitions of different artistic genres and different psychological processes in the creator.

The upper left quadrant in Figure 1, corresponding to negative affect and cosmic assignment of meaning, can be related to the tragic vision, with its alertness to "the great dilemmas, paradoxes, ambiguities, and uncertainties pervading human action and subjective experience. . . . . It requires one to recognize the elements of defeat in victory and victory in defeat" (Schafer, 1976, p. 35). This quadrant is also related to depressive symptoms, alienation, and depressive grandiosity and thus may aid in understanding the role of depressed affect in creativity.

The upper right quadrant in Figure 1, comprising positive affect and cosmic meaning, corresponds to the romantic vision, where "life is a quest . . . .a perilous, heroic, individualistic journey. Its destination or goal combines some or all of the qualities of mystery, grandeur, sacredness, love, and possession by or fusion with some higher power or principle" (Schafer, 1976, p. 31). In relation to styles of psychopathology, this quadrant includes manic, grandiose, and self-referential symptom pictures.

The lower left quadrant in the state space, composed of negative affect and concrete attribution of meaning, corresponds most closely to the ironic vision, which, like the tragic vision, includes a "readiness to seek out internal contradictions." However, rather than "seeing the momentous aspects and implications of events," it "aims at detachment, keeping things in perspective. . . . The ironic

---

[5]Again, nonlinear coupling needs to be introduced into this model. See Footnote 4.

vision may seem to be in the service of standing completely apart from experience and negating its significance," but "essentially it is serious business" (Schafer, 1976, pp. 50–51)[6]. Schizoid symptoms would also fall in this quadrant.

Finally, the lower right quadrant, composed of positive affect and concrete meaning, corresponds to the comic vision, which "seeks evidence to support unqualified hopefulness regarding personal situations in the world. . . . The comic vision maintains itself by emphasizing in a highly selective way the external, familiar, controllable, predictable aspects of situations and people" (Schafer, 1976, p. 26). The syndromes associated with this quadrant may be the disorganized (hebephrenic) subtype of schizophrenia, and perhaps aspects of histrionic personality disorder. This quadrant is also related to the image of the fool or trickster in art and myth.

Returning to the dynamics of the model, given nonlinear coupling among the components (see Footnote 4) along with certain parameter settings and initial conditions, the system shown in Figure 1 could exhibit chaotic motion and self-organization in its behavior. Its possible trajectories would then include phenomena such as rapid transitions between styles; the occurrence of sequences of different styles and of mixed states then becomes much more viable than in static categorical or unidimensional conceptions of creativity and style.

The purpose of this example is to illustrate a transition between static models and dynamic ones. I wish to stress that such a transition can be made in a way that preserves a good deal of existing knowledge. Categorical theories and static classification are worthwhile and important and aid in the construction of dynamic models. An illuminating and generally applicable strategy is to determine what (sometimes opposing) dynamic processes may be involved in a psychological phenomenon (in this case, the creative process) and might underlie relevant static categories. It is possible to work in either direction, starting either with a categorization of states (in this case, the "four visions") or with component processes (in this case, variations in affect and cognition). The notion of the crossing or interaction of two or more relevant dimensions is common to both approaches. Coupled processes can generate phenomena that are classified in two-way tables; the tables can suggest the dimensions that define the processes. Another example of this is a model of how Thematic Apperception Test stories are produced as an interaction of need and press, resulting in an outcome, integrated into a "thema" (Morgan & Murray, 1935).

This suggests a dynamic definition of style. According to Meyer (1987), "Style is a replication of patterning, whether in human behavior or in the artifacts produced by human behavior, that results from a series of choices made

---

[6]The ironic vision is the most difficult to fit to this model. What appears in this quadrant may be closer to the cautionary tale. With its paradoxical combination of seriousness and distance, the ironic vision may represent a hybrid genre, or perhaps be between genres. Additional interesting choices of dimensions that could shed light on the four visions are internal versus external (as in introvert vs. extravert) and individualistic versus community-oriented (see Guisinger & Blatt, 1994). Eminent versus noneminent is another interesting contrast.

CREATIVITY, BIPOLARITY, AND DYNAMICS OF STYLE

within some set of constraints'' (p. 21). In the present model, the constraints are implied by the two dimensions. Choices are conceived here more within a dynamic framework than from the point of view of an efficacious actor, and the role of the will and intention (the praxis) of the artist is left in question.

Genres then emerge as regions in the state space of some system. Because a story also involves movement, these genres may be better considered as phases (including both a position and a velocity for the story). (*Story* here is used to refer to any work of art with a temporal dimension; it is worthwhile to avoid the word *narrative* at this point.) The motion of a story among different moments in different genres defines a directed graph. Regions of state or phase space can similarly define types of interpersonal interactions, artistic products, genres, themes, motifs, and perhaps prototypic styles in general. In the dynamic motion of the creative process and the emergence of the resultant creative products, regions where the story orbits or lingers can be viewed as regions around attractors. When such an attractor is within a region that corresponds to a cell of the original two-way table, the story remains well within a certain genre or set of conventions. The cells in the two-way table are regions around attractors, and style is an attractor in a region of phase space.

Dynamics and Change Within a Single Artistic Product

An important point concerns the fluidity and dynamic nature of styles. It may not be possible to classify a single story or work as belonging to a single genre; it can shift between styles. This is related to the dynamics of a person's personality and each person's particular and recognizable personal style or styles. There may also be a connection between fractals and style; this is manifested in the self-similarity of personality across different situations, temporal scales, and degrees of familiarity with another person. The style of a person, or of a work of art, can often be identified at different scales, in the whole or a detail (McArthur, 1989).

As noted, a story or other creative product can have more than one style or motif, although elements recur and repeat. These shifts between modes in a creative work are related to cusps and phase transitions. Comic relief is a simplified example. When a work of art is viewed as dynamically shifting among themes and genres, there is also the possibility that a creative moment can fall between different genres. R. Richards (1996) and others have suggested that creativity may result from phenomena at the "edge of chaos"; such regions may also represent edge-of-genre phenomena as well as an edge of stagnation. This suggests a related phenomenon of genre-busting. When the world is seen in a new way, however briefly, when the rules of a cognitive or perceptual frame, including those of an existing artistic style or genre, are broken, this can imply a breaking of the societal and personal mores for behaving with others (Schuldberg, 1994). This is related to shattering or disregarding the constraints mentioned earlier in the definition of style. The busting of genres and invention of new ones are of course related to the phenomena of modernism and post modernism and the putative "death of art."

Finally, it is also important to mention a distinction I alluded to earlier: the difference between narrative and nonnarrative forms of expression. In some myths, in the form of some blues songs (Willeford, 1985), in dreams[7], one can enter a story at any point. There is also not necessarily any resolution or any exit; this defines what Frank (1995) termed a "chaos narrative," which, strictly speaking, may not have a narrative structure at all. This is related to the difference between repetition and working through and to the question of whether there is progress, within a work of art or in human life. It raises the question of whether linear or cyclic notions of time (Gould, 1987) best capture motion and trajectory in art and perhaps in everyday life.

CONCLUSION

Positive, negative, and flat affect play complex roles in creativity and the phenomenology of psychopathological syndromes. It is important to realize that both creativity and psychopathological states represent continua and are present as admixtures in phenomenal modes of experience. Mixed emotions and mixed cognitive modes can be considered within a single unified model, without the need to reduce one to the other or subsume one under the other. Social scientists need to make a transition from views of interacting states and crossed categories to pictures of simultaneous, temporal, unfolding processes. Dynamics are important in modeling creative phenomena, and nonlinear dynamics may play a central role in furthering the understanding of creativity, especially in defining genres or styles. In this chapter, I have presented a model of possible connections between dynamic psychological processes and shifting artistic styles.

The time is ripe for the application of dynamic models to phenomena for which either categorical or continuum—but static—descriptions of associations between interesting traits and behavior are well known or represent popular hypotheses. Despite productive empirical research, creativity retains elements of a near-magical, still-mysterious process. Like health, it sometimes confuses and surprises people, as their own moods sometimes take them unawares. Waves of inspiration and stagnation, improvisation, and helpless bewilderment traverse the mental landscape, much as emotional temperature and attributions of meaning fluctuate and shift. Despite their mystery, humans understand these changes, much as they understand the weather. In teaching children, parents are wise to stress flux as well as stability and teach techniques for managing both change and stasis. Humans possess a rich folk vocabulary to describe various forms of life and stylistic variation in themselves, the behavior of people they know well, and even casual acquaintances. They also have the language to share aesthetic

---

[7]Robert Sardello suggests a method of dream interpretations based on this approach.

moments that they savor. Models that use principles of nonlinear dynamics can help illuminate the flux and patterning of these crucial human phenomena.

REFERENCES

Akiskal, H. S., & Akiskal, K. (1988). Reassessing the significance of bipolar disorders: Clinical significance and artistic creativity. *Psychiatry and Psychobiology, 3,* 29s–36s.
Andreasen, N. J. C. (1987). Creativity and mental illness: Prevalence rates in writers and their first degree relatives. *American Journal of Psychiatry, 144,* 1288–1292.
Adreasen, N. C., & Glick, I. D. (1988). Bipolar affective disorder and creativity: Implications and clinical management. *Comprehensive Psychiatry, 29,* 207–217.
Aronow, E., Reznikoff, M., & Moreland, K. (1994). *The Rorschach technique: Perceptual basics, content interpretation, and application.* Boston: Allyn & Bacon.
Callahan, J., & Sashin, J. I. (1987). Models of affect-response and anorexia nervosa. *Annals of the New York Academy of Sciences, 504,* 241–259.
Chapman, L. J., & Chapman, J. P. (1985). Psychosis-proneness. In M. Alpert (Ed.), *Controversies in schizophrenia: Changes and constancies* (pp. 157–174). New York: Guilford Press.
Chapman, L. J., Chapman, J. P., & Raulin, M. L. (1976). Scales for physical and social anhedonia. *Journal of Abnormal Psychology, 85,* 374–382.
Cox, A. & Leon, J. L. (1996, August). *Negative schizotypal traits in the relationship of creativity to psychopathology.* Paper presented at the 104th Annual Convention of the American Psychological Association, Toronto, Canada.
Davis, G. A., & Subkoviak, M. J. (1975). Multidimensional analysis of a personality-based test of creative potential. *Journal of Educational Measurement, 12,* 37–43.
Domino, G. (1970). Identification of potentially creative persons from the Adjective Check List. *Journal of Consulting and Clinical Psychology, 35,* 48–51.
Eckblad, M., & Chapman, L. J. (1986). Development and validation of a scale for hypomanic personality. *Journal of Abnormal Psychology, 95,* 214–222.
Frank, A. W. (1995). *The wounded storyteller: Body, illness, and ethics.* Chicago: University of Chicago Press.
Frith, C. D., & Frith, U. (1991). Elective affinities in schizophrenia and childhood autism. In P.E. Bebbington (Ed.), *Social psychiatry: Theory, methodology, and practice* (pp. 65–89). New Brunswick, NJ: Transaction.
Frye, N. (1957). *Anatomy of criticism: Four essays.* Princeton, NJ: Princeton University Press.
Golden, R. R., & Meehl, P. E. (1979). Detection of the schizoid taxon with MMPI indicators. *Journal of Abnormal Psychology, 88,* 217–233.
Gottschalk, A., Bauer, M. S., & Whybrow, P. (1995). Evidence of chaotic mood variation in bipolar disorder. *Archives of General Psychiatry, 52,* 947–959.
Gough, H. G. (1979). A creative personality scale for the Adjective Check List. *Journal of Personality and Social Psychology, 39,* 1398–1405.
Gough, H. G. , & Heilbrun, A. B. (1980). *The Adjective Check List manual.* Palo Alto, CA: Consulting Psychologists Press.
Gould, S. J. (1987). *Time's arrow, time's cycle: Myth and metaphor in the discovery of geological time.* Cambridge, MA: Harvard University Press.
Guilford, J. P., Christensen, P. R., Merrifield, P.R., & Wilson, R. C. (1978). *Alternate Uses: Manual of instructions and interpretations.* Palo Alto, CA: Mind Garden.
Guisinger, S., & Blatt, S. J. (1994). Individuality and relatedness: Evolution of a fundamental dialectic. *American Psychologist, 49,* 104–111.
Haynal, A. (1985). *Depression and creativity.* Madison, CT: International Universities Press.
Isen, A. M., Daubman, K. A., & Nowicki, G. P. (1987). Positive affect facilitates creative problem solving. *Journal of Personality and Social Psychology, 52,* 1122–1131.

Jamison, K. R. (1990). Manic-depressive illness and accomplishment: Creativity, leadership, and social class. In F. K. Goodwin & K. R. Jamison (Eds.), *Manic-depressive illness* (pp. 332–367). New York: Oxford University Press.

Jamison, K. R. (1993). *Touched with fire: Manic-depressive illness and the artistic temperament.* New York: Free Press.

Kaufmann, G., & Vosburg, S. K. (1997). "Paradoxical" mood effects and creative problem solving. *Cognition and Emotion, 11,* 151–170.

Keefe, J. A., & Magaro, P. A. (1980). Creativity and schizophrenia: An equivalence of cognitive processing. *Journal of Abnormal Psychology, 89,* 390–398.

Ludwig, A. M. (1990). Alcohol input and creative output. *British Journal of Addiction, 85,* 953–963.

McArthur, C. C. (1989, April). Are we fractals? Paper presented at the 50th annual meeting of the Society for Personality Assessment, New York.

Messer, S. B., & Warren, C. S. (1995). *Models of brief psychodynamic therapy: A comparative approach.* New York: Guilford Press.

Meyer, L. B. (1987). I. Toward a theory of style. In B. Lang (Ed.), *The concept of style* (revised and exp. ed., pp. 21–71). Ithaca, NY: Cornell University Press.

Morgan, C. D., & Murray, H. (1935). A method for investigating fantasies: The Thematic Apperception Test. *Archives of Neurological Psychiatry, 34,* 289–306.

Nadasi, C. (1997). *The relationship between creativity, self-actualization, and hypomania.* Unpublished master's thesis, University of Montana, Missoula, MT.

Plimpton, L. M., & Schuldberg, D. (1996, August). *Positive and negative affect, anxiety, and depression in Anhedonia.* Paper presented at the 104th Annual Convention of the American Psychological Association, Toronto, Canada.

Richards, J. M., Holland, J. L., & Lutz, S. W. (1967). Prediction of student accomplishment in college. *Journal of Educational Psychology, 58,* 343–355.

Richards, R. L. (1981). Relationships between creativity and psychopathology: An evaluation and interpretation of the evidence. *Genetic Psychology Monographs, 103,* 261–324.

Richards, R. (1994). Creativity and bipolar mood swings: Why the association? In M. P. Shaw & M. A. Runco (Eds.), *Creativity and affect* (pp. 44–72). Norwood, NJ: Ablex.

Richards, R. (1996). Does the lone genius ride again? Chaos, creativity and community. *Journal of Humanistic Psychology, 36,* 44–60.

Richards, R., Kinney, D. K., Lunde, I., Benet, M., & Merzel, A. P.C. (1988). Creativity in manic depressive, cyclothymes, their normal relatives, and control subjects. *Journal of Abnormal Psychology, 97,* 281–288.

Russ, S. W. (1993). *Affect and creativity: The role of affect and play in the creative process.* Hillsdale, NJ: Erlbaum.

Sabelli, H. C., Carlson-Sabelli, L., & Javaid, J. I. (1990). The thermodynamics of bipolarity: A bifurcation model of bipolar illness and bipolar character and its psychotherapeutic applications. *Psychiatry, 53,* 346–368.

Sass, L. A. (1994). *The paradoxes of delusion: Wittgenstein, Schreber, and the schizophrenic mind.* Ithaca, NY: Cornell University Press.

Schafer, R. (1976). *A new language for psychoanalysis.* New Haven, CT: Yale University Press.

Schildkraut, J. J., Hirschfeld, A. J., & Murphy, J. M. (1994). Mind and mood in modern art, II: Depressive disorders, spirituality, and early deaths in the abstract expressionist artists of the New York School. *American Journal of Psychiatry, 151,* 482–488.

Schuldberg, D. (1988). Abstract: Perceptual-cognitive and affective components of schizotaxia and creativity in a group of college males. *Journal of Creative Behavior, 22,* 73–74.

Schuldberg, D. (1990). Schizotypal and hypomanic traits, creativity, and psychological health. *Creativity Research Journal, 3,* 219–231.

Schuldberg, D. (1993). Personal resourcefulness: Positive aspects of functioning in high-risk research. *Psychiatry: Interpersonal and Biological Processes, 56,* 137–152.

Schuldberg, D. (1994). Giddiness and horror in the creative process. In M. P. Shaw & M. A. Runco (Eds.), *Creativity and affect* (pp. 87–101). Norwood, NJ: Ablex.

Schuldberg, D. (1995, August). *Personal resourcefulness: A preventive factor in risk for positive symptoms?* Poster presented at the 103rd Annual Convention of the American Psychological Association, New York.

Schuldberg, D., & Boster, J. S. (1985). Back to Topeka: Two types of distance in Rapaport's original thought disorder categories. *Journal of Abnormal Psychology, 94,* 205–215.

Schuldberg, D., French, C., Stone, B. L., & Heberle, J. (1988). Creativity and schizotypal traits: Creativity test scores, Perceptual Aberration, Magical Ideation, and Impulsive Nonconformity. *Journal of Nervous and Mental Disease, 176,* 648–657.

Schuldberg, D., & Nichols, W. G. (1990). Using HyperCard to administer a figural test on the Apple Macintosh. *Behavior Research Methods, Instruments, and Computers, 22,* 417–420.

Schuldberg, D., & Norris, K. (1996, August). *Lifetime creativity, vocational adjustment, and hypothetical psychosis-proneness.* Paper presented at the 104th Annual Convention of the American Psychological Association. Toronto, Canada.

Weisberg, R. W. (1994). Genius and madness? A quasi-experimental test of the hypothesis that manic-depression increases creativity. *Psychological Science, 5,* 361–367.

Welsh, G. S., & Barron, F. (1963). *Barron-Welsh Art Scale.* Palo Alto, CA: Consulting Psychologists Press.

Willeford, W. (1985). Abandonment, wish, and hope in the blues. *Chiron, 1985* 173–206.

Index

acceptance, scientific creativity and, 152, 154
active listening, focal attention and, 129
adaptability, 163
  creativity as, 181–183
adjunct processes, 22
  controlled experiments on, 26–27
  correlational studies, 31–32
  measures of, 23
  quasi-experimental studies, 30
adulthood, creative insights and tension, 167–170
adversity, creativity from, 203
aesthetic appreciation. *See also* sublime
  awareness and, 198–199
  creative transformation and, 197–198
  disinterested interest of, 193–194
  flow and, 199–200
  intrinsic and universal properties of, 194–195
  sublime and, 213. *See also* sublime
  usefulness of, 211–212
aesthetic properties
  contribution to evolution of information, 212
  imitation, expression, and form of, 195–196
affect. *See also* affect; positive affect
  artists and architects, 108–109
  creativity and, 57–58, 223
  definition, 21, 127
  theoretical approach to creativity and, 92–95
Affect in Play Scale (APS), 62–63
  creativity prediction, 65

  factor analysis, 69–71
  validity studies, 63–64
affective disorders, clinical and subclinical features of, 217
aggression, scientific creativity and, 149
Alternate Uses Test, 64
  Zeitlin Coping Inventory's relationship to, 71
Amabile, Teresa, 75
anhedonia, 221–222
anterior cingulate gyrus, activation in attention process, 135, 137
anxiety, 94
  creativity and, 180
  decrease in creative thought and, 96
architects
  emotional patterns of, 108–109
  human movement response, 115, 117
  participants in research study of affect in, 114
  personality and creation, 112–113
  response to color in the Rorschacht test, 120–122
  20th century architecture and, 110–111
Aristotle, 98
arousal, positive affect vs. 10–12
artist, creativity and negative affect, 91
artistic creativity
  affective states and, 96–98
  affective traits and, 989–99
artists
  emotional patterns of, 108–109

human movement response, 117
nihilistic influence on 20th century, 110–111
participants in research study of affect in, 114
personality and creation, 112–113
response to color in the Rorschach test, 120–122
art of devastation, 110
Asperger's syndrome, 222
assimilation, adaptation and, 182
attention
  behavioral goal, 137
  interactions of affect and, 128, 135
  listening and role of, 129–130
  processes of, 132N133
auditory perception, auditory imagery and, 138–139

beauty
  concept of, 110–101
  Kant's view on, 191–192, 195
  ubiquity of, 196
behavior, objective experience and, 171
behavioral attention, 137
bipolar disorder, 29, 31, 102, 220
  creative insight and, 96
birth order effect
  achievement and, 181–182
  creativity and, 165
bisociation process, creativity and, 93
boredom, decrease in creative thought and, 96

categorization, 24, 48
  mood and, 27–28
challenge, affective pleasure in, 58
change
  dynamics within an artistic product and, 229
  human agents of, 197–198
  human response to, 197
children. *See also* play
  coping and aesthetic, 205
  coping and play/creativity, 71
  creative *vs.* gifted, 180
  creativity in, xiv
  divergent thinking in kindergarten, 62
  logic, 174
  overjustification effect in, 79
  role of affect in creative process, 85
  stress and creative skills, 163–164, 184
  transitional objects theory and, 184
  verbal fluency and positive affect, 4
choice, impact on creativity, 77
cognitive-motivational perspective, affect and creativity, 95
cognitive perspective
  affect and creativity, 93
  artists/architects, 118–119
cognitive structure
  affect in creativity and, 222–223
  creativity and, 59
  play and development of, 60–62
  scientific creativity, 145
color, feelings and, 120–122
compatibility hypothesis, 96
competition, 162
  sibling, 165
competitiveness, scientific creativity and, 149
conformity, 181
coping
  aesthetic creativity and, 203–205, 212–213
  children play/creativity and, 71
  creativity as a type of, 163, 176
core processes, 22
  controlled experiments on, 25–26
  correlational studies, 30–31
  measures of, 23
  naturalistic studies, 32
  quasi-experimental studies, 28–30
Creative Absolute Rational Ear (CARE), 128–129
  ambiguity and temporality, 131–132
  specifics of, 130–131
creativity. *See also* artistic creativity; scientific creativity
  abreactive, 168
  affect in play scale and, 63–64
  arousal *vs.* positive affect in, 11–12
  cognitive aspects, 48, 59
  coping and, 71
  criteria for, 19–20
  definition, 12, 174
  disequilibrium and, 176–177
  emotional aspects, 49
  everyday, 197–198
  Freud's theory of, 92. *See also* sublimation
  listening and, 138–139
  literature, 178
  mental illnesses and, 98–99
  methods, 49–53
  personal, 182
  psychopathology and, 218
  psychopathology-like traits and normal-range, 218–220
  research on role of affect on, xiii–xiv
  risk taking and, 10

social psychology of, 75
theoretical approach to affect and, 92–95
thought-feeling split in research on, 225–226
creativity processes
  architects and artist, 119–120
  interplay of cognitive and affective factors in, 224
  science and engineering research and development, 144
  types of, 22–23
cyclothymia, 102

danger, themes for high-imagination players, 62, 67
daydream, 60
Deep Listening. *See also* Creative Absolute Rational Ear (CARE)
  description, 129–130
depression
  long-term affective dispositions and, 98
  negative affect, 221
  suicide and, 180–181
Dewey, John, 212
  aesthetic and everyday creativity, 196–198
differences, positive affect and perceived, 4–5
discounting principle, 79
discretion, creativity and, 174–175
disequilibrium, creativity and, 176–177
divergent thinking, 48
  affect in play and, 64
  association of unusual words with, 49
  fantasy and imagination on APS and measure of, 65
  play and, 58, 62
  primary process thinking and, 61
  tension and, 172–173
divergent-thinking problems. *See* adjunct processes
dopamine neurotransmitter, 12–13
drawing, 60
Duncker candle task, 6, 11, 25, 48

education
  art in American, 205–206
  tension in, 166–167
educational process, scientific creativity research and, 155
Einstein, Albert, 99–100
emotion
  ability to experience, 58
  artistic creativity and, 97
  creativity and, 41–42

creativity and cognitive theory of, 94
definition, 21, 108
endocepts in memory, 43–45
functional role in cognition, 53. *See also* emotional resonance model (ERM)
play and mastering of, 60–62
processes, 134–135
scientific creativity and, 99–102
temporal level to affective experience, 96
emotional resonance model (ERM)
  automatic resonance mechanism, 45
  components of, 42
  creativity improvement method and, 51–52
  endocepts in memory, 43–45
  individual differences, 46
  resonance detection threshold, 45–46
environment
  attention and, 130
  impact on creativity, xiv
everyday creativity
  aesthetic and, 196–198, 212
  bipolar characteristics in, 220
expectation, preparation and attentional, 133

failure, 152
fantasy, 58
  APS and, 63
  divergent thinking and, 65
  movement response through, 115
  organization and quality of, 69
fear, role in creativity, 93
feeling
  reunion of thought and, 107
  young people's acceptance of, 156
Feeling and Thought Questionnaire (FTQ), 97
feeling states, 21
flexibility
  cognitive organization and, 6, 8
  positive affect on cognitive, 3–5, 7
  primary process and, 68
  young adulthood's tension and, 168, 171
flow, aesthetic appreciation and, 199–200
Freud, Sigmund, 60–61, 67, 92, 154
  libidinal energy, 200

gap, between cognitive state and immediate experience, 177
gender
  adaptability/creativity correlation and, 182
  differences in divergent thinking and APS, 64
  discounting ability and, 80
  flexibility/divergent thinking and, 68

tension/creativity and, 164 n. 2
genes, aesthetic appreciation, 200
genres, 228
grief, creative expression and, 95
Guilford's Unusual Uses and Consequences test, 93

heuristic processing
  positive affect and, 9
  scientific creativity and, 147–148
hypomania, correlation between manic traits and, 220

ideational fluency tasks, 26–27, 155
illumination, scientific creativity and, 151, 154
imagery, transformative drive in Rorschach, 114
imagination, 64, 69
  attention and, 130
immortality, creative achievement and, 92–93
incubation, scientific creativity and unconscious, 150
insight problems. See also core processes
  as optimizing requirements, 26
  positive mood and, 30
integrative perspective, affect and creativity, 95
intelligence, 64
  architects' intuitive, 119
  creativity and, 163
  creativity vs., 20
  intrapsychic tension of asynchronies in, 172
intuition, 173
  scientific creativity and, 150

job perception, 58

Kant, Emmanuel, 191–192, 195, 198, 212
  sublime, 206–207
knowledge, requirement and scientific creativity, 149, 155

Le Corbusier, 111, 113
life, change and biology in the aesthetic of, 196–197
Lifetime Creativity Scales, 31
listening. See also listening; receptive listening
  process, 135–136
literature
  dynamics of affect and cognitive meaning in creativity, 224–228
  style and genre as attractors, 226–228
logic, 174
Luchin's Water-Jar Test, 68

mania, 30
manic-depressive illnesses, 32
  long-term affective dispositions and, 98
marginality, 167
  innovation and, 170–171
Maslow's needs hierarchy, application to deficiency creativity, 204
means-ends tasks, 28
Mednick, S. A., theory of creativity, 7
memes, aesthetics and, 200–201
memory. See also metaphor
  attention and, 130
  discounting ability and, 79–81
  ERM and individual, 46
  expectation and 133
  imagination and auditory, 138–139
  memory of emotion vs. emotional, 134
  mood interaction with emotional aspects of, 49
  primary process thinking and, 61
  record of emotional experiences, 434–45
  role in creative performance cognitive aspects, 48
mental illnesses, creativity and, 28–31, 98–99
metaphor
  emotion-based associations and, 47
  problem conceptualization with emotion-based, 51
mood. See also emotion
  definition, 20–21
  impact on controlled core processes' experiments, 25
  induction research, 66
  influences on creativity, 48–49, 221
  problem-solving's dimensions and, 33
  remote associates tasks and, 27
  temporal level to affective experience, 96
mood disorders, creativity and, 30–31
motivation
  business leaders' understanding of, 157
  extrinsic vs. intrinsic, 75–78
  immunization against reward's effects on intrinsic, 82–84
  tension and intrinsic, 177
movement response
  architects, 115, 117
  artists, 117
music improvisation, creativity and, 127–128

nature. See also aesthetic appreciation
  beauty and, 100–101
  sublime in, 206–207

negative affect
  creativity and, xiv
  problem solving and, 11
negotiation, positive-affect condition and, 6
neurotic anxiety, creative insight and, 96
nonconformity, 164
novelty, 138
  creativity and, 19–20

overinclusion, mania/schizophrenia and, 30
overjustification, effect, 79, 83

pain, in artists' Rorschach, 121
perception. *See also* attention
  artists/architects perpetual modes, 117–118
  auditory imagery *vs.* auditory, 138
  creativity and, 172
  mood and problem, 33–34
performance, 4
peripheral processes, 22
  controlled experiments on, 27–28
  correlational studies, 32
  measures of, 24
persistence, 4
personal conflict, evolution to growth, 204–205
personality
  artists and architects, 112–113
  characteristics and creativity test scores, 222
  creativity and, 58
  play and development of, 58
  problem-solving and, 33
Plato, 98
  beauty and, 192, 195
play. *See also* Affect in Play Scale (APS)
  creative processes and, 57
  development of cognitive structure and, 60–62
  study of work/, 80–81
pleasure, in architects' Rorschach, 121
positive affect
  arousal *vs.*, 10–12
  children verbal fluency, 4
  cognitive flexibility and, 3–5, 7
  heuristic/systematic processing and, 9
  negotiation and, 6
  perceived differences/similarities and, 4–5
  problem solving and, 3, 6
  risk taking and, 10
preconscious, creative person's access to, 180
preparation, as expression of attention, 133
pressures, scientific creativity and external, 152
pretend play, xiv, 58

elements in, 60
research, 66–67
pride, happiness *vs.*, 94
primary process thinking, 60–61
  APS, 64
  creativity and, 93
  Holt content scores for artists/architects, 116
  positive and negative affect, 67–69
problem construction ability, role of cues in, 175–176
problem recognition, scientific creativity, 152
problem solving. *See also* pride; risk taking
  affective pleasure in, 58
  heuristic's application to, 9
  as a kind of disequilibrium, 176–177
  positive/negative affect and creative, 3, 6, 11–12, 102
  process steps, 50
  release of dopamine and, 12–13
  role of gap in, 177
  theory of mood effects on creative, 32–34
process, mood and problem information, 33–34
professional person, psychograms of artists/architects *vs.*, 122 123
psychoanalytic perspective, affect and creativity, 92
psychopathology, empirical work on creativity and, 218
psychotherapy
  creativity and, 156
  impact on creativity, 91

receptive listening, global attention and, 129
recreation, scientific creativity and, 150
regression, creativity and, 93
rejection
  as a form of failure, 155
  scientific creativity, 152
remote associates tasks, 27, 48
Remote Associates Test, 6, 11, 24
research
  criteria for inclusion of studies in, 24–25
  developmental, 163–165
  methodological design for mood and creativity, 23
  mood induction, 66
  original *vs.* integrative, 170
  play and creativity, 62–64
  pretend play, 66–67
  on role of affect on creativity, xii–xiv
reward
  mechanisms of decreased motivation, 78–79

negative impact on creativity, 76–77
risk taking, positive affect and, 10
Rorschach, 64, 68, 93
   differences between artists/architects and professional persons, 122–124
   protocols of architects and artists, 109, 113–114, 116
   response to color in, 120–122

Sagan, Carl, 100
schizophrenia, 30, 93. *See also* anhedonia
   schizotypy and, 218
schizotypy, 218, 220
Schuman, Robert, 30
scientific creativity. *See also* literature
   aesthetic emotions and, 99–102
   affective states and, 97
   artistic creativity *vs.*, 99, 103, 143
   explication and creative synthesis, 151
   feeling and emotions in, 143–144
   structural model of integrated components of, 145–147
scientist, creativity and affect, 92
Sexual instinct, 199
   aesthetic sensibility and, 200
sexuality
   drive toward illumination and, 154
   role in creativity, 92–93
similarity, positive affect and perceived, 5
social-group perception, 4
Socrates, 98
solution requirement, mood and problem, 33
sound perception. *See also* Deep Listening
   affect and, 127–128
strategy
   mood and problem solving, 33–34
   tactical creativity, 161–162
stress, 163
style, 228–229
sublimation, 92
sublime
   awe and, 207–208
   fingerprints of chaos, 208–210
   forms of infinity, 206–207
   intuitive knowing, 208
   patterns of chaos and human lives, 210

suicidal ideation
   correlation adjunct processes and, 31
   creative person, 180
   systematic processing, positive affect and, 9

task
   affect and type of, 5, 8–9
   ideational fluency, 26–27
   integrative bargaining, 5–6
tension, 120
   adulthood's creative insights and, 167–170
   career and personal needs, 169
   creative thought and, 95
   creativity and, 162–163
   as a cue to problem-solving, 175–176
   in education, 166–167
   top-down processing and integration of, 171–174
thalamus-amygdala circuit, emotional response, 135–136
Thematic Apperception Test, 93
trait
   artistic creativity and affective, 98–99
   temporal level to affective experience, 96
trauma
   abreactive creativity theory and, 168
   creativity and, 165

unconventionality, as a criterion for creativity, 20

validation
   aesthetic experience universal, 199
   creativity and, 20
   scientific creativity, 152
variety enjoyment, 6
Velten procedure, 28
verbal fluency
   means-ends tasks and, 28
   positive affect and children, 4

work, children's perception of, 80–82
Wright brothers, 161–162
writers, 179

Zeitlin Coping Inventory, Alternate Uses Test' relationship to, 71